EAT RIGHT F4R YOUR TYPE

FULLY REVISED AND UPDATED

The Original Individualized
Blood Type Diet Solution

Dr Peter J. D'Adamo
with Catherine Whitney

arrow books

1 3 5 7 9 10 8 6 4 2

Arrow Books
20 Vauxhall Bridge Road
London SW1V 2SA

Arrow Books is part of the Penguin Random House group of companies
whose addresses can be found at global.penguinrandomhouse.com

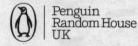

Penguin
Random House
UK

Copyright © 1996, 2016 by Hoop-a-Joop, LLC

Dr. Peter J. D'Adamo has asserted his right to be identified as the author of
this Work in accordance with the Copyright, Designs and Patents Act 1988

This is the revised and updated version of *Eat Right 4 Your
Type* published as a paperback in April 1998 by Century

First published in 2016 by Century
Published in paperback in 2017 by Arrow Books

www.penguin.co.uk

A CIP catalogue record for this book is available from the British Library.

ISBN 9781784756949

Book design by Deborah Kerner

Typeset in 9.79/12.9 pt Caslon LT Stdby Jouve (UK), Milton Keynes
Printed and bound in Great Britain by Clays Ltd, St Ives plc

Penguin Random House is committed to a sustainable future
for our business, our readers and our planet. This book is made
from Forest Stewardship Council® certified paper.

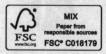

This day is called the feast of Crispian:
He that outlives this day, and comes safe home,
Will stand a tip-toe when this day is named,
And rouse him at the name of Crispian.

Contents

A Diet
for the Twenty-First
Century

THE BLOOD TYPE DIET IS NOW TWENTY YEARS OLD. IT IS A HAPPY ANniversary for me and for the millions of people around the world who have bought *Eat Right for Your Type*, the book that started it all. The most striking fact about *Eat Right for Your Type* is its longevity. It's rare to see a diet book that retains its sales strength after two decades. New diets come and go every season, exploding into the marketplace only to fade before being replaced the next season by something new. And although the Blood Type Diet has often been labeled a "fad" by skeptics, the definition of *fad* is something that inspires intense fashion in the moment but quickly fades. Twenty years in, I think we can agree that the Blood Type Diet is not a fad.

In 1997, I set out to share my life's work in the first edition of this book, and frankly, I didn't know if the world would be receptive to it. At the time, most people didn't even know their blood types. They'd learned in school that blood type was important only if you needed a blood transfusion. I was proposing a radical idea: that blood type is a genetic powerhouse with a primary influence on the immune system, metabolism, and digestive processes and that different blood types have their own food preferences. Rather than being an obscure factor that you need to think about only during an emergency, knowing and understanding your blood type is actually essential to lifelong good health.

I wrote *Eat Right for Your Type* in a simple, clear fashion that every layperson could grasp. My later books would drill deeper into the scientific connections—for those interested in taking it a step further. But the goal of *Eat Right for Your Type* was to introduce the basic idea and diet. Many people were initially drawn to it because the science seemed to explain so many mysteries about their difficulties losing weight or their health complications. So they went out and got their blood typed and tried the diet. And when it worked, they told their friends, and the word spread. And spread. *Eat Right for Your Type* broke all the rules of how to be a diet book blockbuster. It wasn't an instant bestseller, but it gained momentum slowly and steadily right up to the present—with over 7 million books sold in 65 languages around the world. Its success is based not on gimmicks but on evidence and science—and results.

Long before *Eat Right for Your Type* appeared on the *New York Times* bestseller list and sold its first million copies, I could already feel that something significant was happening out there with our readers. I was inundated with emails, letters, and calls. People were emotional about their experience on the diet.

They spoke of a child's chronic ear infections suddenly gone, a mother's lifelong colitis eased, a father's symptoms of rheumatoid arthritis disappearing, a friend not needing his cholesterol or blood pressure medication anymore, and their own weight loss. They spoke of never having felt better, of having more energy, and of no longer being bloated after they ate. They spoke of medical checkups in which changes in their lab results shocked their physicians. Many of those medical doctors, along with naturopathic doctors, adopted the Blood Type Diet for their patients.

On tour speaking to groups, I was regularly approached by readers, some of them tearfully recounting how medical and fitness challenges they'd endured for years had been overcome. They often described how they had tried everything and nothing had helped them lose weight and live a healthy life until they tried the Blood Type Diet. Lifetimes of suffering were being resolved. They were getting positive results—the only measure of success that matters. And the results weren't just short-term, which is the case with most popular diets. People found the Blood Type Diet easy to follow and adopted it as a long-term way of eating and living.

This momentum kept building in spite of a huge backlash, not only from the conventional nutrition community, which had never heard of anything like this, but also from the alternative nutritional community, whose pet theories were being threatened by my methods.

I could paper my walls with all of the articles claiming that the Blood Type Diet doesn't work; most of these were based on deeply flawed studies, inexplicable rancor, or simply an intransigent attitude that something new or unknown couldn't possibly be viable. A 2014 study claiming to debunk the Blood Type Diet was particularly egregious, a study not in search of a result as much as a conclusion. After examining the study this article was based on, we found that none of the participants actually followed the diet as it was written. In one example, experimental subjects ate potato chips, sandwiches, pizza, mac-and-cheese, French fries, and processed meat products while adhering to only 13.7 percent of the guidelines and recommendations of the Blood Type Diet. The study might have debunked something, but it wasn't the Blood Type Diet.

What people in this country eat is big business. There is an institutional and financial stake in keeping the status quo alive and selling outdated concepts like the Food Pyramid or dictating universal commandments about "good" and "bad" foods. The purveyors of this misinformation are registered dietitians, health "experts," and others who have a financial and social stake in the status quo. They preach dietary wisdom as if it were delivered from the mountaintop—*meat is bad, fish is good, fat will kill you, all vegetables are healthful*—whatever the current script dictates. The one thing they don't do (and the reason the Blood Type Diet is such an outlier) is acknowledge that individuals differ, and therefore a diversity of diets makes sense. When I wrote *Eat Right for Your Type*, the word *nutrigenomics* (the way food affects gene expression) had yet to be coined, but it is a historical fact that the Blood Type Diet is the first nutrigenomic diet system. The Blood Type Diet is unique in that it presents a theory of personalized nutrition in a society where people have learned to be comfortable with a one-size-fits-all solution. However, I believe that with our growing understanding of genetics and a more sophisticated knowledge of biochemistry and gut bacteria, it's clear that personalized nutrition is the wave of the future. In this respect, the Blood Type Diet has successfully pioneered a new approach to treating people as individuals.

In the last twenty years, the scientific community has started to catch up with the fact that our blood types are critical predictive markers for disease. New studies appear every year (see Appendix G), linking blood type to yet another medical condition, and a 2016 review went so far as to say, "B group markers such as ABO and Lewis are highly promising targets for novel approaches in the field of personalized medicine." It's remarkable that while the chief tenets of the Blood Type Diet have not changed in two decades, what *has* changed is an increasing acceptance in the medical/scientific community and the population at large of the importance of blood type. The Blood Type Diet was ahead of its time, created in a period before genetic breakthroughs hit the mainstream. But the evolving understanding of biological diversity has only cemented the feasibility of this approach.

My critics still argue that the Blood Type Diet itself has not been subjected to a rigorous double-blind study, considered the gold standard for research. That might be true, but the double-blind study is a paradigm much better suited to a clean get-in, get-out trial of a single therapy or intervention, like a drug or a specific medical procedure. The logistics of testing the theory of eating according to your blood type would be staggering. Thousands of patients would have to be enrolled, their diets carefully regulated. Would people actually stick to the prescribed diet? And even if they followed it to the letter, because it takes so long for health effects to develop in people, the experiment would have to be carried out for years. What would be required to test the Blood Type Diet, a theory that involves hundreds of foods—times four, one separate test for each blood type? If the lack of a large-scale, double-blind, placebo-controlled study of the Blood Type Diet bothers you, you may also want to know that it is generally agreed that upwards of 25 percent of all prescribed pharmaceuticals lack similar proof.

That's not to say we're without evidence. Early on, I created a Blood Type Outcome Registry, where thousands of dieters documented the levels of improvement they'd experienced from their perspective, supplemented and fortified by hard data like lab tests and physician reports from those same individuals. Over the years, we've polled our many thousands of followers on social media and our website, soliciting their experiences on the Blood Type Diet. Repeatedly, our large polls have shown a level of satisfaction with the Blood Type Diet of between 85 and 90 percent. What makes this interesting is not the degree of satisfaction, because that is subjective, but rather the constancy of that number across the four blood type groups—each following a different diet specifically tailored to the requirements of that blood type.

So all I ask is that you become the study, or what we call in medicine an "N of One" (*N* is used to denote the number of participants in a research project). You have nothing to lose. Each of the four basic Blood Type Diets is healthy in its own right. Many popular diets contain similar recommendations to those found in the individual diets—the difference being they're promoted for everyone. The Blood Type Diet simply adds the extra element of knowing which of four basically healthy diets is the most healthful diet for you.

The growth of the Blood Type Diet community has been one of the most rewarding and astonishing developments of this entire journey. With the diet being adopted all over the world, it was a challenge to figure out how to reach all of these people, to offer guidance and support. Twenty years ago the Internet was in its infancy, and online communities were not very common, but we jumped in and created a simple online forum, which in time grew into an online center for educational resources, lists of targeted foods with health-promoting ingredients called nutraceuticals, supplements, training, and support that is among the most sophisticated on the web. Keeping apace with developing web opportunities, the Blood Type Diet's social media presence and smartphone app are designed to help people connect, learn, and more easily follow the diet. A groundbreaking clinic shift at the University of Bridgeport College of Naturopathic Medicine allows me to train new doctors to apply the principles of genetic individuality and the Blood Type Diet to their patients.

With millions of people following the Blood Type Diet, we thought the twentieth year was a perfect time to issue an updated version of the book. This twentieth anniversary edition of *Eat Right for Your Type* has been revised to include new information that will help people better follow the diet, along with cutting-edge research, including a new chapter on losing weight with the Blood Type Diet, edge research on blood type and the microbiome, updated disease connections, and information about tapping into the enormous worldwide support community. And if you still have your doubts, and are at all squeamish about trying the diet, the 10-Day Blood Type Diet Challenge will allow you to judge for yourself in a very short period of time whether this is the diet for you.

Looking back over the last twenty years, I experience a tremendous sense of gratitude. I started this journey as a lone voice, proposing a new way of eating and living. The science, paired with my own clinical experiences, was convincing to me, but I could never have predicted how it would take hold and grow. Thanks to the overwhelming response of the public, who trusted me and then had that trust verified, what was once labeled an odd little diet from a guy nobody had ever heard of is now a force in the nutrition world. That's how change happens.

With this edition my aim is to set the stage for the next twenty years. I invite you to join me on this fantastic voyage.

—Peter J. D'Adamo
January 2017

EAT RIGHT

F4R

YOUR TYPE

(REVISED AND UPDATED)

The Work
of Two Lives

I believed that no two people on the face of the earth were alike; no two people have the same fingerprints, lip prints, or voiceprints. No two blades of grass or snowflakes are alike. Because I felt that all people were different from one another, I did not think it was logical that they should eat the same foods. It became clear to me that since each person was housed in a special body with different strengths, weaknesses, and nutritional requirements, the only way to maintain health or cure illness was to accommodate to that particular patient's specific needs.

James D'Adamo,
my father

YOUR BLOOD TYPE IS THE KEY THAT UNLOCKS THE DOOR TO THE MYS-teries of health, disease, longevity, physical vitality, and emotional strength. Your blood type determines your susceptibility to illness, which foods you should eat, and how you should exercise. It is a factor in your energy levels, in the efficiency with which you burn calories, in your emotional response to stress, and perhaps even in your personality.

The connection between blood type and diet may sound radical, but it is not. We have long known that there was a missing link in our comprehension of the process that leads either to the path of wellness or to the dismal trail of disease. There had to be a reason there were so many paradoxes in dietary studies and disease survival. There also had to be an explanation for why some people were able to lose weight on particular diets, while others were not; why some people retained vitality late in life, while others deteriorated mentally and physically. Blood type analysis has given us a way to explain these paradoxes. And the more we explore the connection, the more valid it becomes.

Blood types are as fundamental as creation itself. In the masterly logic of nature, blood types follow an unbroken trail from the earliest moment of life to the present day. They are the signature of our ancient ancestors on the indestructible parchment of history.

Now we have begun to discover how to use the blood type as a cellular fingerprint that unravels many of the major mysteries surrounding our quest for good health. This work is an extension of groundbreaking findings concerning human DNA. Our understanding of blood type takes the science of genetics one step further by stating unequivocally that every human being is utterly unique. There is no right or wrong lifestyle or diet; there are only right or wrong choices to be made based on our individual genetic codes.

How I Found the
Missing Blood Type Link

MY WORK in the field of blood type analysis is the fulfillment of a lifetime pursuit—not only my own but also my father's. I am a second-generation naturopathic physician. Dr. James D'Adamo, my father, graduated from naturopathic college (a four-year postgraduate program) in 1957 and later studied in Europe at several of the great spas. He noticed that although many patients did well on strict vegetarian and low-fat diets, which are the hallmarks of "spa cuisine," a certain number of patients did not appear to improve, and some did poorly or even worsened. A sensitive man with keen powers of deduction and insight, my father reasoned that there should be some sort of blueprint that he could use to determine differences in the dietary needs of his patients. He rationalized that since blood was the fundamental source of nourishment to the body, perhaps some aspect of the blood could help identify these differences. My father set about testing this theory by blood-typing his patients and observing individualized reactions when they were prescribed different diets.

Through the years and with countless patients, a pattern began to emerge. He noticed that patients who were Type A seemed to do poorly on high-protein diets that included generous portions of meat, but did very well on vegetable proteins such as soy and tofu. Dairy products tended to produce copious amounts of mucous discharge in the sinuses and respiratory passages of Type As. When told to increase their levels of physical activity and exercise, Type A individuals usually felt fatigued and unwell; when they performed lighter forms of exercise, such as yoga, they felt alert and energized.

On the other hand, Type O patients thrived on high-protein diets, and they felt invigorated by intense physical activities, such as jogging and aerobics. The more my father tested the different blood types, the greater his conviction became that each of them followed a distinct path to wellness.

Inspired by the saying "One man's food is another man's poison," my father condensed his observations and dietary recommendations into a book he titled *One Man's Food*. When the book was published in 1980, I was in my third year of naturopathic studies at Seattle's John Bastyr College. During this time revolutionary gains were being achieved in naturopathic education. The goal of Bastyr College was nothing less than to produce the complete alternative physician, the intellectual and scientific equal of a medical internist, but with specialized naturopathic training. For the first time naturopathic techniques, procedures, and substances could be scientifically evaluated with the benefits of modern technology. I waited for an opportunity to research my father's blood type theory. I wanted to assure myself that it carried valid scientific weight. My chance came in 1982, my senior year, when, for a clinical rounds requirement, I began scanning the medical literature to see if I could find any correlation between the ABO blood types and a predilection for certain diseases, and whether any of this supported my father's diet theory. Since my father's book was based on his subjective impressions of the blood types rather than on an objective method of evaluation, I wasn't certain that I would be able to find any scientific basis for his theories. But I was amazed at what I learned.

My first breakthrough came with the discovery that two major diseases of the stomach were associated with blood type. The first was the peptic ulcer, a condition often related to higher-than-average stomach-acid levels. This condition was reported to be more common in people with Type O blood than in people with other blood types. I was immediately intrigued, since my father had observed that Type O patients did well on animal products and protein diets—foods that require more stomach acid for proper digestion.

The second correlation was an association between Type A and stomach cancer. Stomach cancer was often linked to low levels of stomach-acid production, as was pernicious anemia, another disorder found more often in Type A individuals. Pernicious anemia is related to a lack of vitamin B$_{12}$, which requires sufficient stomach acid for its absorption.

As I studied these facts I realized that on the one hand, Type O blood predisposed people to an illness associated with too much stomach acid, while on the other hand, Type A blood predisposed people to two illnesses associated with too little stomach acid.

That was the link I'd been looking for. There absolutely was a scientific basis for my father's observations. And so began my ongoing love affair with the science and anthropology of the blood types. In time, I found that my father's initial work on the correlation among blood type, diet, and health was far more significant than even he had imagined. In the coming years, scientific research would reinforce my initial findings with the publication of many studies linking blood type to nearly every metabolic and immune system condition.

My father's work has lived on in me. When he died in 2013 he was still in private practice, promoting the concepts of individualized nutrition. In one of his later writings, not long before he died, he wrote with his characteristic passion and certainty:

"My clarion call after practicing for 50 years is the same: all people are unique individuals, created by the shared genetics of two parents; molded by their culture, society, and geographic region in which they were raised and live; and directed by their dominant thoughts.

"Most important, a person's blood type—whether it is O, A, B, or AB—is nature's most reliable guide in determining their individualized dietary needs."

Four Simple Keys to Unlock Life's Mysteries

I GREW UP in a family that was mostly Blood Type A, and because of my father's work we ate a basically Mediterranean-style diet consisting of foods such as tofu, seafood, steamed vegetables, and salads. As a child I was often embarrassed and felt somewhat deprived, because none of my friends ate weird foods like tofu. To the contrary, they were happily engaged in another kind of "diet revolution" sweeping the 1950s: their diets consisted of hamburgers, hot dogs, French fries, candy bars, ice cream, and lots of soda pop.

Today, I still eat the way I did as a child, and I love it. Every day I eat the foods that my Type A body craves, and it's immensely satisfying.

In *Eat Right for Your Type* I will teach you about the fundamental relationship between your blood type and the dietary and lifestyle choices that will help you live at your very best. The essence of the blood type connection rests in these facts:

- Your blood type—O, A, B, or AB—is a powerful genetic fingerprint in your DNA, especially when it comes to your diet.
- When you use the individualized characteristics of your blood type as a guidepost for eating and living, you will be healthier, you will naturally reach your ideal weight, and you will slow the process of aging.
- Your blood type is a more reliable measure of your identity than race, culture, or geography. It is a genetic blueprint for who you are, a guide to how you can live most healthfully.
- The key to the significance of blood type can be found in the story of human development and expansion: Type O appeared in our survivalist ancestors: hunter-gatherers; Type A evolved with agrarian society; Type B emerged as humans migrated north into colder, harsher territories; and Type AB was a thoroughly modern adaptation, a result of the intermingling of disparate groups. This evolutionary story relates directly to the dietary needs of each blood type today.

What is this remarkable factor, the blood type?

Blood type is one of several medically recognized variations, much like hair and eye color. Many of these variations, such as fingerprint patterns and DNA analyses, are used extensively by forensic scientists and criminalists as well as those who research the causes and cures of disease. Blood type is every bit as significant as other variations; in many ways, it's a more useful measure than some others. Blood type analysis is a logical system. The information is simple to learn and easy to follow. I've taught the system to numerous doctors, who tell me they are getting good results with patients who follow its guidelines. Now I will teach it to you. By learning the principles of blood type analysis, you can tailor the optimal diet for yourself and your family members. You can pinpoint the foods that make you sick, contribute to weight gain, and lead to chronic disease.

Early on, I realized that blood type analysis offered a powerful means of interpreting individual variations in health and disease. Given the amount of available research data, it is surprising that the effects of blood type on our health have not received the measure of attention that they deserve. But now I am prepared to make that information available—not just to my fellow scientists and colleagues in the medical community, but to you.

At first glance, the science of blood type may seem daunting, but I assure you it is as simple and basic as life itself. I will tell you about the ancient trail of the evolution of blood types (as riveting as the story of human history), and demystify the science of blood types to provide a clear and simple plan that you will be able to follow.

I realize that this is probably a completely new idea for you. Few people ever even think about the implications of their blood type, even though it is a powerful genetic force. The ABO gene not only controls your blood type but also affects many other processes. In particular, genes that regulate stress and digestion use ABO as a switch, turning themselves on or off depending on the specific blood type of the individual.

You may be reluctant to wade into such unfamiliar territory, even if the scientific arguments seem convincing. I ask you to do only three things: Talk to your physician before you begin, find out your blood type if you don't already know it, and try your Blood Type Diet for at least 10 days. Most of my patients experience some results within that time period—increased energy, weight loss, a lessening of digestive complaints, and improvement of chronic problems such as asthma, headaches, and heartburn. Give your Blood Type Diet a chance to bring you the benefits I've seen it bring to millions of people who swear by the diet. See for yourself that blood not only provides your body's most vital nourishment but now proves itself a vehicle for your future well-being.

Your
Blood Type
Identity

Blood Type:

The Real Evolution Revolution

*B*LOOD IS LIFE ITSELF. IT IS THE PRIMAL FORCE THAT FUELS the power and mystery of birth and the horrors of disease, war, and violent death. Entire civilizations have been built on blood ties. Tribes, clans, and monarchies depend on them. We cannot exist without blood— literally or figuratively.

Blood is magical. Blood is mystical. Blood is alchemic. It appears throughout human history as a profound religious and cultural symbol. Ancient peoples mixed it together and drank it to denote unity and fealty. From the earliest times, hunters performed rituals to appease the spirits of the animals they killed by offering up the animal blood and smearing it on their faces and bodies. The blood of the lamb was placed as a mark on the hovels of the enslaved Jews of Egypt so that the Angel of Death would pass over them. Moses is said to have turned the waters of Egypt to blood in his quest to free his people. The symbolic blood of Jesus Christ has been, for two thousand years, central to the most sacred rite of Christianity.

Blood evokes such rich and sacred imagery because it is in reality so extraordinary. Not only does it supply the complex delivery and defense systems that are necessary for our very existence but it provides a keystone for humanity—a looking glass through which we can trace the faint tracks of our journey.

For many decades we have been able to use biological markers such as blood type to map the movements and groupings of our ancestors. By learning how these early people adapted to the challenges posed by constantly changing climates, germs, and diets, we learn about ourselves. Change in climate and available food produced new blood types. Blood type is an unbroken cord that binds us to one another.

Ultimately, the differences in blood types reflect on the human ability to acclimate to different environmental challenges. For the most part, these challenges impacted the digestive and immune systems: a piece of bad meat could kill you; a cut or scrape could develop into a deadly infection. Yet the human race survived. And the story of that survival is inextricably tied to our digestive and immune systems. It is in these two areas that most of the distinctions between blood types are found.

The Human Story

THE STORY OF humankind is the story of survival. More specifically, it is the story of where humans lived and what they could eat there. It is about food—about finding food and moving to find food. We don't know for certain when human evolution began. Neanderthals, the first humanoids we can recognize, may have developed 350,000 to 500,000 years ago. Maybe more.

We do know that human prehistory began in Africa, where we evolved from humanlike creatures. Early life was short, nasty, and brutish. People died a thousand different ways—opportunistic infections, parasites, animal attacks, broken bones, childbirth—and they died young.

Early humans must have had a harrowing time providing for themselves in this savage environment. Their teeth were short and blunt—ill-suited for attack. Unlike most of their competitors on the food chain, they had no special abilities in regard to speed, strength, or agility. Initially, the chief quality humans possessed was an innate cunning, which later grew to reasoned thought.

Early humans ate a rather crude diet of wild plants, grubs, and the scavenged leftovers from the kills of predatory animals. They were more prey than predator, although in time they became very accomplished hunters. Infections and parasitic afflictions were part of daily life, much more common than in our sanitized modern existence. In fact, when paleoanthropologists discover a new human coprolite (a piece of fossilized fecal waste) and analyze it in the lab, they're always amazed at the large number of parasites and worms these early people harbored within their bodies. Many of the parasites, worms, flukes, and infectious microorganisms do not stimulate the immune system to produce a specific antibody to them, a distinct advantage for Type O people because, as we will see, they already had broad protection in the form of the antibodies they carried from birth against foreign antigens. As human groups migrated into new areas, their diets changed in reaction to new environmental conditions; new food sources provoked adaptations in the digestive tract and immune system, necessary for these groups to first survive and later thrive in each new habitat. These biological changes are reflected in the remarkable differences in the worldwide distribution of the blood types, each of which appears to have flourished at critical junctures of human development.

When talking about the anthropology of the blood types it is important to distinguish between two kinds of history: molecular (gene) history and epidemiologic (population) history. Molecular history is the story of the ABO gene—the gene that determines the blood type of an individual—and this history is quite ancient. In fact the history of the ABO gene goes way beyond humans, although *Homo sapiens* (modern humans) are the only known species to possess all four ABO blood types. This is not surprising because the chemicals that make up the ABO blood types are nothing special. They can be found in everything from invertebrates to pond scum. Yet there is an important story to be told here as well. Genes are not static, and we have now begun to understand that they change and alter their function much more rapidly and dynamically than we'd previously thought possible. If you change your habits or diet, your body will turn certain genes on or off to adapt to the change, and sometimes these changes will be passed on to your offspring. This is known as the science of epigenetics.

We must also not make the mistake of thinking that, just because we share the same ABO gene with another species, the ABO gene will do the same exact things in both. For example, in certain species of pigs, having Blood Type O results in a coat of black hair. Obviously not every human who is Type O has black hair. This is because different species link a different variety of other genes to the ABO gene, a phenomenon known as *gene linkage*. As it turns out, we humans link a lot of our digestive functions to our ABO blood type rather than to our hair color.

In molecular history, the picture is a bit different. Although we can say that Type O is the oldest from the standpoint of population movement, Type A appears to be the oldest in the molecular sense, in that the mutations that gave rise to Types O and B appear to stem from it. Geneticists call this the wild-type or ancestral gene. The building blocks that make up DNA are four nucleotide bases—adenine, cytosine, guanine, thymine—referred to by the first letter of their names: A, C, G, and T. The Type B mutation is a simple replacement of one of the letters of the DNA of the ABO gene with another; what geneticists call a single nucleotide polymorphism, or SNP, pronounced *snip*. The Type O mutation is much more fascinating. It resulted from the complete loss of a letter in the ABO DNA, which is like a train that has lost a boxcar and so all the other cars just move up by one. This type of mutation is called a *frame shift* and, perhaps most amazingly, virtually every other known frame shift mutation within the genome is highly lethal. Yet if you are Type O, it *made* you.

Although Type A is the molecular ancestor, it appears to have disappeared in humans a very long time ago, and then "resurrected" itself about 300,000 years ago. This is where we now turn to the population history of blood type, and the story really starts to get interesting.

Over the last two decades I've written a lot of genomic software and have seen quite a few patients, and I can honestly tell you that spending time with people is much more interesting. Genes are an important part of the blood type story, but what your ancestors did with those genes is even more important. That is, the interactions between early humans and their environment, and how those interactions—climate, food supply, microbes and other factors—advanced the development of the blood type factors we still see today.

Much of what follows is about survival, and yes, it's the survival of the fittest. Without adequate knowledge of sanitation and zero knowledge of microbiology, our ancestors were prey to a multitude of infectious ailments. As we will explore in more detail later on in the book, there are major differences between the blood types in how individual immune systems interact with the environment. One of the most important differences involves the antibodies carried by the different blood types. These are the same antibodies that prohibit transfusing blood between certain blood types.

Now, obviously, Mother Nature did not provide us with these antibodies to mess up blood transfusion, although when talking to some physicians one can sometimes get this impression. These antibodies are part of a delicate system of defining friend from foe, self from nonself. Most authorities agree that the basic reason we have anti-other-blood-type antibodies is to act as a sort of firewall against particular germs and pathogens that just happen to also resemble the other blood types. There is compelling evidence for this. Virtually every infectious disease that afflicted our ancient ancestors has a preference for one blood type or another. Mother Nature, it seems, was merely doing what any good gambler does: hedging her bets.

Good gamblers always lead with their best card, which in this case was Type O, the simple reason being that two is a larger number than one. Type O is the only blood type with two different anti-blood-type antibodies. Type O makes anti-A, which is why it cannot take blood from Type A donors; and anti-B, which means Type B blood is a no-go as well. Although this double antibody production does limit your transfusion options, it also produces a form of broad-spectrum immune protection. With its better immune protection Type O got the jump on the other blood types—including Type A, which, as I mentioned, it mutated from—and as the dictator Joseph Stalin is said to have observed, "Quantity has a quality all its own."

In this context, the story of blood type can be summarized this way:

1. Survival, expansion, and ascent of humans to the top of the food chain (Type O to its fullest expression).
2. The change from hunter-gatherer to a more domesticated agrarian lifestyle (advance of the original Type A).

3. The merging and migration of population groups from the African homeland to Europe, Asia, and the Americas (advance of Type B).
4. The modern intermingling of disparate groups (the arrival of Type AB).

Each blood type contains the genetic message of our ancestors' diets and behaviors, and though we're a long way away from early history, many of their traits still affect us. Knowing these predispositions helps us understand the logic of the Blood Type Diet.

O Is for Old

MODERN HUMANS may have emerged out of Africa as recently as 60,000 years ago, although other ancestral humans were certainly well distributed throughout Asia and Europe by that time and had developed hunter-gatherer type technologies and the ability to control fire. At about this same time it is thought that humans developed the phonetic diversity necessary for true speech and communication. These skills propelled the human species to the top of the food chain, making them the most dangerous predators on earth. They began to hunt in organized packs; in a short time, they were able to make improved weapons and advanced tools. These major developments gave them strength and superiority beyond their natural physical abilities.

Skillful and formidable hunters, the early modern humans soon had little to fear from any of their animal rivals. With no natural predators other than themselves, the population exploded. Protein—meat—was their fuel, and it was probably at this point that gene followed function. Besides its double-barreled antibody armory there is one other observation that indicates that we are by and large talking about Type O during this period.

In the 1940s and 1950s the geneticist Arthur Mourant studied the distribution of the ABO blood types across the globe. What made Mourant's work so important was that he studied the blood type distributions of indigenous peoples. Studying blood type distributions in modern populations would be essentially useless, as over the last millennia humans have intermingled to a very great degree.

Mourant's findings were very interesting. In virtually every society where an indigenous population (such as the Inuits or Native Americans) was isolated or otherwise separated from contact with other groups over a long period of time the percentage of Blood Type O skyrocketed, at times reaching over 90 percent of the total population. And all of these populations, where still possible, pursued a hunter-gatherer type of existence.

Genes can alter their function based on changes in the environment: change a habit for long enough and the body will alter the functions of genes needed to metabolize the result of that change. As we will soon see, Type Os possess many of the digestive characteristics needed to make an effective hunter-gatherer.

These early humans thrived on meat, and it took a remarkably short time for them to kill off the big game within their hunting range. Evidence suggests that these Paleolithic hunters were quite healthy: bone fossils indicate that they were taller than their ancestors. This may have led to an explosion in the population, a persistent problem

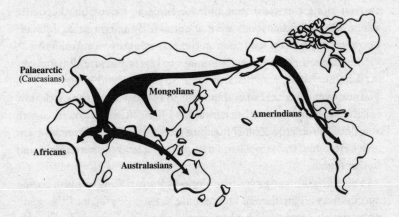

From their base in the ancestral homeland of Africa, early Blood Type O hunter-gatherers wandered throughout Africa and into Europe and Asia in search of new supplies of large game. As they encountered changing environmental conditions, they began to develop modern physical and physiological characteristics.

for hunter-gatherer societies. More mouths to feed and dwindling game reserves prompts migration.

Migration often leads to conflict, especially if you are the person who already occupies the land others are migrating to. Hunters began fighting and killing others who were impinging on what they claimed were their exclusive hunting grounds. As always, human beings found their greatest enemy to be themselves. Good hunting areas became scarce. The migration of the human race began.

Bands of hunters were traveling farther and farther in search of meat. When a shift in the trade winds desiccated what had been fertile hunting land in the African Sahara, and when previously frozen northern areas grew warmer, people began to move out of Africa into Europe and Asia.

This movement seeded the planet with its base population, which was Blood Type O, the numerically predominant blood type even today.

By 20,000 B.C.E. modern humans had moved fully into Europe and Asia, decimating the vast herds of large game to such an extent that other foods had to be found. Searching each new area for anything edible, it is likely that humans quickly became omnivorous, with a mixed diet of berries, grubs, nuts, roots, and small animals. Populations also thrived along the coastlines and the lakes and rivers of the earth, where fish and other foods were abundant. By 10,000 B.C.E., humans occupied every main landmass on the planet, except for Antarctica.

The movement of the early humans to less temperate climates created lighter skins, less massive bone structures, and straighter hair. Nature, over time, acclimated humans to the regions of the earth they inhabited. People moved northward, so light skin developed, which was better protected against frostbite than dark skin. Lighter skin was also better able to metabolize vitamin D in a land of shorter days and longer nights.

Paleolithic hunter-gatherers eventually burned themselves out; their success was an anathema. Overpopulation soon exhausted the available hunting grounds. What had once seemed like an unending supply of large game animals diminished sharply. This led to increased competition for the remaining hunting grounds. Competition led to war, and war to further migration.

It is interesting to note that almost every society carried down in its history a story of creation that involved an early time of paradise followed by an eventual downfall and expulsion. Many experts in the field of folklore believe that these stories all stem from a distant memory of a halcyon time of freedom and abundance, followed by a time of shortage and struggle. It you are Type O, that memory of paradise is locked into your genetic memory.

A Is for Agrarian

THE PERIOD between the decline of Paleolithic existence and the advent of agricultural technology is not very well-defined. However, much like the man with one foot in his boat and one foot on the dock, we can conclude that this intermediate period was somewhat precarious. We can assume a certain hardscrabble, hand-to-mouth existence was the order of the day, perhaps not unlike what we still see to this day in areas of famine. When hungry we will eat, or attempt to eat, almost anything.

However, somewhere in Asia or the Middle East between 25,000 and 15,000 B.C.E. humans began to understand that plant energy could be controlled, and even optimized. This is the beginning of the so-called Neolithic Revolution, with its hallmarks of agriculture and animal domestication. This new technology probably started with a strain of notoriously bitter legumes known as vetches, and moved on to different grains, which in fact started out in nature as simple wild grasses.

As anyone with hay fever can tell you, grasses are among the most allergy-inducing things in nature. In fact, plant food products are typically more allergenic than animal foods. This is a dilemma for the immune system: how can one derive nutrients from foods that also induce allergic reactions? The solution, as in many other dilemmas, is tolerance.

Good design is, in a way, a form of negotiation, and a good negotiation is usually defined as resulting in both parties leaving the table mildly dissatisfied with the final result. If you study the physiology of Blood Type A, it soon appears evident that this is a blood type that tries mightily to get along with others, often perhaps to a fault, as we will soon see.

The cultivation of grains changed everything. Unlike animal proteins, which require a simple, yet powerful, mix of stomach acid and protein-digestion enzymes, plant proteins require a slower, more nuanced approach. You have to first figure out how to render them innocuous to the immune system before you can move on to metabolizing them. Able to forgo their hand-to-mouth existence and sustain themselves for the first time, people established stable communities and permanent living structures. This radically different lifestyle, a major change in diet and environment, resulted in the need for entirely new characteristics in the digestive tracts and immune systems of the Neolithic peoples—changes that allowed them to better tolerate and absorb cultivated grains and other agricultural products. Type A was in the spotlight. Evidence clearly indicates that the advance of farming technology geographically parallels the distribution of Blood Type A in ancient populations.

Settling into permanent farming communities presented new developmental challenges. The skills necessary for hunting together now gave way to a different kind of cooperative society. Agriculture could allow for an almost infinite increase in population and for specialization and division of labor. For the first time, a specific skill at doing one thing depended on the skills of others doing something else. For example, the miller depended on the farmer to bring in crops; the farmer depended on the miller to grind the grain. One no longer thought of food as only an immediate source of nourishment or as a sometime thing. Fields needed to be sown and cultivated in anticipation of future reward. Planning and networking with others became the order of the day. Psychologically, these are traits at which Type As excel—perhaps another environmental adaptation.

Agriculture also required the concentration of resources, leading to the beginning of urban existence. This is again reflected in the distribution of blood type on the world map. Mourant's maps clearly show a high percentage of Blood Type A in the areas of the world with long histories of urban living.

What could have been the reason for this extraordinary rate of growth in the number of Type A individuals? It was survival. Survival of the fittest in a crowded society. Because Type A emerged as more resistant to infections common to densely populated areas, urban industrialized societies quickly became Type A. Even today, survivors of plague and cholera show a predominance of Type A over Type O.

Eventually, the gene for Type A blood spread beyond Asia and the Middle East into Western Europe, carried by people such as the Indo-Europeans, a seminomadic people who penetrated deeply into the pre-Neolithic populations and gave us the foundation for most of our modern languages.

Today, Type A blood is still found in its highest concentration among Western Europeans. The frequency of Type A diminishes as we head eastward through Europe, following the receding trails of the ancient migratory patterns. Type A people are highly concentrated across the Mediterranean, Adriatic, and Aegean seas, particularly in Corsica, Sardinia, Spain, Turkey, and the Balkans. The Japanese also have some of the highest concentrations of Type A blood in eastern Asia, along with a moderately high number of Type B.

Blood Type A surged in response to the dietary changes stemming from the conversion of the Paleolithic hunter-gatherer way of life into the Neolithic urban-agricultural revolution, including the changes in diet and the exposure to new diseases that this lifestyle brought with it. It was almost as if Mother Nature were presenting us with a signpost at a fork in the road as well as a source for innumerable diet controversies: Paleo/high-protein diet to the left, Asian/Mediterranean diet to the right. Two powerful enough formulas by the standards of your typical one-size-fits-all diet book. But, as it turns out, the story of blood type is even richer and more sophisticated.

B Is for Balance

BLOOD TYPE B appears to have reached significant numbers sometime between 10,000 and 15,000 B.C.E., in the area of the Himalayan highlands—now part of present-day Pakistan and India—where it may have initially developed its characteristics in response to climatic changes. It is interesting that many of its physiological characteristics appear to vary with altitude: Studies show that women who are Type B are taller and get their menses earlier the higher up they live.

Of all the ABO blood types, Type B has the most unusual and specific distribution on the world map: a huge swath of territory extending north to south right across the area where Europe meets Asia. Type B is found in increased numbers from Japan, Mongolia, China, and India up to the Ural Mountains. From there westward, the percentages fall until a low is reached at the western tip of Europe.

This was traditionally an area that was home to a mix of Caucasian and Mongolian tribes, and Type B is very characteristic of the great tribes of steppe-dwellers, who once dominated the Eurasian plains.

As the steppe-dwellers swept through Asia, the gene for Type B blood was spread along the way. The groups ranged northward, pursuing a culture dependent on herding and domesticating animals—as their diet of meat and cultured dairy products reflected.

Two distinct groups of Type B sprang up as the pastoral nomads pushed into Asia: an agrarian, comparatively sedentary group in the south and the east, and a nomadic, warlike society conquering the north and the west. The nomads were expert horsemen who penetrated far into eastern Europe: Like a wave at the seashore, Type B blood can be found in many eastern European populations, but dissipates rapidly the farther west we look.

A study of blood group patterns in the United Kingdom showed that Blood Type B, although not common there, was found to be in great concentration along the internal rivers, indicating a path of invasion by and/or commerce with Norsemen who had perhaps picked it up from their raids into present-day Russia.

In the meantime, an entire agriculturally based culture had spread throughout China and Southeast Asia. Because of the nature of the land they chose to till and the climates unique to their areas, these people created and employed sophisticated irrigation and cultivation techniques that displayed an awesome blend of creativity, intelligence, and engineering.

The schism between the warlike tribes to the north and the peaceful farmers to the south was deep, and its remnants exist to this day in southern Asian cuisine, which consists of little if any dairy foods. To many Asian minds, dairy products are the food of the barbarian, which is unfortunate because the diet they have adopted does not suit their Type B blood as well.

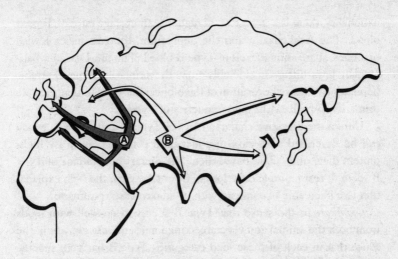

Origins and movements of Type A and Type B. From its beginnings in Asia and the Middle East, the gene for Type A was carried by Indo-European peoples into western and northern Europe. Other migrations carried Type A into northern Africa, where it spread into the Saharan populations. From its origins in the western Himalayan mountains, Type B was carried by Mongolian peoples into southeast Asia and into the Asian flatlands, or steppes. A separate migration of Type B people entered eastern Europe. By this time, sea levels had risen, removing the land bridge between North America and Asia. This prevented any movement of Type B into North America, where the Native American populations continued on as exclusively Type O.

The small numbers of Type B individuals among old and western Europeans represents western migration by Asian nomadic peoples. This is best seen in the east-central Europeans—the Germans and Austrians—who have an unexpectedly high incidence of Type B blood compared to their western neighbors. The highest occurrence of Type B in Germans occurs in the area around the upper and middle Elbe River, which had been nominally held as the dividing line between civilization and barbarism in ancient times.

Modern subcontinental Indians, a Caucasian people, have some of the highest frequencies of Type B blood in the world. The northern Chinese and Koreans have very high rates of Type B blood and very low rates of Type A.

The blood type characteristics of Jewish populations have long been of interest to anthropologists. As a general rule, regardless of their nationality, there is a trend toward higher-than-average rates of Type B blood. The Ashkenazim and the Sephardim, the two major Jewish branches, share strong levels of Type B blood. The pre-Diaspora Babylonian Jews differ considerably from the primarily Type O Arabic population of Iraq (the location of the biblical Babylon) in that they are primarily Type B, with some frequency of Type A.

Unlike the digestive characteristics of Type O and Type A, which can be described with easy-to-understand concepts, such as "high-protein diet" and "plant-based diet," the dietary adaptations of Type B seem to resist simple description. Over the years, the best explanation I've been able to come up with is "idiosyncratic omnivore."

Omnivore in the sense that Type B seems to do well with foods from both the animal and vegetable kingdoms, and *idiosyncratic* in the sense that in each of these food categories Type B has very specific strengths and weaknesses that are experienced only by those who are Type B. Many of the relationships seem to defy logic—such as the notion that chicken is a problem food, while turkey is not, although, for most of us, there would appear to be little difference between the two. We'll explore these fascinating relationships when we introduce the concept of food lectins later in the book.

AB Is for Modern

IN GENETICS it appears that blood type plays by its own rules. As we've seen with Type O, you can have what is normally a lethal mutation and simply wind up with a different blood type. With Type A you can have an ancient gene that, for some unknown reason, decided to exit the stage eons ago and then resurrect itself. With Type B your physiology appears to change as you change altitude. However, with Type AB, Mother Nature may have saved the best for last.

Like most genes, ABO blood type exists in a sort of dominant–submissive relationship. Certain variations, known as alleles, are just stronger than others. For example, given an allele for brown eyes from one parent and an allele for blue eyes from another, you will most likely wind up with brown eyes. Brown eyes are the dominant trait and blue eyes the submissive, or recessive, trait.

Of course, blood type genetics works things out in a unique way. Like other genes, there are dominant alleles (A and B) and a submissive one (O), and from here the math is rather simple: If you receive either a B allele or an A allele from one parent and an O allele from the other, you'll be either Type A or Type B. You can be Type O only if both parents give you an O allele. But because the recessive O is more common than either A or B, there are more Type O individuals in the population.

But what happens if one parent gives you an A allele and the other a B allele? The obvious answer (which is in fact true) is that you become Blood Type AB. But like any good puzzle, it is the *why* that is the most interesting part.

Just like the mutation that creates Type O breaks all the rules for the average mutation, how a person gets to be Type AB turns out to be another rule breaker. In genetic parlance (and the criteria for any good relationship), the A allele and B allele are said to be *co-dominant*. That is, they simply co-exist with each other.

Thus we arrive at the basic essence of Type AB: It is not an adaptation in the sense that the development of O, A, and B were adaptations to climate, diet and disease. Instead, it came into being through the simple circumstance of a population of Type A blood colliding and cohabitating with a population of Type B blood. You might think this is nothing special, but remember our earlier discussions—for a long, long time, Type A resided in one part of the globe, and Type B in a different part. It has only been in the last 1,000 to maybe 2,000 years that there was any kind of real interaction between the two.

Until ten or twelve centuries ago, there was no Type AB blood. Then barbarian hordes sliced through the soft underbelly of many collapsing civilizations, overrunning the length and breadth of the Roman Empire. As a result of the intermingling of these eastern invaders with the last trembling vestiges of ancient European civilization, Type AB blood came to be. No evidence for the occurrence of this blood type extends beyond that time, when a large western migration of eastern peoples took place. Blood Type AB is rarely found in European graves before 900 C.E. Studies on exhumations of prehistoric graves in Hungary show a distinct lack of Type AB into the fourth to seventh century C.E. This would seem to indicate that up until that point in time, European populations of Type A and Type B did not come into common contact, or if so, rarely mingled or intermarried.

Because Type ABs inherit the tolerance of both Type A and Type B, their immune system has an enhanced ability to manufacture more specific antibodies to microbial infections. This unique quality of possessing neither anti-A nor anti-B antibodies minimizes the chances of being prone to allergies and other autoimmune diseases such as arthritis, inflammation, and lupus. There is, however, a greater predisposition to certain cancers because Type AB responds to anything A-like or B-like as "self," so it manufactures no opposing antibodies.

Type AB presents a multifaceted, and sometimes perplexing, blood type identity. It is the first blood type to adopt an amalgamation of immune characteristics, some of which make it stronger, and some of which are in conflict. Perhaps Type AB presents the perfect metaphor for modern life: complex and unsettled.

The Blending Grounds

BLOOD TYPE, geography, and race are woven together to form our human identity. We may have cultural differences, but when you look at blood type, you see how superficial they are. Your blood type is older than your ethnicity and more fundamental than your nationality. The blood types were not a hit-or-miss act of random genetic activity. Each blood type developed as an adaptation to a series of cataclysmic chain reactions, spread over eons of environmental upheaval and change— dietary, environmental, and geographical—that became part of the evolutionary engine that ultimately produced the different characteristics of each blood type.

Some anthropologists believe that classifying humans into races invites oversimplification. Blood type is a far more important determinant of individuality and similarity than is race. For example, an African and a European of Type A blood could exchange blood or organs and have many of the same aptitudes, digestive functions, and immunological structures—characteristics they would not share with a member of their own ethnic group or nationality who was Blood Type B.

Racial distinctions based on skin colors, ethnic practices, geographical homelands, or cultural roots are not a valid way to distinguish among people. Members of the human race have a lot more in common with one another than we may have ever suspected. We are all potentially brothers and sisters. In blood.

Today, as we look back on this remarkable evolutionary revolution, it is clear that our ancestors had unique biological blueprints that complemented their environments. It is this lesson we bring with us into our current understanding of blood types, for the genetic characteristics of our ancestors live in our blood today.

- TYPE O: The most widespread early mutation and most basic blood type, the survivor at the top of the food chain, with a strong and ornery immune system willing to and capable of destroying anyone, friend or foe.
- TYPE A: The first adaptors, forced by the necessity of migration and shortage to adapt to a more agrarian diet and lifestyle.
- TYPE B: The assimilator, the idiosyncratic omnivore, adapting to new climates and the mingling of populations.
- TYPE AB: The enigma, the unique offspring of a rare merger between the opposing forces of tolerance and adaptation.

Our ancestors left each of us a special legacy, imprinted in our blood types. This legacy exists permanently in the nucleus of each cell. It is here that the anthropology and science of our blood meet.

Blood Code:

*The Blueprint
of Blood Type*

*B*LOOD IS A FORCE OF NATURE, THE ÉLAN VITAL THAT HAS SUS-
tained us since time immemorial. A single drop of blood, too small to
see with the naked eye, contains the entire genetic code of a human
being. The DNA blueprint is intact and replicated within us endlessly—
through our blood.

Our blood also contains eons of genetic memory—bits and pieces
of specific programming, passed on from our ancestors in codes we are
still attempting to comprehend. A crucial part of this code rests within
our blood type. Perhaps it is the most important code we can decipher
in our attempt to unravel the mysteries of blood and its vital role in our
existence.

To the naked eye, blood is a homogeneous red liquid. But under
the microscope, blood shows itself to be composed of many different
elements. The abundant red blood cells contain a special type of iron
that our bodies use to carry oxygen and create the blood's characteristic rust color. White blood cells, far less numerous than red, cruise our
bloodstreams like ever-vigilant troops, protecting us against infection.

This complex living fluid also contains proteins that deliver nutrients to the tissues, platelets that help it clot, and plasma that contains
the guardians of our immune system.

The Importance of Blood Type

YOU MAY BE UNAWARE of your own blood type unless you've donated blood or needed a transfusion. Most people think of blood type as an inert factor, something that comes into play only when there is a hospital emergency. But now that you have heard the dramatic story of the roots of blood type, you are beginning to understand that blood type has always been the driving force behind human survival, changing and adapting to new conditions, environments, and food supplies.

Why is our blood type so powerful? What is the essential role it plays in our survival—not just thousands of years in the past, but today?

Your blood type is the key to your body's entire immune system. It controls the influence of viruses, bacteria, infections, chemicals, stress, and the entire assortment of invaders and conditions that might compromise your immune system.

The word *immune* comes from the Latin *immunis*, which denoted a city in the Roman Empire that was not required to pay taxes. (If only your blood type could give you that kind of immunity!) The immune system works to define "self" and destroy "non-self." This is a critical function, for without it your immune system could attack your own tissues by mistake or allow a dangerous organism access to vital areas of your body. In spite of all its complexity, the immune system boils down to two basic functions: recognizing "us" and killing "them." In this respect your body is like a large invitation-only party. If the prospective guest supplies the correct invitation, the security guards allow her to enter and enjoy herself. If an invitation is lacking or forged, the guest is forcibly removed.

Enter the Blood Type

NATURE HAS ENDOWED our immune system with very sophisticated methods to determine if a substance in the body is foreign or not. One method involves chemical markers called *antigens*, which are found on the cells of our bodies. Every life-form, from the simplest virus to humans themselves, has unique antigens that form a part of its chemical fingerprint. One of the most powerful antigens in the human body is the one that determines your blood type. The different blood type antigens are so sensitive that when they are operating effectively, they are the immune system's greatest security system. When your immune system sizes up a suspicious character (that is, a foreign antigen) one of the first things it looks for is your blood type antigen to tell it whether the intruder is friend or foe.

Each blood type possesses a different antigen with its own special chemical structure. Your blood type is named for the blood type antigen you possess on your red blood cells.

IF YOU ARE	YOU HAVE THIS ANTIGEN ON YOUR CELLS
BLOOD TYPE A	A
BLOOD TYPE B	B
BLOOD TYPE AB	A AND B
BLOOD TYPE O	NO ANTIGENS

Visualize the chemical structure of blood types as antennae of sorts, projecting outward from the surface of our cells into deep space. These antennae are made from long chains of a repeating sugar called fucose, which by itself forms the simplest of the blood types, Blood Type O. The early discoverers of blood type called it "O" as a way to make us think of "zero" or "no real antigen." This antenna also serves as the base for the other Blood Types, A, B, and AB.

- BLOOD TYPE A is formed when the O antigen, or fucose, plus another sugar called *N*-acetyl-galactosamine, is added. So fucose plus *N*-acetyl-galactosamine equals Blood Type A.
- BLOOD TYPE B is also based on the O antigen, or fucose, but has a different sugar, named D-galactosamine, added on. So fucose plus D-galactosamine equals Blood Type B.
- BLOOD TYPE AB is based on the O antigen, fucose, plus the two sugars, *N*-acetyl-galactosamine and D-galactosamine. So fucose plus *N*-acetyl-galactosamine plus D-galactosamine equals Blood Type AB.

The Four Blood Types and Their Antigens

key -

CELL

Fucose > basic sugar

N-acetyl-galactosamine > A sugar

D-galactosamine > B sugar

N-acetyl-galactosamine + D-glactosamine > AB sugar

The four blood types and their antigens. Type O is the stalk, fucose; Type A is fucose plus the sugar N-acetyl-galactosamine; Type B is fucose plus the sugar D-galactosamine; Type AB is fucose plus the A sugar and the B sugar.

At this point you may be wondering about other blood type identifiers, such as positive and negative. Usually, when people tell their blood types they say, "I'm A positive." Or "I'm O negative." These variations, or minor blood types, play relatively insignificant roles. More than 90 percent of all the factors associated with your blood type are related to your primary type—O, A, B, or AB. However, one additional influence, secretor status, can be important, and we'll describe it later. For now we will concentrate on your ABO blood type itself.

Antigens Create Antibodies
(Immune System Smart Bombs)

WHEN YOUR IMMUNE SYSTEM SENSES that a foreign antigen has entered the system, the first thing it does is create antibodies to that antigen. These antibodies, specialized chemicals manufactured by the cells of the immune system, are designed to attach to and tag the foreign antigen for destruction.

Antibodies are the cellular equivalent of the military's smart bomb. The cells of our immune system manufacture countless varieties of antibodies, and each is specifically designed to identify and attach to one particular foreign antigen. A continual battle wages between the immune system and intruders that try to change or mutate their antigens into some new form the body will not recognize. The immune system responds to this challenge with an ever-increasing inventory of antibodies.

Most of the antibodies made by the immune system are simple molecules that resemble a basic adjustable wrench, which alters its size to fit the size of the nut that needs to be twisted. Likewise, the immune system adjusts the antibody to fit the shape of the antigen of an invader. These types of antibodies (known as immunoglobulin G, or IgG) simply tag the foreign object. The combination of the invader and this type of antibody alerts the patrolling cells of the immune system, which move to the invader, attach to the antibody, and attack and destroy it.

However, the antibodies that we make as part of our ABO blood type are different. These antibodies (known as IgM) are very large molecules that resemble a snowflake; they have multiple attachment points and are made without stimulation of the immune system. When they encounter an antigen that resembles an opposing blood type, they change their form from a snowflake to something resembling a crab. This allows them to produce a reaction called agglutination (literally, "gluing"). This type of crablike antibody attaches to the foreign antigen and makes it very sticky. When cells, viruses, parasites, and bacteria are agglutinated, they stick together and clump up, which makes it easier for the body to dispose of them. This is why getting a transfusion of the wrong blood type is so deadly. The antibodies you have against the wrong blood type attack the transfused blood and trigger massive agglutination, which leads to shock and possibly death.

The anti-other-blood-type antibodies are the strongest antibodies in our immune system, and their ability to clump—agglutinate—the blood cells of a different blood type is so powerful that it can be immediately observed on a glass slide with the unaided eye. Most of our other antibodies require some sort of stimulation (such as a vaccination or an infection) for their production. The blood type antibodies are different: They are produced automatically, often appearing at birth and reaching almost adult levels by four months of age. Evidence suggests that they are stimulated by the first bacteria that begin to inhabit the newborn's gut and, perhaps not surprising, by the first foods they eat.

As microbes must rely on their slippery powers of evasion, this agglutination is a very powerful defense mechanism. It is rather like handcuffing criminals together; they become far less dangerous than when they are allowed to move around freely. Sweeping the body for odd cells, viruses, parasites, and bacteria, the antibodies herd the undesirables together for easy identification and disposal.

The system of blood type antigens and antibodies has other ramifications besides detecting microbial and other invaders. More than a hundred years ago, Karl Landsteiner, a brilliant Austrian physician and scientist, also found that blood types produced antibodies to other blood types. His revolutionary discovery explained why some people could exchange blood, while others could not. Until Landsteiner's time, blood transfusions were a hit-or-miss affair. Sometimes they "took," and sometimes they didn't, and nobody knew why. Thanks to Landsteiner, we now know which blood types are recognized as friend by other blood types, and which are recognized as foe.

Landsteiner learned that

- BLOOD TYPE A carries anti-B antibodies. Type B is rejected by Type A.
- BLOOD TYPE B carries anti-A antibodies. Type A is rejected by Type B.

Thus Type A and Type B cannot exchange blood.

- BLOOD TYPE AB carries no antibodies. The universal receiver, it accepts any other blood type. But because it carries both A and B antigens, it is rejected by all other blood types.

Thus Type AB can receive blood from everyone, but can give blood to no one. Except another Type AB, of course.

- BLOOD TYPE O carries anti-A and anti-B antibodies. Type A, Type B, and Type AB are rejected.

Thus Type O can't receive blood from anyone but another Type O. But free of A and B antigens, Type O can give blood to everyone else. Type O is the universal donor.

IF YOU ARE	YOU CARRY ANTIBODIES AGAINST
BLOOD TYPE A	BLOOD TYPE B
BLOOD TYPE B	BLOOD TYPE A
BLOOD TYPE AB	NO ANTIBODIES
BLOOD TYPE O	BLOOD TYPES A AND B

But there is much more to the agglutination story. It was also found that many foods agglutinate the cells of certain blood types (in a way similar to rejection) but not others, meaning a food that may be harmful to the cells of one blood type may be beneficial to the cells of another. It's not surprising that many of the antigens in these foods have A-like or B-like characteristics. This discovery provided an entirely different scientific link between blood type and diet. Remarkably, however, its revolutionary implications would lie dormant, gathering dust for most of the twentieth century—until a handful of scientists, doctors, and nutritionists began to explore the connection.

Lectins: The Diet Connection

A CHEMICAL REACTION OCCURS between your blood and the foods you eat. This reaction is part of your genetic inheritance. It is amazing but true that today, in the twenty-first century, your immune and digestive systems still maintain a memory, a certain favoritism, for foods that your blood type ancestors ate and adapted to.

We know this because of a factor called lectins (from the Latin, "I choose"). Lectins are abundant and diverse proteins found in foods that have agglutinating properties affecting your blood and tissues. Lectins are a powerful way for organisms in nature to attach themselves to other organisms in nature. Lots of germs, and even our own immune systems, use this superglue to their benefit. For example, cells in our liver's bile ducts have lectins on their surfaces to help them snatch up bacteria and parasites. Bacteria and other microbes have lectins on their surfaces as well, which work rather like suction cups, so that they can attach to the slippery mucosal linings of the body. Often the lectins used by viruses or bacteria can be blood type specific, making them a stickier pest for people of that blood type.

So too with the lectins in food. Simply put, when you eat a food containing protein lectins that are incompatible with your blood type antigen, the lectins can attach to the walls of the digestive tract, initiate inflammation, and even penetrate the gut lining and escape into the circulation.

Here's an example of how a lectin agglutinates in the body. Let's say a Type A person eats a plate of lima beans. The lima beans are digested in the stomach through the process of acid hydrolysis. However, the lectin protein is resistant to acid hydrolysis. It doesn't get digested, but stays intact. It may interact directly with the lining of the stomach or intestinal tract, causing inflammation or blocking the absorption of nutrients, or it may even get absorbed into your bloodstream along with the digested lima bean nutrients. Different lectins target different organs and body systems.

Once the intact lectin protein interacts with your tissues, it virtually has a magnetic effect on the cells in that region. It clumps the cells together, which targets them for destruction, as if they too were foreign invaders. This clumping can cause irritable bowel syndrome, disrupt the balance of healthy bacteria in the gut, and even block the absorption of other foods. Some authorities on the subject have even speculated that the lectin-rich diets consumed in third-world and developing countries might be responsible for much of the anemia seen in these populations.

Lectins: A Dangerous Glue

YOU MAY HAVE HEARD the story of the bizarre assassination of Georgi Markov in 1978 on a London street. Markov was killed while waiting for a bus by an unknown Soviet KGB agent. Initially, the autopsy could not pinpoint how it was done. After a thorough search, a tiny gold bead was discovered embedded in Markov's leg. The bead was found to be permeated with a chemical called ricin, which is a toxic lectin extracted from castor beans. Ricin is so potent an agglutinin that even an infinitesimally small amount can cause death by swiftly converting the body's red blood cells into large clots, which block the arteries. Ricin kills instantaneously. It is so instantly deadly that ricin poisoning has been attempted as a terrorist tool—so far unsuccessfully— and a letter containing ricin is believed to have been sent to President Barack Obama. Ricin also made an appearance on the popular TV series *Breaking Bad*.

Fortunately, most lectins found in the diet are not quite so life threatening, although they can cause a variety of other problems, especially if they are specific to a particular blood type. For the most part, our immune systems protect us from lectins. Ninety-five percent of the lectins we absorb from our typical diets are sloughed off by the body, but at least 5 percent of the lectins we eat are filtered into the bloodstream, where they react with and destroy red and white blood cells. The actions of lectins in the digestive tract can be even more powerful. There they often create a violent inflammation of the sensitive mucus of the intestines, and this agglutinative action may mimic food allergies. Even a minute quantity of a lectin is capable of damaging a huge number of cells if the particular blood type is reactive.

This is not to say that you should suddenly become fearful of every food you eat. After all, lectins are widely abundant in legumes, seafood, grains, and vegetables. It's hard to bypass them. The key is to avoid the lectins that agglutinate your particular cells—determined by blood type. For example, gluten, the most common lectin found in wheat and other grains, binds to the lining of the small intestine, causing substantial inflammation and painful irritation in some blood types— especially Type O.

Lectins vary widely, according to their source. For example, the lectin found in wheat has a different shape from the lectin found in soy, and attaches to a different combination of sugars; each of these foods is dangerous for some blood types, but beneficial for others.

Nervous tissue as a rule is very sensitive to the agglutinating effect of food lectins. This may explain why some researchers feel that allergy-avoidance diets may be of benefit in treating certain types of nervous disorders, such as hyperactivity. Russian researchers have noted that the brains of schizophrenics are more sensitive to the attachment of certain common food lectins. In fact, a Swedish study linked the decline of new schizophrenia cases in Sweden in the years 1940–45 with the lack of bread due to the wartime blockade of wheat shipments. Lectins are also implicated in leptin resistance, a factor in obesity.

Injections of the lentil lectin into the knee joint cavities of nonsensitized rabbits resulted in the development of arthritis that was indistinguishable from rheumatoid arthritis. Many people with arthritis feel that avoiding the nightshade vegetables such as tomatoes, eggplant, and white potatoes seems to help their arthritis. That's not surprising because most nightshades are very high in lectins.

Food lectins can also interact with the surface receptors of the body's white cells, programming them to multiply rapidly. These lectins are called mitogens because they cause the white cells to enter mitosis, the process of cell division. They do not clump blood by gluing cells together; they merely attach themselves to things, like fleas on a dog. Occasionally an emergency room physician will be faced with a very ill but otherwise apparently normal child who has an extraordinarily high white blood cell count. Although pediatric leukemia is usually the first thing to come to mind, the astute physician will ask the parent, "Was your child playing in the yard?" If the answer is yes, "Was he eating any weeds or putting plants in his mouth?" Often it will turn out that the child was eating the leaves or shoots of the pokeweed plant, which contains a lectin with the potent ability to stimulate white cell production.

Finally, if and when lectins penetrate the body's gut defenses and reach the systemic circulation, they can attach to receptors on cells originally designed to receive signals from the body's hormones. Sometimes the lectin can sit on the receptor and block the intended hormone

Blood Type–Specific Food Lectins

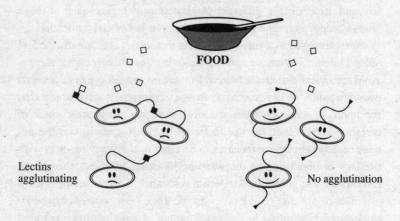

FOOD

Lectins
agglutinating

No agglutination

Each blood type antigen possesses a unique shape; thus, many lectins interact with only one specific blood type because of its form. In the lima bean example, food lectins interact with and agglutinate Type A cells (on the left) because they fit the shape of the A antigen. The antigen for Type B blood (on the right), a different sugar molecule with a different shape, is not affected. Conversely, a food lectin (such as buckwheat) that can specifically attach to and agglutinate cells of Blood Type B would not fit Type A blood.

from attaching and exerting its effects; other times the lectin can actually stimulate the receptor, making the cell think that the hormone was produced, when in fact it wasn't. From this information, it's possible to conclude that cases of hormonal imbalance could be cured by the simple expedient of intelligent eating.

Your Personal Ecosystem

YOUR DIGESTIVE TRACT is a hotbed of activity, with a level of interactions rivaling that of a small city. It is estimated that the human digestive tract may contain up to 100 trillion microorganisms, and the human gut may host up to a thousand different species of bacteria. More and more, we hear and read about the importance of the microbiome: the ecological community of friendly and unfriendly microorganisms that share our body space—for both good and ill.

New studies are revealing how the gut microbiome has co-evolved with us and how it manipulates and complements our biology in ways that are mutually beneficial. We are also starting to understand how friendly bacteria operate to improve the integrity and function of the digestive system—and, indeed, the entire human body. For example, consider the microbial profile of an obese person. Obesity appears as the result of a complicated mix of factors such as genetics, environment, diet, and lifestyle, resulting in an imbalance of the equilibrium between energy expenditure and storage in the form of an overabundance of fat. The makeup and interactions of microorganisms and bacteria in the gut are widely recognized as a potential factor in human obesity.

The science of the microbiome is a hot topic in health circles. But clearly not every individual has the same ecosystem. That's where blood type enters the picture. Your blood type antigens are very prominent in your digestive tract. Because of this, many of the bacteria in your digestive tract actually use your blood type molecule as a preferred food supply. Talk about eating right for your blood type! In fact, the blood type's influence is important among intestinal bacteria, almost half of which show some Blood Type A, B, or O specificity.

Simply put, people of different blood types have different gut bacteria. Certain bacteria are 50,000 times more likely to turn up in people with one blood type than another. This originated from our ancestors whose digestive tracts developed to accommodate one type of diet over another, and whose blood types controlled the ability to reject or co-exist with certain bacteria but not others. Our blood type can actually seed our gut by encouraging the growth of only those bacteria strains that can use our blood type antigens as a source of food, while our anti-blood-type antibodies attack bacteria that carry antigens resembling those of a different blood type.

Human feces contain enzymes produced by the bacteria of the microbiome that degrade the ABO blood type antigens lining the digestive tract and convert it to an energy source for their own use. The population of fecal bacteria that produces blood type–degrading enzymes is highly correlated with the blood type of the host. Because many foods have blood type–like antigens, it stands to reason that those foods will be favored by your microbial system.

Harmful lectins in foods can encourage the growth of problematic strains of bacteria, impairing absorption, damaging the intestinal lining, and causing "leaky gut." That is why the first line of support for healing your digestive tract and building a healthy microbiome is eating the right foods for your blood type.

Secretor Versus Non-Secretor

Up until now we've discussed the role of your blood type antigen as a marker on your cells and tissues. However, in reality there are two forms of the blood type antigen, the one we've been discussing up until this point called the "bound" form that is found in our blood, and another form that floats around in our secretions (tears, digestive juices, perspiration, semen, etc.) called the "unbound" form. Everyone has the ability to make the bound form, where the blood type antigen is attached, and many of us can produce the unbound form as well—but a significant minority are missing the gene for this and cannot. The ability to produce both the bound and unbound form identifies you as a secretor. The inability to produce the unbound form means that you are a non-secretor. Secretors make up about 80 percent of the population; non-secretors, 20 percent.

You might be familiar with the idea of secretor status if you know about law enforcement. For example, a semen sample taken from a rape victim can be used to help convict the rapist if he is a secretor and his blood type matches the blood type identified in the semen. However, if he is in the small population of non-secretors, his blood type cannot be identified from any fluids except the blood because his body does not produce the unbound form of the blood type antigen. (From a practical standpoint, DNA testing makes this less an issue than it once was, although a blood type match is a quick-and-dirty way to know you're on the right track.)

People who do not secrete their blood type antigens in other fluids besides blood are called non-secretors. Being a secretor or a non-secretor is independent of your ABO blood type; it is controlled by a different gene. Thus, one person could be a Type A secretor, and another a Type A non-secretor.

Because secretors have the ability to produce both bound and unbound versions of the blood type antigen, they have more places to put these antigens; thus they have what is referred to as more blood type "expression" in their bodies than non-secretors. This gives them a distinct advantage, especially with the activity of lectins on gut bacteria, because the free-floating blood type antigens that secretors manufacture can act as a kind of decoy and sop up harmful lectins before they have a chance to interact with the blood type antigens attached to the tissues and cells. Secretors have a stronger defense against harmful lectins than do non-secretors. It is likely that secretor status was a further adaptation to our immune system, which evolved as additional threats from the environment—foreign bacteria, pollutants, and pathogens—produced more sophisticated challenges.

Many of the peculiar relationships we share with the microbial world can be understood and predicted by factoring in both ABO blood type and secretor status. For example, non-secretors are much more likely to be carriers of *Candida albicans* yeast and to have problems with persistent *Candida* infections, especially if they are Blood Type O. And in one study, among individuals with type 2 diabetes, 44 percent of non-secretors of all blood types were oral carriers of this yeast. Inflammatory problems of the digestive tract, allergies, carbohydrate intolerance, and autoimmune problems are also more frequent among non-secretors.

Finding out whether you are a secretor is not as easy as finding out your ABO blood type. The most common way to determine secretor status involves testing saliva for the presence of blood type activity. (To order this test, see Appendix F.) Knowing your secretor status gives you one more tool to healthy living. This is especially important if you have a medical condition or struggle with your weight. If you are in the minority of people who are non-secretors, you might want to follow the Blood Type Diet all the more closely.

How to Detect
Your Harmful Lectins

I OFTEN have the experience of hearing patients insist that they are following the Blood Type Diet to the letter and staying away from all the lectins targeted for their blood type—but I know differently. When I challenge their assurance, usually they will drop all signs of protest and ask in amazement, "How did you know?"

I know because the effects of lectins on different blood types are not just a theory. They're based on science. I've tested virtually all common foods for blood type reactions, using both clinical and laboratory methods. I can purchase isolated lectins from foods such as peanuts, lentils, soy, or wheat from chemical laboratories, and the results are often visible under the microscope: I can see them agglutinating cells in the affected blood type. However, I caution you against dropping foods on slides of your blood to see what happens. Many lectins have subtle effects that can be identified only with more sophisticated testing under controlled conditions. Do-it-yourself testing will just yield innumerable false-positive and false-negative results.

Here is a simple quiz to help you identify whether your current diet may be too high in reactive lectin-containing foods problematic for your blood type:

- Do you suffer from digestive cramps, bowel inflammation, or irritable bowel?
- Do you experience bloating 30 to 60 minutes after meals?
- Do you suffer from joint pain, achiness, and stiffness, often worse after eating?
- Do your symptoms increase 30 to 60 minutes after consuming sugar?
- Have you been told you have fibromyalgia?
- Do you suffer with hay fever or seasonal allergies?
- Do you experience cloudy thinking 30 to 60 minutes after meals?
- Do you suffer with acne, rosacea, psoriasis, or eczema?
- Do you suffer from low thyroid function?

- Do you experience fatigue, which increases over the course of the day?
- Are you experiencing weight gain even after reducing your calorie intake?
- Are you experiencing difficulty gaining weight despite consuming more calories?
- Do you experience allergic symptoms after eating?
- Do you experience congestion or nasal stuffiness, persistent throat-clearing, or post-nasal drip 30 to 60 minutes after meals?
- Does your red blood cell count or white blood cell count run low or low-normal?
- Do you have an autoimmune disorder?
- Women: Do you experience painful menses or migraine headaches with menses?
- Women: If menopausal, are you experiencing excessive symptoms (hot flashes, etc.)?
- Men: Are you experiencing erectile dysfunction?
- Men: Have you been told you have an enlarged prostate?
- Children: Has the child been diagnosed with a learning disability?

If you can answer yes to four or more of these questions, it is very likely that the consumption of food lectins is contributing to your current health situation and that following the prescribed diet for your blood type offers a safe, proven way to correct it. If you've answered less than four, congratulations! However, still do the work. Intelligent eating using the Blood Type Diet is your best insurance against experiencing these uncomfortable and unpleasant effects again.

A Blood Type Lesson: The Rabbi's Story

OVER THE YEARS, I have witnessed many transformations as a result of the Blood Type Diet. But few so moved and inspired me as my experience many years ago with a wise, older Brooklyn rabbi.

In early 1990, I received an urgent phone call from a New York City doctor who respected my work. He asked if I could come to see one of his patients, a renowned Hasidic rabbi who was bedridden.

"Rabbi Jacob is a very special man," he told me. "It should be quite an experience for you—and, I hope, for him, too." He went on to tell me that the rabbi, seventy-three, had a long history of diabetes, which was poorly controlled by injectable insulin therapy. A massive stroke had left him partially paralyzed.

When I arrived to see him in his Brooklyn home, I found that Rabbi Jacob was, indeed, an impressive man who gave off an air of deep spiritual understanding and quiet compassion. Obviously once tall and strongly formed, now the rabbi lay withered and exhausted in his bed, his luxuriant white beard almost falling to his chest. In spite of his medical condition, his eyes were clear, kind, and filled with life. His main interest was getting out of bed so he could go on about his work. But I could see he was in terrible pain. Even before the stroke, he told me, his legs had been giving him problems. Poor circulation had caused swelling and inflammation in both legs and caused him to experience excruciating jolts of "pins and needles" when he tried to walk. Now his left leg was not responding to his bidding.

I wasn't surprised to learn that Rabbi Jacob was Blood Type B. Although this blood type is relatively uncommon in America, it is very common among Hasidic Jews, the majority of whom emigrated from Eastern Europe.

I realized that to help the rabbi, I must first learn something about the way he lived and the foods he ate. Food is intimately bound to ritual in Jewish tradition.

I sat down with Rabbi Jacob's wife and daughter, both of whom were unfamiliar with naturopathic treatments. But they wanted to help the rabbi, and they were eager to learn.

"Tell me about the rabbi's diet," I said.

"He usually eats the same foods every day," his daughter told me. Those foods consisted of boiled chicken; cholent, a meat-and-bean stew; and kasha varnishkes, which is buckwheat combined with bowtie noodles. "So, how is the kasha dish made?" I innocently asked. There was a quick conversation back and forth between mother and daughter in Yiddish, punctuated with lovely smiles at me, and gales of laughter.

"Well," said the daughter in perfect New York English, "first you cook up the kasha—the buckwheat—then you stir it in with the bow ties. Then you serve it, say blessings, and eat."

"Do you season the kasha at all?" I again innocently asked. Another outbreak of Yiddish. Then the rabbi's daughter began. "Kasha, Doctor, well . . . you take all the fat you pulled off the chicken while you were koshering it, you put it in a heavy saucepan with just a *bissel* [tiny bit] of chopped onion, and you cook it down. You render off the fat as it cooks down, and you've got beautiful pure chicken fat. We give it to the little ones on a piece of fresh challah bread with some salt. It's so delicious you could die!"

Yes, yes, you could, I thought darkly.

"Anyway," the rabbi's daughter continued, "you take some of the *gribenes*, which is what's left when you cook the fat away. It's all nice and dark and crispy with the caramelized onions, and you put this on the side along with the kasha for a little treat. It tastes better than potato chips. The rabbi loves it! The chicken fat you've rendered you mix into the kasha and noodles. Oh, it's just delicious. Delicious!"

I learned that these are very common Hasidic dishes, and they made up the family's typical Sabbath meal. But it was more than just a weekly ritual for the rabbi. A pious man who spent most of his time in prayer, the rabbi thought little of food and simply ate the same meal twice daily, day after day.

Although part of a centuries-old tradition, the rabbi's diet was not a good choice for people with Type B blood. The lectins in foods such as chicken, buckwheat and beans (not to mention the *gribenes*!) were causing the cells of his blood to agglutinate, and that was probably a major factor in his stroke. These particular lectins can also block the effects of insulin, which explains why Rabbi Jacob's diabetes became increasingly difficult to control.

I understood that Hasidic Jews obeyed the laws of *kashrut*—kosher—ancient dietary principles first laid out in the Old Testament of the Bible. According to these dietary laws, a number of foods are forbidden, and dairy and meat are never eaten at the same meal. In fact, there are separate pots, pans, dishes, and cutlery for dairy and meat in kosher homes. And separate sinks to wash all of these things, as well.

So I approached the matter of dietary changes carefully with the two women, not wanting to disrupt the ritual and religious associations that meant so much. I was also careful not to suggest foods that I knew to be considered unclean in their tradition.

Fortunately, there were allowable substitutes. I asked Rabbi Jacob's wife to vary the family diet, restricting the rabbi's typical dishes to once a week for the actual Sabbath meal. For his other meals I asked her to prepare lamb, fish, or turkey instead of chicken; rice or millet instead of kasha; and to vary the beans used to prepare the cholent. Finally, I prescribed several vitamin and herbal combinations to speed his recovery.

Over the next year, the rabbi made wonderful progress. Within eight weeks he was walking and doing moderate exercise, which greatly helped improve his circulation. He showed remarkable vigor for a man of his age, and shook off the effects of his stroke. At six months he was switched from injectable to oral insulin therapy—a remarkable achievement considering he had been on injectable insulin for many years. There were no further episodes of stroke, and Rabbi Jacob's diabetes was finally under control.

Treating the rabbi gave me a new appreciation for just how ancient and fundamental the wisdom of the blood types is. It also illustrated that foods chosen for religious or cultural reasons may not always be the healthiest for a person in that culture. A 5,000- or 6,000-year-old tradition may be time-honored, but many of the characteristics of our blood types are thousands of years older.

As you study your Blood Type Diet, take a lesson from the rabbi. The Blood Type Diet is not an attempt to superimpose a rigid formula on what you eat, or to rob you of the foods that are important to your culture. Rather, they are a way to fully support your most basic identity—to lead you back to the essential truths that live in every cell of your body and to link you to your historical, evolutionary ancestry.

THREE

Blood Type
and
Weight Loss:

The Individualized Key

THE BLOOD TYPE DIET OFFERS YOU A SIMPLE PROMISE: IF YOU EAT AC-
cording to the biochemical script that's coded in your blood and genes,
you can lose weight and achieve a level of health and fitness you might
never have imagined. Instead of being at war with your body, you can
live in harmony with your unique biology.

If you're a veteran of the diet wars, this is the best possible news for
you because you've probably found the dieting process ridden with con-
flicts as you try to force compliance with eating plans that don't make
you feel better and ultimately fail.

Why is lasting weight loss such an elusive goal, even for the most motivated dieters? Each year brings a new weight loss trend to the forefront—
gluten-free, Paleo, vegan, no-carb, macrobiotic, fasting cleanses, and
so on. In every case these approaches are heralded as the weight loss
panacea, but it never quite works out that way. Upward of 50 million
Americans go on a new diet each year. Failure rates are estimated at 95
percent—and that's a conservative number.

There are plenty of theories about why diets fail, including lack of
willpower, poor portion control, and low compliance. It's a convenient
excuse for promoters of diet theories to blame the dieters when they
fail. But it's ludicrous to believe that 95 percent of dieters are lazy and

unmotivated; to the contrary, dieters are the most motivated people around.

What is rarely discussed is the main reason people don't lose weight on diets. Virtually every diet program begins with the premise that it is formulated to work for everybody. Think about it for just a moment—how can that be? You don't have to be a biochemist or a geneticist to understand that individuality is an essential part of our human code. And as we have seen, blood type is one of the most potent markers of biologic individuality.

I'd like to dispel once and for all the myth that any single diet approach works for every individual. The biggest breakthrough of the Blood Type Diet is that it is a truly individualized approach, harnessing your unique biochemical attributes, while avoiding the pitfalls.

My patients always want inside information about all of the latest popular diets: Does a low-carb diet really work? What about calorie restriction? Veganism? Raw food? Paleo? Are any of these approaches right for them? My answer is a variation of yes and no. Yes, some aspects of a particular diet might work for them, depending on their blood type; and no, a one-size-fits-all diet can't be a solution for everyone. Most popular diets are not entirely bad, but they're formulaic—and a single formula just doesn't cut it in a world of individuality.

I'm now in my third decade of private practice, and have seen theories and trends come and go. When I started, we were in the middle of the fat-phobic 1980s and people wanted nothing to do with protein and fat. Try as I might, I could not convince many Type O patients to work with a higher-protein and healthy-fat diet: They wanted to eat like Type A. Thirty years later, it's been reversed. The Type A patients want to go on a Paleo diet and eat like Type O.

Many aspects of the Paleo, low-carb, and gluten-free diets work well for Blood Type O and to some extent for Blood Type B. By severely limiting carbohydrates, high-protein diets force the burning of fats for energy and the production of ketones, which indicates that the body is in a "fat-burning" mode. It doesn't surprise me that the patients who tell me they have lost weight on high-protein diets are usually Type O and Type B, although most of these diets eliminate dairy foods, which are beneficial for Type B. I don't know of a popular diet that comes close to satisfying the needs of Blood Types B and AB, with their idiosyncratic lectin issues with foods like corn and chicken. Even when they're generally feasible, Paleo and low-carb diets don't account for the blood type–specific lectins in certain vegetables, fruits, and nuts that can be a stumbling block—although, thanks perhaps to the earlier versions of this book, some Paleo authors now factor lectins into their recommendations. Some Paleo dieters tip the scales too far in one direction by overconsuming protein. Good-quality carbohydrates that are right for your blood type help the body to better utilize the protein you eat.

I don't see many Type As who do well on Paleo or low-carb diets; their systems are biologically unsuited to metabolize meat as efficiently as Type O and Type B. In fact, years ago, I read an online transcript of an interview with the head nurse who worked with one of the great low-carb doctors. Asked about the Blood Type Diet, she was perhaps a bit more frank than her employer would have liked. Try as they might, she said, they always had trouble getting their diet to work for Type As. Nor do Type ABs lose weight on high-protein diets because these diets lack the balance of A-like foods that Type ABs require.

On the other hand, the principles of a macrobiotic diet, which encourage the consumption of natural foods such as vegetables, rice, whole grains, fruits, and soy, might be best suited for Type A dieters, providing they eat the recommended grains and legumes and avoid those that contain harmful lectins. Type As and, to a lesser extent Type ABs, make good vegetarians, with certain caveats.

Several diets have hopped on the sugar-busting trend, advancing the simplistic notion that carbohydrates (thus sugars) should be avoided. Other diet approaches are simply metabolically unsustainable and even harmful. For example, although I'm a big fan of plant antioxidants, I am not a proponent of juice-type cleansings. Many people ask me about this popular trend, attracted to the idea of "detoxing" their liver and kidneys. On the surface, it sounds good. However, when I look at the support material, it is usually quite clear that the designers of these sorts of detoxes don't really know very much about detoxification, a process the body is already adept at, given the right support and genetics. In fact, studies on the effects of foods on the body's detox mechanisms always indicate that whole foods are the most powerful and have the most profound effect on the microbiome. Although there might be an initial weight loss—because cleansing diets are often in the range of 1,000 calories a day—in the long run these types of diets do more harm than good.

Even if a diet is generally right for you, unless it is individualized you could be tripped up. *The bottom line is that the best weight loss diet is an individualized nutritional approach.* Because the Blood Type Diet is tailored to the cellular composition of your body, specific foods will promote weight gain or weight loss for you, even though they may have a different effect on a person of another blood type. In that respect, there are no good or bad foods—just foods that are right or wrong for your blood type.

A national television program once conducted an experiment to test the weight loss potential of the Blood Type Diet. Type O Loren was placed on a diet that featured lean organic meats and vegetables. Type A Miguel was placed on a diet that favored whole grains, vegetables, and soy foods. At the end of two weeks Type O Loren had lost seven pounds, and Type A Miguel had lost eight pounds. The results caused a flurry of amazement because a striking anomaly in the typical diet rigidity had occurred. Two very different diets had delivered equally satisfying results.

If you eat right for your blood type, you will lose weight. And you'll feel good in the process—not deprived, not sick, not lethargic but as if a key clicked into the lock. The science is clear—and so are the testimonials from hundreds of thousands of people who have shared their success stories.

A Personalized Approach Works

I UNDERSTAND how much anxiety people feel around food and how worrisome it can be to embark on a new diet. The typical trajectory of the modern weight loss diet goes something like this: initial excitement and enthusiasm, followed by hopeful early results, followed by emerging difficulties, followed by a crushing fear of falling off the diet, followed by succumbing and abandoning the diet, followed by weight gain. This is such a common formula that you could patent the whole process. The Blood Type Diet follows a different trajectory—one that involves far less suffering and much more success.

I have often said that the Blood Type Diet is not a weight loss diet per se. It's a diet for optimal health and performance. The natural outcome of that, of course, is weight loss if you need to lose weight. This is not a gimmick to squeeze off a few pounds but a restoration of your body's natural set point. The primary weight-related benefit is that this diet helps your body find and maintain its ideal weight. For some, this means losing weight naturally. For others, this may involve gaining or retaining muscle.

It's interesting to me that so many top fashion models have adopted the Blood Type Diet. You might think, "Well, of course!" What better exemplifies the cultural obsession with being thin than fashion models? But what these women (and sometimes men) have said is that in eating and exercising right for their blood types, they have gained levels of fitness and well-being that allowed them to succeed in a very strenuous occupation. For them, the Blood Type Diet is a rejection of the starvation method in favor of a way of life that allows them to look and feel their best. Many of them have told me that this is an enormous breakthrough in a profession often characterized by desperation and unhealthy diets.

Fitness expert Justin Gelband, who works with many Victoria's Secret models, became a proponent of the Blood Type Diet when he saw how much more fit, energized, and balanced his clients were when they ate right for their types. He noticed that they felt better, their skin looked clearer, they had better digestion, and their metabolisms were more efficient. Gelband had been one of those people who didn't believe in diets. He'd seen firsthand how much physical and emotional devastation they could cause. But this was different. It was an eating plan that worked *with* his clients' bodies, not against them. I was gratified to hear the testimonials, but not surprised. The Blood Type Diet has exactly the same effect, no matter who you are.

Right for Your Type

MOST PEOPLE who embark on a weight loss diet think of it as a temporary process of restricting the foods they eat. They gear up for a period of sacrifice and denial. Weight loss is a game they play with themselves, hoping to beat their cravings. It's a miserable way to look at it, which is why most diets don't feel *natural*. Repeatedly, people who follow the Blood Type Diet describe the way it feels "right" for them. Maybe they notice that their digestion is smoother—less bloating after meals, more regularity, the disappearance of heartburn, more energy, all happening simultaneously as they are losing weight. Even when weight loss is their primary goal, they find themselves happiest about how good they feel.

Weight loss doesn't exist in a vacuum. Achieving your healthiest weight happens when your body itself is healthy. This is a fact that many weight loss diets ignore, but the biochemical process is clear. The dynamics of weight loss are related to the changes your body makes when you follow your genetically tailored diet.

In the beginning, as your body makes the dramatic shift of eliminating foods that are poorly digested or toxic, the first thing it does is try to flush out the toxins that are already there. Those toxins are deposited mainly in the fat tissue, so the process of eliminating toxins also means eliminating fat.

Depending on your blood type, the lectin activity of certain foods may do the following:

- Inflame the digestive tract lining.
- Interfere with the digestive process, causing bloating.
- Slow down the rate of food metabolism, so you don't efficiently burn calories for energy.
- Compromise the production of insulin.
- Upset the hormonal balance, causing water retention (edema), thyroid disorders, and other problems.

For example, after consuming any number of foods containing wheat, both Blood Types O and A can experience bloating and other digestive problems. This may be more than a simple food intolerance. The walls of the stomach and intestines are lined with sensitive receptors that interact with, and respond to, the lectin in wheat. At first, you may experience that wheat lectin interaction as only a mild digestive problem or a dull, listless feeling after consuming foods not right for you. Over time, the result is a steadily deteriorating state of health, loss of energy, and weight gain.

The good news is, by removing these targeted foods and replacing them with foods more suitable for your blood type, you begin to experience the benefits of a leaner, cleaner, more energetic body.

As we've seen, increasingly studies are showing that changes in the microflora content of the digestive tract can be linked to metabolic illnesses, including type 2 diabetes and obesity. Many lectins in foods upset the balance of intestinal flora, contributing to insulin resistance, and so to weight gain. Blood type and secretor status play important roles in conditioning the overall characteristics of the digestive tract, including influencing the appearance and frequency of many strains of bacteria.

The hormone insulin controls your body's ability to metabolize food and use it for energy. When you eat, your pancreas releases insulin into your bloodstream, which regulates the metabolism of carbohydrates and fats by promoting the absorption of glucose from the blood to skeletal muscles and fat tissue. When your system is properly balanced, everything works fine—principally because once insulin has accomplished its job, a feedback message is sent to the brain, which then informs the pancreas to cut off insulin production. With no new insulin being produced, the circulating insulin gradually dwindles and the cycle starts again.

If your body is unable to use the insulin produced for this purpose, the result is a condition called insulin resistance. Insulin resistance almost always occurs for people who are overweight. With insulin resistance, the normal amount of insulin secreted is not sufficient to move glucose into the cells—thus the cells are said to be "resistant" to the action of insulin. Over time, this sends your blood sugar levels up. That can set you up for type 2 diabetes as well as heart disease, but it doesn't have to. Exercise and a good diet can help you stay healthy.

Dietary lectins have been shown to interact with insulin on the body's fat cells, which can impair its proper signaling and function. Insulin resistance can be triggered when you eat foods containing lectins that react improperly with your tissues, often in ways controlled by your blood type. Some lectins have insulin-like effects on fat cell receptors, which signal fat cells to store calories as fat. In this situation, the fat cell is permanently paralyzed, capable only of storing fat and incapable of releasing it. This explains why certain people gain weight on a high-carbohydrate diet: It is not the calories in the food or the percentages of fat, protein, and carbohydrate that are causing the weight gain—after all, most carbohydrates are low in calories compared to fats—but rather the lectins in the food itself, which mimic the effects of naturally occurring hormones and result in weight gain.

Optimal Fitness

ONE OF THE MOST COMMON QUESTIONS people ask me about the Blood Type Diet is whether calories matter. The answer is that they do and they don't. If all diets were simply a matter of calorie restriction, the major benefit gained by dieting according to your blood type—the maintenance of active tissue mass—would be lost. When your diet is based solely on calorie restrictions, you'll lose body fat, but it's a fool's errand because you'll also lose active tissue mass (muscle and organ tissue), which is the part of the body that burns calories. Losing weight by losing body fat is great, but losing weight by losing active tissue mass is counterproductive. If you eat correctly for your blood type, you will actually gain active tissue mass, increasing your basal metabolic rate, allowing excess fat to be burned away without losing any muscle. So, if you follow the Blood Type Diet, your weight loss will be consistent. You'll also maintain or increase your active tissue mass.

When your body is working properly, you build muscle mass naturally through daily activity and regular exercise combined with diet. One of your body's natural cycles involves occasionally breaking muscle proteins down to be used for energy, a process called protein turnover. Your body is in a continuous cycle of anabolic (muscle building) and catabolic (breaking muscle down) changes, seeking a natural balance between these two alternating processes—with a preference toward anabolic. You literally feed and encourage either of these states mostly through the dietary choices you make.

Many people on typical weight loss diets are under the mistaken impression that eating light meals with fewer calories can help them lose weight. The reverse is actually true in the long term. Studies show that the weight you lose on these diets, along with any temporary fat loss, is typically muscle. Severely curtailed low-calorie diets can cause your body to go into starvation and conservation mode. These kinds of diets or even long periods during the day without eating can actually create a catabolic state of muscle burning to conserve energy. Muscle is metabolically active tissue, requiring a great deal of caloric energy just to maintain it. Maintaining a high percentage of active tissue is particularly important when you are trying to lose weight. Because calorie-restrictive diets do nothing to increase active tissue mass, your metabolic rate remains unchanged or declines, leaving you predisposed to regain the weight you lost—and often more—as soon as you resume normal eating.

Thus eating too little or too infrequently will have the exact opposite result than the one you intend. With fewer meals, your body slows its metabolism, making the food you do eat harder to metabolize. The more frequent, smaller, nutrient-rich meals you eat, the more efficient your metabolism will become. In fact, this has been measured. Using your resting (basal) metabolism as the starting point, the additional caloric expenditure that it takes to digest, absorb, and process the food you eat is called the thermic effect of feeding (TEF).

It is not surprising that different foods have different effects on TEF, which is yet another reason to choose a personalized diet right for your type. One significant study demonstrated that during the normal 6-hour resting metabolism period, we typically burn about 270 calories. When eating a single meal of carbohydrates alone or fat alone, the energy burned during this 6-hour period reached 290 calories (an additional 20 calories). It is interesting that when eating protein alone, the subjects in this study burned 310 calories during the 6-hour period (an additional 40 calories). It appears that protein alone had double the thermogenic potential of fat or carbs alone.

The body requires protein to maintain and build muscle. But which type and how much protein is right for you? Your Blood Type Diet is the ideal guide not only to the protein sources ideally suited for you but also to the ideal amounts. Generally, studies show that smaller meals, spaced 2 to 3 hours apart, with a quality protein source in each mini-meal, provide the muscle tissue the nutrition it requires to thrive.

Stress-Weight Cycle

IN YOUR BLOOD TYPE DIET you will also find very specific recommendations for exercise and stress management that are crucial for weight loss. You probably know that too much stress is bad for you. In its most simplified sense, stress is what you feel when the demands on your life exceed your ability to meet them. Did you also know that stress promotes weight gain? Furthermore, like the food you eat, your stress responses and therefore exercise requirements differ according to your blood type.

The old adage about exercise—"no pain, no gain"—is the polar opposite of the blood type–specific recommendation. Your stress responses and therefore your exercise recommendations differ according to your blood type. These are outlined in your Blood Type Diet, and you will see that they too contain important differences.

So, exercise right, but don't overdo it. If you overdo it, especially on an exercise regimen that is wrong for your blood type, you can actually experience the irony of being a somewhat "healthier" version of your still overweight self.

What Is Your Ideal Weight?

THE NUMBER on your scale is only one part of the equation. There are two measurements, in addition to the scale, that will help you judge your ideal weight—waist circumference and body mass index (BMI).

Waist Circumference

This is a measurement of abdominal fat, a reliable sign of unhealthy weight leading to obesity, diabetes and heart problems. An unhealthy waist circumference is above 35 inches for women and 40 inches for men. Measure in a standing position, placing a tape measure around your waist, just above the hip bones.

Body Mass Index (BMI)

This is a simple measure of body fat based on height and weight. You can calculate your BMI by dividing your weight in kilograms by the square of your height in meters. For Americans and other folks who are nonmetric, you'll have to do some simple conversions, so grab a calculator:

1. To convert height in inches to height in meters, divide by 39.37. If you're 72 inches tall, your height in meters is 1.83 (72 ÷ 39.37).
2. To convert weight in pounds to kilograms, divide by 2.2. If you weigh 150 pounds, your weight in kilograms is 68.2 (150 ÷ 2.2).
3. To calculate BMI, multiply height in meters by itself and then divide weight in kilograms by the result. In our example, first multiply your weight by itself (1.83 x 1.83) to get 3.35. Then divide your weight by the result (68.2 ÷ 3.35) to get your BMI, which is 20.4 in this case.

Once you have your BMI, you need to analyze the results:

BMI	MEANING
UNDER 18.5	UNDERWEIGHT
18.5–24.9	NORMAL
25.0–29.9	OVERWEIGHT
30.0 AND ABOVE	POTENTIALLY OBESE

The BMI is a useful indicator of weight status in most people, but for certain folks, such as athletes, it is too simplistic, as it assumes all extra weight is fat; however, in athletes the extra weight is often muscle instead. Thus many authorities are moving away from using BMI as any definitive measure of obesity. Adding a waist circumference gives a bit more clarity to the picture, since waist girth is almost always fatty tissue. You may also go to your doctor, or to your gym and have your percentage of body fat measured. This will tell you how much of your body is composed of lean muscle and bone versus fat. Both of these are good indicators of weight as a health risk.

Your Individualized Weight Loss Key

YOUR BLOOD TYPE DIET, as detailed later in the book, provides all the specifics you need to eat right. But focusing on weight loss, here's a quick-and-dirty rundown on how your blood type gains and loses weight.

Blood Type O

The main weight gain factors for Blood Type O are

Insulin resistance
Intestinal dysbiosis
Thyroid hormone imbalance
Inflammation

Your genetic inheritance offers you the opportunity to be strong, lean, productive, long-lived, and tenacious. When a Type O's wiring gets crossed, as a result of a poor diet, lack of exercise, unhealthy behaviors, or elevated stress levels, you're more vulnerable to negative metabolic effects, including insulin resistance, sluggish thyroid activity, and weight gain. As a Blood Type Os, you may also be predisposed to certain illnesses, such as thyroid disorders, which can impact weight control. It is not uncommon for Type O to experience thyroid instability, and you often exhibit insufficient levels of iodine, an element critical for proper thyroid activity. Imbalanced thyroid function can cause many negative health effects such as weight gain, fluid retention, hair loss, and fatigue.

The key to your optimal diet is embedded in the historical imprint of your blood type. Blood Type O is wired for action, and this quality is reflected in your metabolism, your digestion, and your immune system. When you eat a diet of lean, chemical-free meats and healthy fruits and vegetables, your body maintains a lean physique and you have lots of energy. On the other hand, grains—wheat gluten, especially—compromise your natural state and lead to weight gain and other metabolic complications. A restriction of grains, bread, legumes, and beans is part of the Type O weight loss strategy.

You will succeed by incorporating plenty of high-quality protein in your diet. This increases active tissue mass and raises your metabolic rate. A high-protein diet will boost your weight loss and burn off any excess fat.

How can Blood Type O lose weight by eating meat? The secret is in your genetic memory of the Paleolithic paradise. Your genetic ancestors' reliance on meat, an early key to the survival of the species, is coded into a variety of genes controlled by your blood type. You possess a secret weapon not available to all blood types: higher levels of stomach acid that allow you to efficiently digest and metabolize meats and fats. In particular, you have three times the normal level of an enzyme called intestinal alkaline phosphatase (IAP), which helps break down protein and fat, allowing for easier digestion and metabolism.

One of the most controversial aspects of the Blood Type Diet has been the recommendation that Blood Type O individuals—and to some extent Blood Type B individuals—consume red meat as a key component of their diets. Many current nutritional guidelines demonize meat because of a legitimate concern over saturated animal fats, which are implicated in heart disease, cancer, and other ailments. But consider the typical meat made available in most grocery stores or restaurants: This is often fatty meat loaded with chemicals and is the furthest thing in the world from the healthy, lean, organic meats recommended for Blood Type O. Some high-protein, low-carb diets encourage the indiscriminate consumption of lots of meat protein from many sources—including ham and bacon—in an effort to create a state called ketosis, where the body burns what is known as "brown fat." The consumption of large amounts of meat protein may initially cause significant weight loss, but in the end it's unhealthy and counterproductive, placing an enormous strain on the liver and kidneys and taxing the heart as well. Ultimately, once the diet has ended, the weight will return.

One recommendation made in the original version of this book, twenty years ago, was to use only sources of animal protein that are organic, grass-fed, and free range. Two decades ago this caused quite a stir, as at the time, there were virtually no places to find grass-fed meats. Now, of course, they are common fare in supermarkets and restaurants.

I am not suggesting that Blood Type Os travel to their nearest steak house and chow down on a sixteen-ounce rib eye. Much of the meat consumed today is too fatty, shot through with hormones, antibiotics, and other chemicals. The meat I recommend for Blood Type O is lean, organic, and free of chemicals and is consumed in reasonable portions, with all visible fat removed.

Your Blood Type O ancestors' primary path to survival depended on maintaining a high state of active tissue mass and a low percentage of body fat. That's your nature as well—as long as you maintain the right diet for your type. You are vulnerable to insulin resistance and weight gain when you veer from this path, eating foods with dietary lectins that prevent their being used as a source of energy. These foods signal your body to send those calories to the storage shed and lock the door to utilization. The result is that your energy levels become depleted, and stored fat causes fluid retention and a sluggish metabolism.

The most problematic dietary factor in weight gain for Type O is the gluten found in wheat germ and whole wheat products. It acts on your metabolism to create the exact opposite of the state of ketosis. Instead of keeping you lean and in a high-energy state, the gluten lectins inhibit your insulin metabolism, interfering with the efficient use of calories for energy. Eating gluten is like putting the wrong type of gasoline in your car. Instead of fueling the engine, it clogs the works. I have seen overweight Type Os, who had been unsuccessful with other diets, quickly lose weight solely by eliminating wheat from their diets.

But if weight loss is your primary goal, wheat gluten isn't the only culprit. Certain beans and legumes, especially lentils and kidney beans, contain lectins that are deposited in your muscle tissues, making them more alkaline and less "charged" for physical activity. Type Os are leaner when their muscle tissues are in a state of slight metabolic acidity. In this state, they use calories more rapidly.

Blood Type O also has a tendency to have low thyroid hormone, a condition called hypothyroidism. This can result from imbalances in your gut flora—your microbiome. Excessive levels of yeast (*Candida*) overgrowth or certain strains of non-blood-type-friendly bacteria in the gut can actually cause the immune system to attack the thyroid by mistake. I've seen many cases of autoimmune thyroid disease resolved in Type O patients by a simple change in diet. The Type O diet features foods that support thyroid function and discourage the growth of antagonistic bacteria in the gut.

Type O individuals also have a tendency toward inflammatory conditions. The reasons are not completely understood, but may have to do with their double-barreled anti-blood-type antibodies, or as previously discussed, imbalances in their microbiome. Scientists have found that inflammation is directly related to weight gain in that it compromises the hormone leptin, which is responsible for energy balance. So a Type O weight loss plan is also an anti-inflammatory plan.

In addition to moderating food portions and choosing leaner meats for maximum weight-control benefits, Type O needs to highlight certain foods for their beneficial effects and avoid others for their hindering effects. Here's a quick guide:

TYPE O WEIGHT LOSS PROBLEM FOODS

TRIGGER INFLAMMATION	*Wheat, corn, cow's milk and cow's milk products, kidney beans, lentils, bacon, navy beans, potatoes, tomatoes, corn oil, food additives (guar gum, carrageenan), peanut oil*
ENCOURAGE DYSBIOSIS (GROWTH OF ANTAGONISTIC BACTERIA IN THE GUT)	*Cow's milk, corn, potatoes, rhubarb, oranges*
TRIGGER LEAKY GUT	*Tomatoes, corn, cow's milk, vinegar, coffee, aloe, barley*
IMPAIR PROPER THYROID FUNCTION	*Cabbage, Brussels sprouts, cauliflower, mustard greens*
INTERACT WITH METABOLIC HORMONES	*Wheat, kidney beans, navy beans*

TYPE O WEIGHT LOSS SUPERFOODS

REDUCE INFLAMMATION	*Omega-3-containing fish (cod, halibut, red snapper, trout), walnuts, hazelnuts, flaxseed oil, parsnips, peas, pineapple*
ENCOURAGE GROWTH OF HEALTHY MICROBIOME IN THE GUT	*Onions, string beans, broccoli, escarole, chicory, Swiss chard, kale*
INCREASE ACTIVE TISSUE MASS	*Beef, lamb, veal, mutton, buffalo*
ENCOURAGE PROPER THYROID FUNCTION	*Turmeric, sea vegetables (kelp, dulse)*
REPAIR LEAKY GUT	*Chicory, onions, peas, prunes, maitake mushrooms, beet greens, collard greens, fava beans*

Blood Type A

The main weight gain factors for Blood Type A are

Ineffective animal protein breakdown
Poor metabolism of saturated fats
Adrenal hormone stress imbalance
Tendencies toward higher blood and cell viscosity
Bacterial overgrowth

The chief factor in the development of the digestive characteristics of Blood Type A, the adaptation to a plant-protein-based diet, can be traced to the struggle for survival long ago, when a previous golden age gave way to a time of turbulence and uncertainty. As the local pool of game was exhausted, humans ventured farther afield, came in contact with new flora and fauna, and adapted and experimented. The cultivation of grains and livestock changed everything. For the first time, people were able to forgo the hand-to-mouth lifestyle of the hunter-gatherer and establish stable communities. Over time the adaptations that produced Blood Type A were based on the need to fully utilize nutrients from carbohydrate sources. These biological adaptations can still be observed today in Type A's digestive structure. You typically have higher levels of intestinal starch-splitting digestive enzymes, permitting a slower and more efficient digestion of carbohydrates. Your microbiome is also better suited to a plant-based diet.

In some respects, your dietary profile is almost the opposite of Type O. When you eat red meat, it is poorly digested and not properly absorbed, because your lower stomach acid and lack of fat-busting enzymes prevent proper metabolism. Because the Blood Type A digestive tract developed as an adaptation to a more agrarian, plant-based lifestyle, your optimal weight loss diet is rich in whole grains, vegetables, and plant proteins.

In the 1950s it was observed that Type A typically produces less hydrochloric acid (HCl) in the stomach in response to animal protein. Along with the proteolytic enzymes, HCl breaks down proteins into smaller and smaller fragments until they return to their original amino acid building blocks. Insufficient HCl can result in an incomplete breakdown of proteins, forcing the digestive tract and immune system to deal with large "half-baked" macromolecules that may be more allergenic than nutritious. Type A also manufactures much lower levels of intestinal alkaline phosphatase (IAP), a molecule involved in digesting the fats that accompany animal proteins. One study showed that Type A has as little as one-third the level of IAP as Type B, while another showed that the presence of the Type A antigen in the digestive tract actually turned IAP off.

The incomplete results of this compromised digestion can result in the production of a class of toxic molecules and damage to the delicate lining of the blood vessels. Many of these toxins can act as growth factors—molecules that signal the cell to store energy as fat. In many ways, Type A is also the exact opposite of Type O when it comes to metabolism. While animal proteins rapidly increase the active tissue mass in Type O, increasing the metabolic rate, they have a very different effect on Type A. Perhaps you have already noted that when you eat red meat, you feel sluggish and less energized than when you eat plant proteins. Consumption of animal proteins can also result in the blood becoming more thick and viscous, impairing circulation and increasing the risk of cardiovascular disease. Type O turns animal protein into muscle; Type A ultimately stores meat as fat. If you are a Type A accustomed to eating a lot of meat in your diet, switching to the Blood Type Diet will be dramatic. You'll lose weight rather rapidly in the beginning as you eliminate the foods you digest poorly.

One big caveat to Type A's vegetarian-based diet is the necessity of eliminating all processed and highly refined foods because you are especially sensitive to the effects of the chemicals that are predominant in such foods.

Although you can eat modest amounts of cultured dairy, such as yogurt—it's even beneficial—on the whole, dairy will provoke an imbalanced microbiome. That's because one of the sugars in milk is galactose, the Blood Type B antigen. Large amounts of galactose in the diet encourages strains of bacteria that metabolize galactose, bacteria better suited to Blood Type B than Blood Type A. In addition, many dairy foods are very high in saturated fats, the kind that compromise the heart and lead to obesity and type 2 diabetes, all primary factors for Blood Type A. However, many Type As tolerate soy milk and its associated by-products quite well, and these have the added benefit of providing not only a significant amount of protein but positive blood sugar regulation as well as protecting the delicate artery lining from damage.

Wheat is a mixed factor in the Type A Diet. While Type As may eat wheat, they have to be careful not to eat too much of it or it may increase inflammation. If you've eaten a diet high in wheat before beginning the Blood Type Diet, you may need to stay clear of wheat products for the first two or three weeks of the diet. This will give your digestive tract a bit of a breather and allow it to repair and regenerate. Once the gut lining is strong and viable, you should be able to tolerate reasonable amounts of wheat in the diet as long as you do not have solid medical evidence that you are gluten intolerant. Gluten intolerance is determined by a gene that is independent of blood type, so if your doctor has found that you have a problem with gluten you'll still need to find alternatives.

Research done in the 1970s showed that Type A has a tendency to more viscous (thicker) blood, a trait that is often accelerated with stress and disease. This is due to the fact that Blood Type A has higher levels of clotting Factor VIII. Factor VIII is critical to proper blood clotting, and under even normal circumstances Type A has levels of Factor VIII that are 30 percent greater than in the other blood types. Factor VIII is involved in the genesis of arteriosclerosis because it is part of the inflammation on the lining of the blood vessels that begins the process. A diet rich in animal protein increases Factor VIII and contributes to cardiovascular disease. In addition to the higher viscosity in the blood, I've found a distinct tendency in Type A toward higher viscosity in the cells. Using a device called a bioimpedance analyzer, we've tested thousands of patients to determine the percentages of water inside and outside the cells. Overweight Type A individuals always have greater percentages of water outside the cell (extracellular water) versus inside the cell (intracellular water). The preferred values are 55 to 60 percent intracellular and 40 to 45 percent extracellular. A dehydrated cell is a dysfunctional cell. For example, in a properly hydrated cell a molecule acting as a chemical messenger takes about 4 minutes to travel from the cell nucleus to the target site. In a dehydrated cell, this can take several hours. This has big consequences concerning metabolism, where cellular responses must be quick and effective.

Blood Type A should heed the recommendations for stress reduction in the diet. In addition to the effect of stress on blood cell viscosity, another area of concern for Type A is controlling a stress hormone known as cortisol—one of the chemicals responsible for the fight-or-flight response. Among its other damaging effects, studies have shown a direct link between high cortisol and weight gain. Increased cortisol depresses the activity of leptin, which is needed for energy regulation and appetite. Studies have shown that unlike Type Os, who have a quick spike in cortisol in response to stress, Type As and Bs experience a lower elevation in cortisol, but this elevation persists for a much longer time—and this is the trait that is associated with the most danger. Poor sleep habits, overwork, and a stressful environment all contribute to adrenal hormone imbalance and weight gain.

In addition to eating a wide variety of healthy, good-fat foods and balancing vegetables and grains, Type A needs to highlight certain foods for their beneficial or hindering effects. Here's a quick guide:

TYPE A WEIGHT LOSS PROBLEM FOODS

INEFFECTIVE ANIMAL PROTEIN AND FAT BREAKDOWN	*Red meats (beef, lamb, veal), pork, organ meats, crustaceans (lobster, crab), shellfish, tropical and industrial oils, high-fat cheeses*
TENDENCIES TOWARD HIGHER BLOOD AND CELL VISCOSITY	*Vinegar, oranges, cow's milk products, distilled liquors, guar gum*
BACTERIAL OVERGROWTH	*White and sweet potatoes, black pepper, navy beans, oranges, kidney beans, lima beans, whey*

TYPE A WEIGHT LOSS SUPERFOODS

INTELLIGENT PROTEIN CHOICES	*Soy, sardines, snapper, snails, acceptable legumes, beans, nuts*
INCREASE CELL VISCOSITY	*Lemons, water, pineapple, blueberries, blackberries, green tea, acceptable oils (olive, flaxseed, walnut)*
CONTROL AND BALANCE MICROBIOME	*Escarole, dandelion, chard, rapini (broccoli rabe), fava beans, prunes, mushrooms (silver dollar)*

Blood Type B

The main weight gain factors for Blood Type B are

Lectin sensitivity
Liver detox dysfunction
Hyperassimilator tendencies
Imbalanced microbiome

I often describe Blood Type B as idiosyncratic, meaning that you carry a mixture of characteristics that sometimes resemble Blood Type

O, but oftentimes are uniquely your own. As a Type B, you have the genetic potential for great malleability and the ability to thrive in changeable conditions. Unlike Blood Types A and O, which are at opposite ends of every spectrum, your position is fluid, with the ability to move in either direction along the continuum. It's easy to see how this flexibility served the interests of early Type Bs who needed to balance the twin forces of the animal and vegetable kingdoms. At the same time, it can be extremely challenging to straddle two poles, and Type Bs tend to be sensitive to anything that threatens to knock them off kilter. However, like a delicate and carefully crafted Stradivarius violin, when healthy, Type Bs manage to achieve that exquisite equilibrium between what would normally be considered opposing forces.

Blood Type B is extremely lectin sensitive, and when I talk to Type Bs who have lost weight on the Blood Type Diet, removing chicken from their diet is almost always the first thing they mention. Often they will also remark that up until the point when they gave it up they had never noticed how bad it made them feel. This might seem paradoxical to health-conscious readers because not only is chicken ubiquitous in many ethnic diets but it is often considered leaner and healthier than other meats. Unfortunately, this is not so if you're Blood Type B.

The lectins in foods such as corn, wheat, lentils, buckwheat, and peanuts also impede weight loss. If they're in your diet, you will have a hard time losing weight. Each of these foods has a different lectin, but all of them affect the efficiency of your metabolic process, resulting in fatigue, fluid retention, and a severe drop in blood sugar after eating a meal, called hypoglycemia.

Why this is the case is not completely clear. We do know that many lectins capable of passing through the gut lining will first pass through the liver before reaching the systemic circulation. The detoxification areas of the liver are richly sprinkled with galactose and galactose-like sugars, which, as you may remember, also resemble your blood type. Because the liver is the major metabolic organ in the body, these lectins may play some role in the liver issues that are such a factor for Type B.

One possible mechanism has more than a little irony. It has to do with the liver's process of detoxification. Normally, the products of our digestive assimilation pass from the gut to the liver via the portal vein.

This circulation acts much like a border station between two nations because not everything we assimilate from our gut, such as virus particles and bacteria, is necessarily good for us. To sort this out, the liver has a team of customs agents known as Kupffer cells, scavenger cells that go around and swallow up dangerous or risky elements from the diet. However, in certain instances the liver's guardians can be tricked into overreacting to a small number of bad guys but then letting an even larger number of them go by completely unmolested—like a border guard who is so fixated on a tourist with too many souvenirs that she ignores a shipment from a drug cartel. In addition to the obvious metabolic and immune issues, a common consequence of this is often profound fatigue and hypoglycemia (low blood sugar).

My patients with hypoglycemia often ask me if they should follow the standard advice of eating several small meals a day in order to keep their blood sugar levels from dropping. I discourage this practice as I find that the major problem is not *when* they eat, but *what* they eat. Certain foods trigger a drop in blood sugar—especially for Type B. When you eliminate these foods and begin eating the right diet for your type, your blood sugar levels should remain normal after meals. The problem with "grazing"—eating many small meals throughout the day—is that it interferes with your body's natural hunger signals, and you may begin to find that you are hungry all the time, which is not a very helpful situation if you're trying to lose weight.

Another area of potential problems for Type B involves over-assimilation to nutrients from the diet. You've probably observed this phenomenon: two people eat the same food; one gains weight, but the other stays the same or even loses weight. So much for the simple calorie-counting theory! We now know that this outcome is real, and we may even know the cause. And like an increasing amount of health issues, it stems from the microbiome. We've discussed how blood type is a major influence on the strains of bacteria that inhabit our gut, the microbiome, and although research on the microbiome is still in its infancy, we know that certain strains of bacteria in the gut can produce enzymes that actually act to enhance the breakdown of foods. One class of these enzymes is the glucosidases, in particular an enzyme called alpha-glucosidase. Alpha-glucosidase helps digest starches into simple sugars. Many strains of bacteria produce alpha-glucosidase, and it would appear that many of these strains like to reside in the gut of Type B.

Having an excessive amount of alpha-glucosidase activity in your gut marks you as a hyperassimilator—someone who will extract nutrients from elements in the diet that normally just pass through unprocessed, like digestive-resistant starches and fiber. Where the normal assimilator will not convert these into sugars (and calories), the hyperassimilator will. I have observed this as a trait most commonly in Type B and have found that when I treat obese or overweight Type B patients with agents that inhibit alpha-glucosidase, after a few days of digestive turmoil (mostly gas and bloating) they rapidly begin to lose weight.

Of all the blood types, Type B can benefit the most from a variety of dairy foods, with cultured dairy products ranking the highest. It is interesting that there is some evidence that whey, one of the abundant proteins in milk, is a moderate alpha-glucosidase inhibitor. Whey also has a well-researched reputation as a useful adjunct to increase muscle tissue, which helps increase the metabolic rate. Bear in mind that some folks may have problems with dairy products due to an insufficient amount of lactase, the enzyme required to break down milk sugar. This is a genetic tendency independent of your blood type, so you'll have to navigate this challenge using your own personal experience.

TYPE B WEIGHT LOSS PROBLEM FOODS

LECTIN SENSITIVITY	*Chicken, corn, buckwheat, wheat, sesame, amaranth, soy, rye*
LIVER DETOX DYSFUNCTION	*Lentils, black beans, black-eyed peas, mung beans, artichokes, aloe*
HYPERASSIMILATOR TENDENCIES	*Peanuts, tomatoes, soy, cashews, corn, cornstarch, black pepper, poppy seeds, pinto beans, maltodextrin, rhubarb*
IMBALANCED MICROBIOME	*Sorghum, peanuts, sucrose, dextrose, carrageenan, distilled liquor, acacia (gum arabic)*

TYPE B WEIGHT LOSS SUPERFOODS

BLOCK LECTIN SENSITIVITY	*Cultured dairy products, ricotta cheese, kefir, cottage cheese, mozzarella, farmer cheese, feta cheese, paneer*
BUILD ACTIVE TISSUE MASS	*Halibut, cod, mackerel, sardines, lamb, rabbit*
IMPROVE LIVER FUNCTION	*Mustard greens, beet greens, green tea, licorice root tea, parsnips, curry powder, gingerroot*
BLUNT HYPERASSIMILATOR TENDENCIES	*Mushrooms (silver dollar, enoki, maitake), whey, blueberries, Brussels sprouts, blackberries, grapes*
BALANCE MICROBIOME	*Brewer's yeast, molasses, cabbage*

Blood Type AB

The main weight gain factors for Blood Type AB are

Bacterial overgrowth/dysbiosis
Cell-signaling issues
Stress
Lectin sensitivities

The Hapsburg dynasty had an interesting motto that could easily apply to the metabolism of Type AB: "Leave the waging of wars to others! But you, happy Austria, marry." When it comes to gaining weight, Type AB reflects the marriage of A and B genes, a harmonious alliance that provides new benefits and a few unexpected problems. I visualize Type AB as what Charles Forte once called the "excluded middle." Any characteristic of Type A or Type B will either be "more or less" true—or its opposite will be "more or less" true—for Type AB.

For example, Type AB has Type A's more-or-less adaptation to plant proteins, along with Type B's more-or-less adaptation to meats. So, from a functional standpoint, Type AB can be frustratingly difficult to characterize. Another example: Type AB women are taller than average, but Type AB men are shorter than average. Throw in the rarity of this blood type, which makes up only 2 to 3 percent of most populations, and you know why I often refer to it as "the enigma."

Let's begin with what we do know. Type AB has both the A and B antigens and lacks any anti-other-blood-type antibodies. Having both antigens and no antibodies means that both A-like and B-like foods and bacteria are generally well tolerated, though at times perhaps to a fault. This tolerance can lead to problems with bacterial overgrowth and a poorly regulated population of microorganisms in the gut called dysbiosis. On occasion this overgrowth can become large enough that the microbial population in the large intestine, an area normally loaded with bacteria, floods over into the upper reaches of the small intestine, an area normally sterile. This produces a condition known as small intestinal bacteria overgrowth (SIBO), which is quite common, especially in Type AB.

SIBO is not hard to diagnose. One simple method tests for high levels of hydrogen in the breath. We give the patient a bit of a sugar preparation, called lactulose, and over four hours record the breath hydrogen readings. High readings in the early stages indicate that there is fermentation in the upper gastrointestinal tract, while positive readings in the later stages indicate that there is fermentation in the middle to lower gastrointestinal tract. Anywhere there is fermentation, you can bet there are also plenty of bacteria.

One quick way to get Type AB on the road to effective weight loss is to deal with SIBO. There are three basic approaches: Minimize the source of undigested or malabsorbed food in the gut; rebuild the gut flora; and (my least favorite option) kill everything and let the body sort it out, which is never truly successful by itself.

Stress has a big effect on the proper working of the Type AB metabolism. Unlike Types A and B, who appear to have problems removing cortisol, Type AB tends to stress in ways very similar to Type O, reacting to tension and pressure by the excessive conversion of dopamine into norepinephrine. Norepinephrine is part of the fight-or-flight response, so we think of it mostly as having to do with our brain and central nervous system. However, a large amount of it is also produced in the gut, and studies have shown it to encourage the growth of many different microorganisms in the gut, including the ulcer-causing bacteria *Helicobacter pylori*.

Many of the lectins that can contribute to metabolic problems for Types A and B cause similar problems in Type AB, although here again we see the law of the excluded middle: soy contains a problematic lectin for Type B, but a beneficial lectin for Type A. In this case, Type AB acts like Type A. Corn is neutral for Type A but contains a problematic lectin for Type B. In this case Type AB acts like Type B.

However, being Type AB has other benefits. Because your immune system doesn't have opposing blood type antibodies, it has to rely on other methods to pick up the slack. Most of the time you rely on a very efficient population of lymphocytes (white blood cells) known as killer cells. Keeping your killer cells energized and happy is a great way to moderate the inherent tolerance of Type AB (letting foreign invaders go undetected) and build a more effective immune system that gets the job done.

Another benefit to the Type AB metabolism lies in perhaps one of the smallest molecules in the body, a chemical called nitric oxide (NO), which appears and disappears in the tissues so rapidly that it was discovered to be biologically important only in the early 1990s. NO is involved in so many physiological and disease processes that it would take the remainder of this book to explain them. It has very powerful effects on the immune system, nervous system, and circulatory system. For our purposes, suffice it to say that NO is involved in cross talk between different systems of the body. Type AB seems to work with it very well and its actions can be easily optimized by diet. This friendship may be the result of a link between the ABO gene and the gene that controls the regulation of the amino acid arginine, which is part of the cycle that produces NO. Studies show that Type AB infants who receive NO as therapy to increase blood flow seem to require less therapeutic NO than infants of the other blood types.

TYPE AB WEIGHT LOSS PROBLEM FOODS

LECTIN SENSITIVITY   *Chicken, corn, haddock, flounder,*
                                   kidney beans, mung beans, garbanzos
                                   (chickpeas), sesame, sunflower seeds,
                                   lima beans, black beans, fava beans,
                                   black-eyed peas, buckwheat

OVERGROWTH TENDENCIES	*Oranges, Camembert cheese, bananas, distilled liquor, dextrose, sucrose, fructose, guar gum, guava, mangoes, carrageenan, cornstarch, sago, adzuki beans, radishes, rhubarb, sorghum, Jerusalem artichokes*
STRESS/IMMUNE IMBALANCE	*Sorghum, sucrose, dextrose, carrageenan, distilled liquor, acacia (gum arabic), coffee, aspartame, pork*

TYPE AB WEIGHT LOSS SUPERFOODS

BLOCK LECTIN SENSITIVITY	*Yogurt, feta cheese, farmer cheese, mozzarella cheese*
BUILD ACTIVE TISSUE MASS	*Turkey, cod, eggs (chicken), tuna, salmon, sardines, grouper, tofu, tempeh*
IMPROVE CELL SIGNALING	*Watermelon, curry powder, figs, garlic, onions, cranberries, green tea, eggplant, cherries, plums, olive oil, peanuts, walnuts, walnut oil, blackberries*
BALANCE MICROBIOME	*Mushrooms (silver dollar, portobello, enoki, maitake), miso, cabbage, kefir, amaranth, dandelion greens, watercress, brewer's yeast*

Each blood type has its own reactions to certain foods. In the next chapter, you will find highly specific guidelines for every food as well as recommendations for exercise and supplementation. After you familiarize yourself with your Blood Type Diet, turn to Chapter Nine to jump-start a weight loss program with the 10-Day Blood Type Diet Challenge.

FOUR

The Blood Type Solution:

Before You Begin

YOUR BLOOD TYPE DIET LETS YOU ZERO IN ON THE HEALTH AND nutrition information that corresponds to your exact biological profile. Armed with this new information, you can now make choices about your diet, exercise regimen, and general health that are based on the dynamic natural forces within your own body.

So let's get down to business. Here are some basic steps to take before you begin your Blood Type Diet.

1. Learn your blood type. It's easy. If you're a blood donor or have served in the military, you know your blood type. Otherwise, you can use a simple home kit, which you can order. (See Appendix F.)
2. If you want an additional level of information that will aid your compliance, learn your secretor status. See Appendix F for information about ordering the Secretor Status Collection Kit.
3. Write down your primary goals for the Blood Type Diet and articulate how you will measure success. For example:

Weight loss
Blood sugar normalization

Lower cholesterol
Lower triglycerides
Clearer thinking
Normal blood pressure
Reduced allergy or allergy symptoms
Reduced asthma symptoms
More energy
Better sleep cycle
Chronic pain reduction or resolution
More muscular strength
Fewer seasonal colds and flu
Less bloating and digestive discomfort

4. Take stock of where you're at, using basic measurements: Measure your BMI and waist circumference, along with your weight before you begin (see Chapter Three). If you suffer from a chronic medical condition, it's a good time to record your status, including blood tests.

The Blood Type Diet is not a panacea. But it is a way to restore the natural protective functions of your immune system, reset your metabolic clock, and clear your blood of dangerous agglutinating lectins. It is the best thing you can do to halt the rapid cell deterioration that produces symptoms of aging. And if you have medical problems, this plan can make a critical difference. Depending on the severity of any medical conditions and on the level of compliance with the plan, every person will realize some benefits. That has been my experience, and the experience of my colleagues who use this system with people of all ages and conditions around the world. It makes perfect scientific sense.

In this chapter, I introduce the elements you will find in your Blood Type Diet plan. They are the following:

- The Blood Type Diet
- The Supplement Advisory
- The Stress-Exercise Profile
- The Personality Question

After you read this chapter and review your Blood Type Diet, I suggest you read Part III to get a fuller picture of the specific health and medical implications your plan has for you.

The Blood Type Diet

YOUR BLOOD TYPE DIET is the restoration of your natural genetic rhythm. The groundwork for the Blood Type Diet was prepared for us many thousands of years ago. Perhaps if we had continued to follow the inherent, instinctual messages of our biological natures, our current condition would be very different. However, human diversity and the sweeping forces of technology intervened.

As we know, because of advantages fighting infections, most early humans were Type O hunters and gatherers who fed on animals, insects, berries, roots, and leaves. The range of dietary choices was extended when humans learned how to raise animals for their own use and how to cultivate crops. But it was not necessarily a smooth and orderly process because not every society adapted well to this change. In many of the early Type O societies, such as the Missouri Valley Indians, the change from a meat-eating diet to an agrarian diet was accompanied by changes in skull formation and the appearance for the first time of dental cavities. Their systems were simply not suited to the newly introduced foods. In other societies, the change from Paleolithic to Neolithic diets appeared to result in shorter statures and less bone density.

Even so, for a long period of time, the traditional agrarian diet provided ample nutrients to avoid malnutrition and support large populations. This changed as advances in agricultural and food processing techniques began to alter foodstuffs even further, increasingly removing them from their natural state. For example, the refining of rice with new milling techniques in twentieth-century Asia caused a scourge of beriberi, a thiamine-deficiency disease, which resulted in millions of deaths.

A more current example is the change from breast-feeding to bottle-feeding in developing countries. The reliance on highly refined, processed infant formula has been responsible for a great deal of malnutrition, diarrhea, and a lowering of the natural immune factors passed on through mother's milk.

Today, it is well accepted that the foods we eat have a direct impact on the state of our health and general well-being. But confusing, and often conflicting, information about nutrition has created a virtual minefield for health-conscious consumers.

How are we to choose which recommendations to follow, and which diet is the right diet? The truth is, we can no more choose the right diet than we can choose our hair color or gender. It was already chosen for us many thousands of years ago.

Without a doubt, much of the confusion is the result of the simplistic one-diet-fits-all premise I spoke of earlier. Although we have seen with our own eyes that certain people respond very well to particular diets while others do not, we have never made a commitment—in science or nutrition—to study the specialized characteristics of populations or individuals that might explain the variety of responses to any given diet. We've been so busy looking at the characteristics of food that we have failed to examine the characteristics of people.

Your Blood Type Diet works because you are able to follow a clear, logical, scientifically based dietary blueprint based on your cellular and genetic profile.

Each of the Blood Type Diets includes twelve food groups:

- Meats and poultry
- Seafood
- Dairy and eggs
- Oils and fats
- Nuts and seeds
- Beans and legumes
- Grains and cereals
- Vegetables
- Fruit
- Beverages, teas and coffee
- Herbs and spices
- Condiments, sweeteners and additives

Each of these groups divides foods into three categories: highly beneficial, neutral, and avoid. Think of the categories this way:

- Highly Beneficial is a food that acts like a medicine. It advances your health or protects you from possible maladies.
- Neutral is a food that acts like a food. It provides required macronutrients and caloric energy.
- Avoid is a food that acts like a poison. It induces biological disorder or increases your chances of disease based on differences between the blood types.

There are a wide variety of foods in each diet, so don't worry about limitations. When possible, show preference for the highly beneficial foods over the neutral foods, but feel free to enjoy the neutral foods that suit you; they won't harm you, and they contain nutrients that are necessary for a balanced diet.

At the top of each food category, you will see a chart that looks like this:

BLOOD TYPE O		WEEKLY ▪ IF YOUR ANCESTRY IS		
Food	Portion	African	Caucasian	Asian
All seafood	4–6 oz.	1–4x	3–5x	4–6x

The portion suggestions according to ancestry are not meant as firm rules. My purpose here is to present a way to fine-tune your diet even more, according to what we know about the particulars of your ancestry. Although people of different ethnicities and cultures may share a blood type, there are also geographic and cultural variations. For example, many people of Asian ancestry were not traditionally exposed to dairy products or may not have enough copies of the genes that make the enzyme needed to digest dairy, so they may need to incorporate dairy more slowly into their diets as they adjust their systems to it. The portions are not etched in stone: If you are large-framed and tall, you'll want to steer more to the larger serving and if small-framed and shorter, you'll want the smaller serving. Use the refinements if you think they're helpful; ignore them if you find that they're not. In any case, try to formulate your own plan for portion sizes.

For each Blood Type Diet you'll find three sample menus and several recipes to give you an idea of how you might incorporate the diet into your life. Each blood type has its own reactions to certain foods; these are outlined in your Blood Type Diet. In the first few weeks you'll need to experiment with the guidelines.

The entertainer Liberace was once quoted as saying, "Too much of a good thing is wonderful." However, this may not be true of the Blood Type Diet. I've found that many people assume that the best approach is to religiously eat only highly beneficial foods. While this may be okay for a jump-start, the diet is meant to include a sufficient amount of nutrient-rich neutral foods. The best approach is to eliminate all the foods on your avoid list and reduce those neutral foods for which you can substitute beneficial alternatives. That will leave you with a balanced diet and a healthier method of weight loss.

The Role of Supplements

YOUR BLOOD TYPE DIET also includes recommendations about vitamin, mineral, and herbal supplements that can enhance the effects of your diet. This is another area in which there is great confusion and misinformation. Popping nutritional supplements is a popular thing to do these days. It's hard not to be seduced by the vast array of remedies overflowing the shelves of your local health food store and advertised online. While there are many ethical manufacturers of dietary supplements, there are others that have no compunction about cutting costs by using low-quality ingredients. A higher-priced formula from a reliable manufacturer may not look as attractive as a lower-priced product you find on the Internet, but be assured there are many hidden factors in that higher cost, such as microbial assays, stability studies, and ingredient standardization. Beware of supplements claiming miracle cures for diseases. Advertising of cures for arthritis and inflammation, heart disease, dementia, cancer, and other serious chronic diseases is not only despicable but also illegal. In my opinion, when used intelligently and with the same degree of personalization as your diet, supplements can have a role in a healthy lifestyle. As with food, nutritional supplements don't always work the same way for everyone. Every vitamin, mineral, and herbal supplement plays a specific role in your body.

You may be unfamiliar with the term *phytochemicals*. Modern science has discovered that many of these phytochemicals, found in plants often called weeds or herbs, are sources of high concentrations of biologically active compounds. Many phytochemicals—which I prefer to think of as food concentrates—are antioxidants, and several of them are many times more powerful than vitamins. It is interesting that, unlike vitamins, phytochemical antioxidants exhibit a remarkable degree of tissue preference. For example, milk thistle (*Silybum marianum*) and the spice turmeric (*Curcuma longa*) both have an antioxidant capability hundreds of times stronger than that of vitamin E, and they have a great degree of preference for liver tissue. These plants are very beneficial for disorders characterized by inflammation of the liver, such as hepatitis and cirrhosis. The health of your gut bacteria will also be enhanced with prebiotics and probiotics, found in food and some supplements—preferably, specific to your blood type.

Your specialized program of vitamins, minerals, and phytochemicals will round out the dietary aspect of your program.

The Stress-Exercise Connection

IT IS NOT ONLY the foods you eat that determine your well-being. It is also the way your body uses those nutrients for good or ill. That's where stress comes in. The concept of stress is very prominent in modern society. We often hear people remark, "I'm so stressed" or "My problem is too much stress." Indeed, it is true that unbridled stress reactions are associated with many illnesses. Few people realize, though, that it is not the stress itself but our reaction to the stress in our environment that depletes our immune systems and leads to illness. This reaction is as old as human history. It is caused by a natural chemical response to the perception of danger. The best way to describe the stress reaction is to get a mental picture of how the body responds to stress.

Imagine this scenario: You are a man living in a hunting-gathering society. You lie bundled in the dark night, pressed together with your kind, sleeping. Suddenly, a huge animal appears in your midst. Do you grab a weapon and try to fight? Or do you turn and run for your life?

The body's response to stress has been developed and refined over thousands of years. It is a reflex, an animal instinct, our survival mechanism for dealing with life-or-death situations. When danger of any kind is sensed, we mobilize our fight-or-flight response, and we either confront what is alarming us or flee from it—mentally or physically.

Now imagine another scenario: You are in a work cubicle in the offices of a hectic penny stock trading firm. Phones ring constantly, your co-workers are sullen and unsupportive, and more and more work gets dumped into your in-box. Finally, to top it off, you've just seen a memo that several firings will be occurring next week.

The first scenario highlights a type of primordial response to stress. It is produced by a flood of chemicals called catecholamines that cause the adrenal glands to go into overdrive. Your pulse quickens. Your lungs suck in more oxygen to fuel your muscles. Your blood sugar soars to supply a burst of energy. Digestion slows. You break into a sweat. All of these biological responses happen in an instant, triggered by stress. They prepare you—in the same way they prepared our ancient ancestors—for fight or flight. It is a violent biochemical swing in response to an immediate danger. However, like all turbulence, it passes very quickly, which is good, as this type of response is not designed for long-term use.

When the danger passes, your body begins to change again. It starts to calm down and compose itself after the furor caused by the release of so many chemicals. And then, if whatever caused the initial stress is resolved, all of the reactions disappear, and everything is once again copacetic with the body's complex response system. If whatever caused the initial stress continues, the body's ability to adapt to the stress becomes exhausted and the bodily systems eventually shut down.

The second scenario, involving ongoing stress, is quite different.

Unlike the tidal wave of fight-or-flight, this type of stress is low level and ever present. This is the stress of modern living, and it produces a different chemical profile. Unlike the fight-or-flight response of pre-historic humans, which produces a burst of catecholamines, the second type of stress produces a slower chemical response that revolves around the hormone cortisol. This hormone is produced by the adrenal glands according to natural cycles that tend to correlate with the body's internal clock (circadian rhythm). Under stressful situations, cortisol stimulates the production of new glucose from glycogen stores in the liver. Cortisol also blocks the movement of glucose into the cells. All of this means that with high cortisol levels, you will have quite a bit of glucose flying around the bloodstream. A good thing when you are running away from a hungry lion. Not exactly the best thing when you are stressed in everyday life.

Unlike our ancestors, who faced intermittent acute stresses, such as the threat of predators or starvation, we live in a highly pressured, fast-paced world that imposes chronic, prolonged stress. Even though our stress response may be less acute than that of our ancestors, the fact that it is happening continuously may make the consequences even worse. Experts generally agree that the stresses of contemporary society and the resultant diseases—of the body, the mind, and the spirit—are very much a product of our industrialized culture and unnatural style of living.

What is the outcome? Stress-related disorders cause 50 to 80 percent of all illnesses in modern life. We know how powerfully the mind influences the body and the body influences the mind. The entire range of these interactions is still being explored. Problems known to be exacerbated by stress and the mind-body connection are ulcers, high blood pressure, heart disease, migraine headaches, arthritis and other inflammatory diseases, asthma and other respiratory diseases, insomnia and other sleep disorders, anorexia nervosa and other eating disorders, and a variety of skin problems ranging from hives to herpes and from eczema to psoriasis. Stress is disastrous to the immune system, leaving the body open to myriad opportunistic health problems.

Your personal response to stress has a surprisingly strong link to your blood type.

Catecholamines: Short-Term Stress

Studies have shown that Type O has a stress response that centers on fight-or-flight. The reasons are a bit complicated, so I'll describe it simply here. Dopamine is a major neurotransmitter made by the brain that plays an important role as a chemical messenger and central element in what is called the brain's reward-motivated behavior. Most types of rewards increase the level of dopamine in the brain, and most addictive drugs increase dopamine activity and levels. Dopamine is converted to another neurotransmitter, called norepinephrine (also known as noradrenaline), by an enzyme known as dopamine beta-hydroxylase (DBH).

You can visualize this as two buckets, one high, one low, connected by a tube. The upper bucket is dopamine, the lower bucket norepinephrine, the tube connecting them is DBH. If you're Type O you have a very, very large tube (a lot of DBH), which means that under stress lots of dopamine flows from the upper bucket to the lower one (norepinephrine). Dopamine tends to make us happy and content while norepinephrine tends to make us anxious and prepared for fight-or-flight. A surprising amount of norepinephrine is made in the gut where, in excess, it can disrupt digestion and assimilation and even the balance of the flora.

So under even mild stress, Type O will have to work harder at maintaining dopamine and blunting norepinephrine. Fortunately, there are lifestyle and dietary habits that can accomplish this. For example, vigorous exercise tends to block DBH and narrow the tube a bit, as does a high-protein diet. Wheat, unfortunately, tends to widen the tube, draining dopamine and causing the norepinephrine bucket to overflow.

This higher level of catecholamines can increase feelings of anger and aggression, perhaps explaining why ironically "Type A *behavior*" is in fact associated with Type O blood.

Ever in the middle of things, it is interesting to note that Type Bs appear to have less active DBH (narrower tubes connecting dopamine to norepinephrine) so they tend to have an easier time keeping their dopamine levels up. Perhaps this explains their enviable tendencies toward equanimity.

Cortisol: Long-Term Stress

It's amazing to see the lengths to which scientists will go to stress out research subjects. In one study designed to measure the levels of cortisol during stress, they made subjects attempt to copy text while looking at their writing in a mirror as they simultaneously listened to a tape loop of a baby crying. When they compared the results by the blood types of the subjects, they made an interesting discovery. Type O (and to a lesser degree Type AB) subjects had a powerful initial spike in their cortisol levels, followed by a rapid drop. Types A and B, on the other hand, had a lower spike, but the elevated levels persisted and persisted.

As we've seen, this prolonged cortisol response is the really dangerous one, and to explain, I'll provide a simple example. Should a person, perhaps due to a motorcycle accident, sustain a traumatic head injury, it is normal procedure in the ER to administer astronomical amounts of corticosteroids in an attempt to reduce the swelling of the brain. Paradoxically, this super-high dose of steroids has virtually no side effects, because it is given over such a short period of time. On the other hand, all of the negative side effects of cortisone medication—immune suppression, weight gain, and cardiovascular disease—take place when you take low doses of cortisone over very long periods of time. The same treatment can heal when administered over a short period and harm when administered over a long time.

That's the same scenario with cortisol. A brief spike is fine, perhaps even desirable. Prolonged elevations cause problems with metabolism, immunity, sleep, and the actions of many, many other genes. This is a real problem for Type As, as they have been shown to have higher incidence of cardiovascular disease and problems associated with lower immunity. If you are Type A and have issues with your metabolism in addition to sleep disturbances, it's likely your cortisol levels are to blame. Fortunately, there are lifestyle habits and dietary changes that can correct this. Perhaps the simplest approach is to begin a program of yoga or tai chi. Both have been shown in reliable studies to reduce cortisol levels.

Many of our internal reactions to stress are ancient tunes being called up and played by our bodies—the environmental stresses that shaped the metabolism of the various blood types. The cataclysmic changes in locale, climate, and diet imprinted these stress patterns into the biochemical memory of each blood type and even today determine our internal response to stress.

Although each of us reacts to stress in a unique way, no one is immune to its effects, especially if it is prolonged and unwanted. Not all stress is bad for you. Certain stresses, such as physical or creative activity, produce pleasant emotional states, which the body perceives as an enjoyably heightened mental or physical experience.

Your Blood Type Diet includes a description of your own blood type stress patterns, along with the recommended course of exercise that will turn stress into a positive force. This element provides a crucial complement to your diet.

The Personality Question

WITH ALL of these fundamental connections at work, it is not surprising that people might speculate about less tangible characteristics that might be attributed to blood type—such as personality, attitudes, and behavior.

The idea that certain inherited traits, mannerisms, emotional qualities, and life preferences are buried in our genetic makeup is well accepted, although we are only at the very beginning of understanding how this inheritance plays out scientifically. Personality is a mixture of nature and nurture, with nurture probably being the major influence.

Although research has been done linking blood types to personality types, most of it is old, not very good, and subject to the biases common in the time the research was conducted—typically in the 1950s and 1960s. Still, the connection intrigues us because it makes some sense that there might be a causal relationship between what occurs at the cellular level of our beings and our mental, physical, and emotional tendencies as expressed by our blood type. Certainly there must be a link between what we know about the chemical differences between how each blood type responds to stress and at least some elements of personality. For example, higher cortisol levels are associated with obsessive-compulsive disorder (OCD), a condition also known to be more common in Type A. Depression (both unipolar and bipolar) is in part associated with low dopamine levels and has been shown to be more common in Type O.

The belief that personality is determined by one's blood type is held in high regard in Japan. Termed *ketsuekigata*, Japanese blood type analysis is serious business. Corporate managers use it to hire workers, market researchers use it to predict buying habits, and many people use it to choose friends, romantic partners, and lifetime mates. Vending machines that offer on-the-spot blood type analysis are widespread in train stations, department stores, restaurants, and other public places. There is even a highly respected organization, the ABO Society, dedicated to helping individuals and organizations make the right decisions, consistent with blood type.

The leading proponent of the blood type–personality connection is a man named Toshitaka Nomi, whose father first pioneered the theory. In 1980, Nomi and Alexander Besher wrote a book called *You Are Your Blood Type*, which has sold millions of copies in Japan. It contains personality profiles and suggestions for the various blood types—right down to what you should do for a living, whom you should marry, and the dire consequences that might befall you if you should ignore this advice.

It makes for fun reading—not unlike astrology, numerology, or other methods of finding your place in the uncertain scheme of things. I think, however, that most of the advice in the book should be taken with a grain of salt. I don't believe that a soul mate or a romantic partner should be chosen by blood type. I am Type A and I am deeply in love with my wife, Martha, who is Type O. I would hate to think that we might have been kept forever apart because of some psychic incompatibility in our blood types. We do just fine, even though mealtimes can be a little chaotic.

So, what is the value of this speculation, and why am I including it here? It's very simple. Although I think the Japanese *ketsuekigata* is extreme, I can't deny that there is probably an essential truth to the theories about a relationship between differences in physiology and the characteristics of our personalities.

Modern scientists and doctors have clearly acknowledged the existence of a biological mind-body connection, and we've already demonstrated the relationship between your blood type and your response to stress earlier in this chapter. The idea that your blood type may relate to your personality is not really so strange. Indeed, if you look at each of the blood types, you can see a distinct personality emerging—the inheritance of our ancestral strengths. Perhaps this is just another way for you to play to those strengths.

There is as yet not enough hard evidence to justify any sweeping conclusions about the use of blood type to determine personality, but a world of information is waiting to be annexed and explored. For example, a variation in genes known as COMT (catechol O-methyltransferase) appears to result in some rather striking differences in personality and appears to even influence whether we can experience the placebo effect. COMT does have some links to the ABO gene, so perhaps history remains to be written in regard to blood types and personality.

It is possible that in this century we will finally be able to examine some master plan, a map that will show us how to get from here to there within ourselves. But perhaps not. There is so much we don't understand, so much we may never understand, but we can speculate, reflect, and consider the many possibilities. That is why we have, as a species, developed such acute intelligence.

These elements—diet, weight management, dietary supplementation, stress control, and personal qualities—form the essential elements of your individual Blood Type Diet. Refer to them often as you begin to familiarize yourself with the specific qualities of your blood type.

But before you go any further, I suggest you do one more thing if you haven't already: Find out your blood type!

PART II

Your Blood Type Diet

FIVE

Blood Type

O

Diet

TYPE O: *The Hunter*

- MEAT EATER
- HARDY DIGESTIVE TRACT
- OVERACTIVE IMMUNE SYSTEM
- INTOLERANT TO DIETARY AND ENVIRONMENTAL ADAPTATIONS
- RESPONDS BEST TO STRESS WITH INTENSE PHYSICAL ACTIVITY
- REQUIRES AN EFFICIENT METABOLISM TO STAY LEAN AND ENERGETIC

The Type O Diet

TYPE O THRIVES on intense physical exercise and animal protein. The digestive tract of Type O retains the memory of ancient times. The high-protein hunter-gatherer diet and the enormous physical demands placed on the system of early Type Os probably kept most primitive humans in a mild state of ketosis—a condition in which the body's metabolism is altered. The body metabolizes proteins and fats into ketones, which are used in place of sugars in an attempt to keep glucose levels steady. The combination of ketosis, calorie deprivation, and constant physical activity made for a lean, mean hunting machine—the key to the survival of the human race.

Dietary recommendations today generally discourage the consumption of too much animal protein because saturated fats have been proven to be a risk factor for heart disease and cancer. Of course, much of the meat consumed today is shot through with fat and tainted by the indiscriminate use of hormones and antibiotics. "You are what you eat" can take on an ominous meaning when you're talking about the modern meat supply. Fortunately, organic and free-range meats are widely available. The success of the Type O diet depends on your use of lean, chemical-free meat and fish along with an abundance of fresh vegetables and fruit.

Type O doesn't find dairy products and grains quite as friendly as do most of the other blood types because its digestive system still has not adapted to them fully. After all, you don't have to chase down and kill a bowl of wheat or a glass of milk! These foods did not become staples of the human diet until much later in the course of our evolution.

NOTE: Longtime readers will notice a difference in the values of a small number of foods between this edition and the original version of *Eat Right for Your Type*. That is because beginning with the publication of *Live Right for Your Type*, I made a distinction in some foods between secretors and non-secretors. The original version of *Eat Right for Your Type*, which preceded *Live Right for*

Your Type, "homogenized" these differences. Like all of my subsequent books, this edition of *Eat Right for Your Type* uses the secretor values as the base values for the A, B, AB, and O blood types.

KEY

‡ Enhances carbohydrate metabolism, helps with weight loss

↑ Increases microbiome diversity, discourages microbial imbalance

↓ Decreases microbiome diversity, encourages microbial imbalance

Meats and Poultry

BLOOD TYPE O		WEEKLY ■ IF YOUR ANCESTRY IS		
Food	*Portion**	*African*	*Caucasian*	*Asian*
LEAN RED MEATS	4–6 oz. *(men)* 2–5 oz. *(women and children)*	5–7X	4–6X	3–5X
POULTRY	4–6 oz. *(men)* 2–5 oz. *(women and children)*	1–2X	2–3X	3–4X

*The portion recommendations are merely guidelines that can help refine your diet according to ancestral propensities.

Eat lean, chemical- and pesticide-free beef, lamb, beef liver, and venison as a primary protein source. These are your preferred meats, although chicken, turkey, and other neutral poultry products are allowed. The more stressful your job or demanding your exercise program, the higher the grade of protein you should eat. In Type O these are the optimal types of protein for building active tissue mass (calorie-burning tissue) such as muscle, but beware of portion sizes. Try to consume no more than 6 ounces at any one meal (4 to 6 ounces is about the size of the palm of your hand).

Type O can efficiently digest and metabolize meats because it has high stomach acid levels and fat-busting enzymes in abundance. However, Type O must be careful to balance meat proteins with the appropriate vegetables and fruits to provide needed fiber, antioxidants, and micronutrients.

It's very important that Type O choose grass-fed and antibiotic-, hormone-, and pesticide-free meats. These choices are high in conjugated linoleic acid (CLA), a very healthful fatty acid—actually the only trans fat that is good for you. Emphasize eye of round, top round, top sirloin, sirloin tip, brisket, and 95 percent lean ground cuts. These have less of the pro-inflammatory fats.

Optimally, you should look for free-range and grass-fed meats. Grass-fed meat is a natural source of omega-3 fatty acids, whereas grain-fed meat has virtually no omega-3. Be sure poultry is certified organic and is antibiotic- and pesticide-free. Always choose free-range poultry. Select poultry products from the back of the fridge where the temperature is coldest.

Pork naturally contains toxins (biogenic amines) and should be avoided, even organic pork.

Highly Beneficial

BEEF ↑ ‡	CALF, LIVER ↑	SWEETBREADS ↑
BEEF, HEART ↑	LAMB ↑ ‡	VEAL ↑ ‡
BEEF, LIVER ↑	MARROW SOUP	VENISON ↑
BEEF, TONGUE	MOOSE ↑	
BUFFALO, BISON ↑ ‡	MUTTON ↑ ‡	

Neutral

Bear	Chicken	Duck
Bone soup (allowable meats)	Chicken liver	Goat
	Cornish hen	Goose

Grouse	Partridge	Squirrel
Guinea hen	Pheasant	Turkey
Horse	Rabbit	
Ostrich	Squab	

Avoid

| Duck liver | Ham ↓ | Quail |
| Goose liver | Pork and bacon ↓ | Turtle |

Seafood

BLOOD TYPE O		WEEKLY ▪ IF YOUR ANCESTRY IS		
Food	*Portion*	*African*	*Caucasian*	*Asian*
ALL SEAFOOD	4–6 oz.	1–4x	3–5x	4–6x

Seafood, the second most concentrated animal protein, is well suited for Type O. Seafood can be an excellent protein source. Richly oiled cold-water fish, such as cod and mackerel, are excellent for Type O because they contain the much-needed anti-inflammatory omega-3 fatty acids and help build active tissue (muscle) almost as effectively as red and organ meats. Make sure that your fish is fresh caught, not farm raised, and free of industrial toxins (dioxins, xenobiotics, and heavy metals), which accumulate in the fat. Ask for fish that is nearest to the ice or from the back of the refrigerator where the temperature is coldest.

Highly Beneficial

BASS, BLUE GILL ↑	PERCH ↑	SWORDFISH ↑
BASS, SEA, LAKE ↑	PERCH, OCEAN ↑	TILEFISH ↑
BASS, STRIPED ↑	PIKE ↑	TROUT, RAINBOW
COD ↑ ‡	RED SNAPPER ↑ ‡	(WILD) ↑ ‡
HALIBUT ↑ ‡	SHAD ↑	YELLOWTAIL ↑
MACKEREL,	SOLE ↑	
SPANISH	STURGEON ↑	

Neutral

Anchovy
Beluga
Bluefish
Bullhead
Butterfish
Carp
Caviar
Chub
Clam
Crab
Croaker
Cusk
Drum
Eel
Flounder
Grouper
Haddock
Hake
Halfmoon fish
Harvest fish
Herring (fresh/
 pickled/smoked)
Lobster
Mackerel,
 Atlantic

Mahi-mahi
Monkfish
Mullet
Mussels
Ocean pout
Opaleye fish
Orange roughy
Oyster
Parrotfish
Pickerel, Walleye
Pilchards
Pompano
Porgy
Rosefish
Sailfish
Sailfish roe
Salmon, Atlantic
 (wild)
Salmon, Chinook
Salmon roe
Salmon,
 smoked (lox)
Salmon, sockeye
Sardine

Scallop ↑
Scrod
Scup
Sea bream
Shark
Shrimp
Skate
Smelt
Snail, escargot
Sole, gray/Dover
Sucker
Sunfish,
 pumpkinseed
Tilapia
Trout, sea/steelhead
 (wild)/brook
Tuna, bluefin/
 skipjack/yellowfin
Turbot,
 European
Weakfish
Whitefish
Whiting

Avoid

Abalone, sea ear,
 mutton fish ↓
Barracuda
Catfish

Conch
Frog
Muskellunge
Octopus

Pollock, Atlantic
Squid, calamari

Dairy and Eggs

Food	Portion	African	Caucasian	Asian
BLOOD TYPE O		WEEKLY ▪ IF YOUR ANCESTRY IS		
EGGS	1 EGG	0	4–8X	5–8X
CHEESES	2 OZ.	0	0–3X	0–3X
MILK	4–6 OZ.	0	0–1X	0–2X

If you're Type O you should severely restrict your consumption of dairy products, a suboptimal protein source for your type. Your system is ill-designed for their proper daily metabolism, and dairy foods can also exacerbate inflammatory conditions and cause weight gain. The sugars commonly encountered in dairy products can also disrupt the Type O microbiome, inhibiting weight loss and leading to digestive problems.

Generally, Type O can eat eggs up to eight times a week. Use eggs from free-range chickens, preferably those advertised as being "DHA rich." DHA is a fatty acid that is increasingly being viewed as essential for proper nerve and immune system health.

Highly Beneficial
PECORINO CHEESE ↑
ROMANIAN URDA ↑

Neutral

Butter ↑
Egg white, chicken
Egg whole, chicken
Egg whole, duck

Egg yolk, chicken
Farmer cheese
Feta cheese
Goat cheese

Ghee, clarified
  butter ↑
Mozzarella cheese,
  all types

Avoid

American cheese ↓
Blue cheese
Brie cheese
Buttermilk
Camembert cheese ↓
Casein ↓
Cheddar cheese ↓
Colby cheese ↓
Cottage cheese ↓
Cream cheese ↓
Edam cheese ↓
Egg, goose
Egg, quail
Emmental, Swiss cheese ↓

Gorgonzola cheese ↓
Gouda cheese
Gruyère cheese ↓
Half-and-half ↓
Ice cream
Jarlsberg cheese
Kefir ↓
Manchego ↓
Milk, cow (skim or 2%)↓
Milk, cow (whole) ↓
Milk, goat ↓
Monterey Jack cheese ↓
Muenster cheese ↓

Neufchâtel cheese ↓
Paneer cheese ↓
Parmesan cheese
Provolone cheese ↓
Quark cheese ↓
Ricotta cheese ↓
Romano cheese
Roquefort cheese ↓
Sherbet
Sour cream ↓
Stilton cheese ↓
String cheese ↓
Swiss cheese
Whey protein ↓
Yogurt ↓

Oils and Fats

BLOOD TYPE O		WEEKLY ▪ IF YOUR ANCESTRY IS		
Food	*Portion*	*African*	*Caucasian*	*Asian*
OILS	I TABLESPOON	1–5x	4–8x	3–7x

Type O responds well to many oils. They can be an important source of nutrition and an aid to elimination. You will increase their value in your system if you limit your use to the monounsaturated varieties, such as olive oil and flaxseed oil. These oils have positive effects on the heart and arteries, and may even help reduce blood cholesterol.

Always try to buy high-quality oils, preferably cold pressed when appropriate. Oils do go bad, so make a point of never buying more than you can use within two months.

Highly Beneficial

CAMELINA OIL ↑   OLIVE OIL ↑

FLAXSEED,   RICE BRAN OIL

   LINSEED OIL ↑ ‡

Neutral

Almond oil   Canola oil   Perilla seed oil

Apricot kernel oil   Chia seed oil   Pumpkin seed oil

Black currant   Cod liver oil   Sesame oil

   seed oil   Hemp seed oil   Walnut oil

Borage seed oil   Macadamia oil

Avoid

Avocado oil   Evening   Peanut oil

Castor oil   primrose oil   Safflower oil

Coconut oil   Lard   Soy oil

Corn oil ↓   Margarine   Sunflower oil

Cottonseed oil   Palm oil   Wheat germ oil

Nuts and Seeds

BLOOD TYPE O	WEEKLY ▪ IF YOUR ANCESTRY IS			
Food	*Portion*	*African*	*Caucasian*	*Asian*
NUTS AND SEEDS	6–8 NUTS	2–5X	3–4X	2–3X
NUT BUTTERS	I TABLESPOON	3–4X	3–7X	2–4X

Type O can find a good source of supplemental vegetable protein in some varieties of nuts and seeds, while avoiding those with harmful lectins. However, these foods should in no way take the place of high-quality proteins available in meats and seafoods.

Because nuts can sometimes cause digestive problems, be sure to chew them thoroughly or use nut butters, which are easier to digest, especially if you have colon problems, such as diverticulitis.

Highly Beneficial

CAROB	FLAXSEED ↑ ‡	PUMPKIN SEED ↑
CHESTNUT, CHINESE ↑	HEMP SEED	WALNUT ↑ ‡

Neutral

Almond ↑	Filbert, hazelnut	Safflower seed
Almond butter ↑	Hickory ↑	Sesame butter,
Almond cheese ↑	Macadamia nut	tahini ↑
Almond milk	Pecan	Sesame flour
Butternut	Pecan butter ↑	Sesame seed ↑
Chia seed	Pine nut, pignoli ↑	Watermelon seed

Avoid

Beechnut	Litchi/lychee	Poppy seed
Brazil nut	Peanut	Sunflower butter
Cashew	Peanut butter	Sunflower seed
Cashew butter	Peanut flour	
Chestnut, European	Pistachio nut	

Beans and Legumes

BLOOD TYPE O	WEEKLY ▪ IF YOUR ANCESTRY IS			
Food	*Portion*	*African*	*Caucasian*	*Asian*
ALL RECOMMENDED BEANS AND LEGUMES	1 CUP, DRY	1–2X	1–2X	2–6X

Type O doesn't utilize beans particularly well. In general, beans inhibit the metabolism of other more important nutrients, such as those found in meat, and a number of them contain lectins that are harmful to Type O. There are a couple of highly beneficial beans that are exceptions and actually strengthen the digestive tract and the balance of the microbiome. Even so, eat beans in moderation, as an occasional side dish.

Highly Beneficial

ADZUKI BEAN
BLACK-EYED PEA

Neutral

Black bean ↑
Broad bean, fava
Butter bean ↑
Butternut ↑
Cannellini
  bean
Garbanzo bean,
  chickpea
Great Northern
  bean ↑
Green bean
Haricot-vert

Jicama↑
Lima bean
Mung beans,
  sprouts
Natto ↑
Pea, green, yellow,
  snow
Snap bean
Soybean
Soybean cheese
Soybean
  granules, lecithin

Soybean meal
Soybean, sprouted
Soybean,
  tempeh ↑
Soybean, tofu
Soy flakes
Soy milk
Soy miso
String bean
White bean
Yellow bean

Avoid

Copper bean ↓
Kidney bean ↓
Lentil, all types ↓

Lentil, sprouted
Navy bean ↓
Pinto bean ↓

Pinto bean, sprouted
Soybean pasta ↓
Tamarind bean

Grains and Cereals

BLOOD TYPE O	DAILY ▪ IF YOUR ANCESTRY IS			
Food	Portion	African	Caucasian	Asian
BREADS, CRACKERS	1 SLICE	0–4X	0–2X	0–4X
MUFFINS	½ MUFFIN	0–2X	0–1X	0–1X
GRAINS	½ CUP	0–3X	0–3X	0–3X
PASTAS	½ CUP	0–3X	0–3X	0–3X

There are few grains or cereals that could be classified as highly beneficial for Type O. They are the real Achilles' heel of Type O. Many of the most common varieties cause inflammation, exacerbate digestive problems, and confuse hormones. Because Type O does not tolerate wheat products at all, you should eliminate them completely from your diet. They contain lectins that react with both your blood and your digestive tract and interfere with the proper absorption of beneficial foods. Wheat products are also a primary culprit in Type O weight gain because the glutens in wheat germ can interfere with Type O metabolic processes. Inefficient or sluggish metabolism causes food to convert to energy more slowly and to be stored as fat.

Most pasta is made with semolina wheat, so you'll need to select very carefully if you want an occasional pasta dish. Pastas made from buckwheat, Jerusalem artichoke, or rice flour are better tolerated by Type O. However, make sure that these products are 100 percent what they advertise. For example, many types of Jerusalem artichoke pasta have very little Jerusalem artichoke in them, but instead use it as a flavoring along with a base of semolina.

The exceptions are 100 percent sprouted breads, which are usually found in the freezer section of your local market or health food store. These sprouted seed breads are assimilable for Type O because the gluten lectins (principally found in the seed coats) are destroyed by the sprouting process. However, be advised: Some breads advertised as sprouted are only partially sprouted. Read the labels and verify that the bread is made up of 100 percent sprouted ingredients before buying.

Good neutral grains for Type O include spelt, an ancient grain that is higher in protein and more easily digestible, and amaranth, which is gaining popularity as a nutritious, high-protein grain. Be aware, though, that spelt does contain gluten.

If you are a non-secretor, avoid oats, which are neutral for other Type Os.

Highly Beneficial

ARTICHOKE FLOUR, PASTA	FLAXSEED BREAD (CONTAINING	LARCH FIBER ↑
ESSENE, MANNA BREAD	ALLOWABLE GRAINS) ↑	

Neutral

Amaranth ↑
Black bean flour
Buckwheat, kasha,
  soba ↑
Cream of rice
Fonio ↑
Garbanzo bean
  (chickpea) flour
Job's tears
  (*Coix* spp.) ↑
Lima bean flour
Malanga, tannia,
  Xanthosoma
Millet ↑

Oat, oatmeal, flour,
  bran ↑
Quinoa ↑
Rice bran ↑
Rice flour (brown,
  white)
Rice, basmati
Rice, brown
Rice, puffed, rice
  cakes
Rice, white
Rice, wild ↑
Rye ↑
Rye flour ↑

Sago palm
Soybean flour
Spelt, whole grain,
  flour, noodles
Spelt flour, noodles
Tapioca, manioc,
  cassava, yucca
Taro, Tahitian, poi,
  dasheen
Teff ↑
Wheat, whole grain
  kamut

Avoid

Barley ↓
Cornflakes ↓
Cornmeal, hominy,
  polenta, all corn
  grains ↓
Cream of wheat
Emmer
Familia
Farina
Faro ↓

Gluten flour
Graham flour
Grape-Nuts
Grits
Kamut
Lentil flour, dahl ↓
Mastic gum ↓
Papadum
Puffed wheat
Seven grain

Shredded wheat
Sorghum
Wheat, bran, germ ↓
Wheat, bulgur ↓
Wheat, durum,
  semolina,
  couscous ↓
Wheat, whole grain,
  whole wheat flour ↓
White flour, sprouted

Vegetables

BLOOD TYPE O	DAILY ▪ ALL ANCESTRAL TYPES	
Food	*Portion*	
RAW	I CUP, PREPARED	3–5X
COOKED OR STEAMED	I CUP, PREPARED	3–5X

There are a tremendous number of vegetables available to Type O, and they form a critical component of the diet. You cannot, however, simply eat all vegetables indiscriminately. Several classes of vegetables cause big problems for Type O. For example, certain vegetables from the Brassica family—cabbage, Brussels sprouts, cauliflower, and mustard greens—can disrupt the microbiome and even inhibit thyroid function, which is often already somewhat compromised in Type O.

Leafy green vegetables rich in vitamin K, like kale, collard greens, romaine lettuce, broccoli, and spinach are very good for Type O.

Alfalfa sprouts contain components that, by irritating the digestive tract, can aggravate Type O hypersensitivity problems. The molds in domestic and shiitake mushrooms and in fermented olives tend to trigger allergic reactions in Type O.

The nightshade vegetables, such as eggplant and potatoes, can induce inflammation in Type O because of their lectins. Corn lectins can disrupt the proper function of insulin, often leading to diabetes and obesity. All Type Os should avoid corn—especially if there is a weight problem or a family history of diabetes.

Tomatoes are a special case. Heavily laced with powerful lectins, called panhemagglutinins (meaning they agglutinate all blood types), tomatoes are trouble for Type A and Type B digestive tracts. However, Type O can eat tomatoes. They become neutral in your system.

Highly Beneficial

ARTICHOKE	GINGER	PARSNIP ↑
BEET GREENS ↑ ‡	GRAPE LEAVES ↑	PUMPKIN ↑
BROCCOFLOWER ↑	HORSERADISH ↑	SEA VEGETABLES,
BROCCOLI ↑ ‡	JERUSALEM	IRISH MOSS
CANISTEL ↑	ARTICHOKE	SEA VEGETABLES,
CHICORY ‡	KALE ↑ ‡	KELP, KOMBU,
COLLARD	KELP	NORI, BLADDER-
GREENS ↑ ‡	KOHLRABI	WRACK ↑ ‡
DANDELION	LETTUCE, ROMAINE	SEA VEGETABLES,
GREENS	OKRA	WAKAME
ESCAROLE ‡	ONIONS, ALL	SPINACH ↑ ‡
FENUGREEK	PARSLEY	SWEET POTATO

SWISS CHARD ↑ ‡   TURNIP
TURNIP   GREENS ↑ ‡

Neutral

Arugula

Asparagus

Asparagus pea

Bamboo shoot

Beet

Bok choy, pak choi

Broccoli, Chinese

Broccoli leaves

Broccoli rabe,
  rapini

Brussels sprouts

Cabbage

Carrot

Cassava

Celeriac

Celery

Chayote, pipinella,
  vegetable pear

Chervil

Chili pepper

Chinese kale,
  kai-lan

Cilantro

Coriander

Daikon radish

Dill

Eggplant ↑

Endive ↑

Fennel

Fiddlehead fern

Garlic

Hearts of palm

Jicama ↑

Lettuce, Bibb,
  Boston, green
  leaf, iceberg,
  mesclun

Mushroom,
  abalone, black
  trumpet, enoki,
  maitake, oyster,
  portobello, straw,
  tree

Olive, Greek,
  green, kalamata,
  Spanish

Oyster plant, salsify ↑

Pepper, green, orange,
  purple, yellow

Peppers, chili,
  jalapeño

Pimiento

Poi

Radicchio

Radish sprouts

Radish

Rutabaga

Sauerkraut

Scallion

Shallot

Squash

Tomatillo

Tomato

Water chestnut,
  matai

Watercress

Yam ↑

Zucchini

Avoid

Alfalfa sprouts

Aloe vera ↓

Capers ↓

Cauliflower ↓

Corn, popcorn ↓

Cucumber ↓

Leek ↓

Mushroom,
  shiitake,
  white, silver
  dollar ↓

Mustard greens

Olive, black ↓

Pickles, all

Potato, blue, red,
  yellow, white ↓

Quorn ↓

Rhubarb

Spirulina

Taro

Yucca

Fruit

BLOOD TYPE O	DAILY ▪ ALL ANCESTRAL TYPES	
Food	*Portion*	
ALL RECOMMENDED FRUITS	1 FRUIT OR 3–5 OZ.	3–4X

Many wonderful fruits are available on the Type O diet. Fruits are not only an important source of fiber, vitamins, and minerals but they can be an excellent alternative to breads and pasta for Type O. If you eat a piece of fruit rather than a slice of bread, your system will be better served— and at the same time you'll be supporting your weight-loss goals.

It may surprise you to find some of your favorite fruits on the avoid list, and some odd choices on the highly beneficial list. The reason that plums, prunes, and figs are so beneficial to your blood type is that most dark red, blue, and purple fruits tend to cause an alkaline rather than an acidic reaction in your digestive tract. Oranges can be a problem due to their effects on bacterial growth in the gut. Grapefruit is an acceptable substitute. Most of the berries are okay, but stay away from blackberries, which contain a lectin that reacts with Type O cells. And despite the breathless claims of its many proponents that it can cure everything from cancer to Alzheimer's disease, Type O may want to steer mostly clear of coconut and coconut oil—the chemical makeup tends to unbalance what we are trying to accomplish with the consumption of high-protein foods.

All fruits should be thoroughly washed with a mild soap and rinsed for at least 2 minutes before they are eaten.

Highly Beneficial

BANANA ↑	FIG ↑	MANGO ↑
BLUEBERRY	GUAVA	PLUM ‡
CHERRY	MAMEY SAPOTE,	PRUNE ‡
DURIAN ↑ ‡	MAMEY APPLE ↑	

Neutral

Acai berry	Grape	Peach
Apple	Huckleberry	Pear
Apricot	Jack fruit	Persian melon
Boysenberry ↑	Kumquat ↑	Persimmon
Breadfruit ↑	Lemon ↑	Pineapple
Canang melon	Lime	Pomegranate
Casaba melon	Lingonberry	Prickly pear ↑
Christmas melon	Loganberry ↑	Quince
Cranberry ↑	Loquat	Raisin
Crenshaw melon	Mangosteen	Raspberry
Currant	Mulberry	Sago palm
Date ↑	Musk melon	Spanish melon
Dewberry	Nectarine	Starfruit, carambola
Elderberry ↑	Noni	Strawberry
Goji, wolfberry	Papaya	Watermelon
Gooseberry ↑	Passion fruit ↑	Youngberry
Grapefruit	Pawpaw	

Avoid

Asian pear	Cantaloupe	Kiwi
Avocado	Coconut meat	Orange ↓
Bitter melon	Honeydew	Plantain ↓
Blackberry ↓	melon ↓	Tangerine ↓

Beverages, Teas and Coffee

Vegetable juices are preferable to fruit juices for Type O because of higher nutrient content. If you drink fruit juice, choose low sucrose and fructose varieties. Limit high-sugar juices, such as apple juice and apple cider.

Pineapple juice can be particularly helpful in avoiding water retention and bloating, both factors that contribute to weight gain. Black cherry is also a beneficial, alkalinizing juice.

There are very few acceptable general beverages for Type O. You're pretty much limited to the innocuous effects of seltzer, club soda, and tea.

Beer is okay in moderation, but it's not a good choice if you want to lose weight. Modest quantities of red wine are allowed, but not on a daily basis.

The problem that coffee poses for Type O is in the increased levels of stomach acid it produces and its long-term effects on norepinephrine levels. Type O has plenty of stomach acid all on its own, and doesn't need more. If you are a coffee drinker, perhaps you can begin to gradually cut down on the amount you consume each day. Your ultimate goal should be to eliminate coffee altogether. The common withdrawal symptoms, such as headache, fatigue, and irritability, won't occur if you wean yourself gradually. Green tea is a healthy alternative to other caffeinated beverages, with metabolic and immune-enhancing properties.

Highly Beneficial

BLACK CHERRY
   JUICE
BLUEBERRY JUICE
CAYENNE TEA
CHERRY JUICE
CHICKWEED TEA
CLUB SODA
DANDELION TEA
FENUGREEK TEA
GINGERROOT TEA

GREEN TEA,
   KUKICHA,
   BANCHA, ↑
   GENMAICHA
GUAVA JUICE
HOPS TEA
LINDEN TEA
MANGO JUICE
MULBERRY TEA
PARSLEY TEA

PEPPERMINT TEA
PINEAPPLE JUICE
PRUNE JUICE
ROSE HIPS TEA
SARSAPARILLA TEA
SELTZER WATER
SLIPPERY ELM TEA
VEGETABLE JUICE
   (FROM HB
   VEGETABLES)

Neutral

Apple cider
Apple juice
Apricot juice
Beet juice
Cabbage juice
Carrot juice
Catnip tea
Celery juice
Chamomile tea
Coconut water
Cranberry juice

Dong quai tea
Elderberry juice
Elder tea
Ginseng tea
Goji berry juice
Grape juice
Grapefruit juice
Hawthorn tea
Horehound tea
Lemon and
   water

Lime juice
Licorice root tea
Milk, almond ↑
Milk, rice
Milk, soy
Mullein tea
Nectarine juice
Noni juice
Papaya juice
Pear juice ↑
Peppermint tea

Pineapple
   juice
Pomegranate
   juice
Raspberry
   leaf tea
Sage tea
Skullcap tea
Spearmint tea
Thyme tea
Tomato juice

Vegetable juice (from acceptable vegetables)

Valerian tea
Vervain tea
Watermelon juice

White birch tea
White oak tea
Wine, red

Yarrow tea
Yerba mate tea

Avoid

Alfalfa tea
Aloe juice
Aloe tea
Beer ↓
Black tea, all forms
Blackberry juice ↓
Burdock tea
Coconut milk

Coffee
Coltsfoot tea
Corn silk tea
Cucumber juice ↓
Echinacea tea
Gentian tea
Goldenseal tea
Liquor, distilled ↓

Orange juice ↓
Red clover tea
Rhubarb tea
Saint John's wort tea
Senna tea
Shepherd's purse tea

Soda, pop (such as colas and diet colas)
Strawberry leaf tea
Tangerine juice ↓
Wine, white
Yellow dock tea

Herbs and Spices

Your choice of herbs and spices can actually improve your digestive and immune systems. For example, sea vegetables and kelp-based seasonings are very good for Type O. They are rich sources of iodine and are a unique source of fucose, a naturally protective sugar for the Type O digestive tract. However, if you are sensitive to iodine or taking thyroid medication you'll want to check with your doctor first.

Bladderwrack, a type of kelp, tends to counter the hyperacidity of the Type O digestive tract, reducing the potential for ulcers. The abundant fucose in bladderwrack protects the intestinal lining of the Type O stomach, preventing ulcer-causing bacteria from adhering. Kelp is also highly effective as a metabolic regulator for Type O, and is an important aid to weight loss.

Parsley is soothing to your digestive tract, as are certain warming spices, like curry and cayenne pepper. Many of these spices are antimicrobial and help balance the microbiome. Note, however, that black and white pepper are irritants to the Type O gut and can induce unwanted permeability.

Highly Beneficial

CAROB	GINGER	PEPPER, CAYENNE
CURRY ‡	HORSERADISH	PEPPER, RED
DULSE ‡	KELP	FLAKES ↑
GARLIC	PARSLEY ↑	TURMERIC ‡

Neutral

Allspice	Chervil	Dill	Sage
Almond extract	Chili powder	Fennel	Salt, sea salt
Anise	Chives	Licorice root	Savory
Apple pectin	Chocolate	Marjoram	Senna
Arrowroot	Cilantro	Mustard, dry	Spearmint
Basil	Cinnamon	Oregano	Tarragon
Bay leaf	Clove	Paprika	Thyme
Bergamot	Coriander	Peppermint	Vanilla
Caraway	Cream of tartar	Rosemary	Wintergreen
Cardamom	Cumin	Saffron	

Avoid

Guarana	Nutmeg
Mace	Pepper, black ↓

Condiments, Sweeteners and Additives

There are no highly beneficial condiments, sweeteners, and additives for Type O. If you must have mustard or salad dressing on your foods, use them in moderation, and stick to the low-fat, low-sugar varieties.

Although Type O can have tomatoes occasionally, avoid ketchup, which also contains ingredients like vinegar and sugar.

All pickled foods are indigestible for Type O. They severely irritate the Type O stomach lining. My recommendation is that you try to wean yourself from condiments, and replace them with healthier seasonings such as olive oil, lemon juice, and garlic.

Sweeteners such as honey and sugar will not harm you, nor will chocolate. However, on average we consume an enormous amount of sugar, which is quite harmful. These should all be strictly limited to occasional use as condiments. Avoid corn syrup as a sweetener.

Neutral

Agar	Gelatin, plain	Mustard, wheat	Stevia
Agave syrup ↑	Honey	free, vinegar	Sugar, brown,
Apple butter	Jam, jelly (from	free ↑	white
Apple cider	acceptable	Rice syrup	Umeboshi plum,
vinegar	fruit)	Salad dressing,	vinegar
Apple pectin	Lecithin	low-fat	Vegetable
Baking soda	Maple syrup	from	glycerine
Barley malt ↑	Mayonnaise	acceptable	Yeast, baker's ↑
Brown rice syrup	Miso ↑	ingredients	Yeast,
Carob syrup	Molasses	Soybean sauce,	nutritional ↑
Fructose	Molasses,	tamari, wheat	
Fruit pectin	blackstrap	free	

Avoid

Acacia (gum arabic)	Invert sugar	Sodium carboxy-
Aspartame	Ketchup ↓	methyl cellulose ↓
Carrageenan ↓	MSG	Sucanat
Cornstarch	Mayonnaise,	Sucrose
Dextrose ↓	tofu, soy	Tragacanth gum ↓
Fructose	Methyl cellulose ↓	Vinegar, all types ↓
Guar gum	Mustard, with	Worcestershire
High-fructose corn	vinegar and	sauce ↓
syrup ↓	wheat	
High-maltose corn	Pepper, white	
syrup,	Pickle relish ↓	
maltodextrin ↓	Polysorbate 80 ↓	

Meal Planning for Type O

Asterisk (*) indicates the recipe is provided.

THE FOLLOWING sample menus and recipes will give you an idea of a typical diet beneficial to Type O. They were developed by Dina Khader, MS, RD, CDN, a nutritionist who has used the Blood Type Diet successfully with her patients.

These menus are moderate in calories and balanced for metabolic efficiency in Type O. The average person will be able to maintain weight comfortably and even lose weight by following these suggestions. However, alternative food choices are provided if you prefer lighter fare or wish to limit your caloric intake and still eat a balanced, satisfying diet. (The alternative food is listed directly across from the food it replaces.)

Occasionally you will see an ingredient in a recipe that appears on your avoid list. If it is a very small ingredient (such as a dash of pepper), you may be able to tolerate it, depending on your condition and whether you are strictly adhering to the diet. However, the meal selections and recipes are generally designed to work very well for Type O.

As you become more familiar with the Type O diet recommendations, you'll be able to easily create your own menu plans and adjust favorite recipes to make them Type O friendly.

STANDARD MENU ▪	WEIGHT-CONTROL ALTERNATIVES ▪

SAMPLE MEAL PLAN 1

Breakfast

2 slices toasted Essene bread with organic almond butter	1 slice toasted Essene bread with all-natural, low-sugar jam
6 ounces vegetable juice	
banana	
green tea or herbal tea	

Lunch

*Organic Roast Beef, 6 ounces	*Organic Roast Beef, 2 to 4 ounces
*Spinach Salad	
apple or pineapple slices	
water or seltzer	

Midafternoon Snack

*1 slice Quinoa Applesauce Cake	sliced carrot and celery sticks
green tea or herbal tea	

sliced fruits
rice cakes with a
   drizzle of honey

Dinner

*Lamb and Asparagus Stew
steamed broccoli   steamed artichoke with
sweet potato   lemon juice
blueberries, kiwi, mixed fresh
   fruit—grapes, peaches
seltzer or herbal tea
(beer or wine allowed)   avoid beer and wine

SAMPLE MEAL PLAN 2

Breakfast

2 slices Essene bread   1 slice Essene
   with sweet butter, jam, or   bread with
   apple butter   apple butter
2 poached eggs   1 poached egg
6 ounces pineapple juice
green tea or herbal tea

Lunch

chicken sandwich—sliced   broiled chicken breast
   breast of chicken   endive and tomato
1 slice spelt bread or salad greens
2 plums
water or seltzer

Midafternoon Snack

pumpkin seeds and walnuts,   6 ounces vegetable juice
   or rice cakes with almond butter, 2 Finn Crisp crackers
   or figs, dates, prunes   or rice cakes with natural,
seltzer, water, or herbal tea   low-sugar jelly

Dinner
*Arabian Baked Fish   *Baked Fish
*String Bean Salad
steamed collard greens tossed
    with lemon juice
green tea or herbal tea
(beer or wine allowed—but not   avoid beer and wine
    every day)

SAMPLE MEAL PLAN 3

Breakfast
*Maple-Walnut Granola   puffed rice with soy milk
    with milk
1 poached egg
8 ounces pineapple or prune juice
green tea or herbal tea

Lunch
4 to 6 ounces lean ground   4-ounce ground beef
    beef patty   patty (no bread)
2 slices Essene bread
mixed green salad—romaine,
    parsley, red onion, carrots,
    cucumber
olive oil and lemon juice dressing
water or herbal tea

Midafternoon Snack
*2 Carob Chip Cookies   mixed fruit
green tea or herbal tea

Dinner
*Kifta with grilled vegetables
brown rice with dab of butter   endive salad
herbal tea
(beer or wine allowed)   avoid beer and wine

Recipes

ORGANIC BEEF ROAST

1 organic, preferably grass-fed beef roast (about 3 pounds)
Salt, pepper, and allspice to taste
6 cloves garlic
Extra-virgin olive oil
Bay leaves

Remove visible fat and place roast in baking pan. Season and cut gashes, inserting cut garlic cloves, and bay leaves. Brush the meat with extra-virgin olive oil.
Place uncovered roast in 350 degree F. oven for 90 minutes, or until meat is tender.
Serves 6.

QUINOA APPLESAUCE CAKE

1¾ cups quinoa flour
1 cup currants or other (allowed) dried fruit
½ cup chopped pecans
½ teaspoon baking soda
½ teaspoon aluminum-free baking powder
½ teaspoon salt
½ teaspoon ground cloves
½ cup unsalted, sweet butter or ½ cup organic canola oil
1 cup Sucanat sugar or maple sugar
1 large organic egg
2 cups unsweetened organic applesauce

Preheat oven to 350 degrees F. Sprinkle ¼ cup of the flour over the currants and nuts and set aside. Blend the baking soda, baking powder, salt, and cloves with the remaining quinoa flour.

Separately mix together butter or oil, sugar, and egg. Combine all ingredients, adding the fruit and nuts at the end. Spoon into an oiled 8 x 8-inch cake pan and bake for 40 to 45 minutes or until the cake tester inserted in the center comes out clean.

LAMB-ASPARAGUS STEW

1 pound fresh asparagus spears
½ pound free-range lamb meat, cubed
1 medium onion, chopped
3 tablespoons organic, sweet, unsalted butter
1 cup water
Salt, pepper, and allspice to taste
Juice of 1 lemon

Cut asparagus spears in 2-inch lengths, discarding tough portion at bottom. Wash and drain.

Sauté meat and onions in butter until light brown. Add water, salt, and spices. Cook until tender. Add asparagus. Simmer for 15 minutes or until tender. Add lemon juice.

Makes 2 servings.

SPINACH SALAD

2 bunches fresh spinach
1 bunch scallions, chopped
Juice of 1 lemon
¼ tablespoon olive oil
Salt and pepper to taste

Wash spinach well. Drain and chop. Sprinkle with salt. After a few minutes, squeeze excess water. Add scallions, lemon juice, oil, salt, and pepper. Serve immediately.

Makes 6 servings.

ARABIAN BAKED FISH

1 large halibut or whitefish (3 to 4 pounds)
Salt and pepper to taste
¼ cup lemon juice
2 tablespoons olive oil
2 large onions, chopped and sautéed in olive oil
2 to 2½ cups tahini sauce

Preheat oven to 400 degrees F.

Wash fish and dry thoroughly. Sprinkle with salt and lemon juice.

Let stand for 30 minutes. Drain fish. Brush with oil and place in baking pan. Bake for 30 minutes.

Cover with sautéed onions and tahini sauce. Sprinkle with salt and pepper. Return to oven and bake until fish is easily flaked with a fork (from 30 to 40 minutes).

Serve the fish on a platter and garnish with parsley and lemon wedges.

Makes 6 to 8 servings.

TAHINI SAUCE

1 cup organic tahini
Juice of 3 lemons
2 cloves of garlic, crushed
2 to 3 teaspoons salt
¼ cup dried, organic parsley flakes or
fresh parsley, chopped finely
Water

In a bowl, mix tahini with lemon juice, garlic, salt, and parsley.

Add enough water to make a thick sauce.

BAKED FISH

1 large whitefish (2 or 3 pounds) or other fish
Lemon juice and salt to taste
¼ cup oil
1 teaspoon cayenne
1 teaspoon cumin (optional)

Preheat oven to 350 degrees F.

Wash fish. Sprinkle with salt and lemon juice. Let stand for 30 minutes. Drain.

Coat fish with oil and spices and place in a baking pan. To prevent fish from drying, wrap with lightly oiled foil. Bake for 30 to 40 minutes, or until fish is tender and easily flaked.

Makes 4 to 5 servings.

WITH STUFFING *(OPTIONAL)*

⅓ cup pine nuts or shredded almonds
2 tablespoons sweet, unsalted butter
1 cup parsley, chopped
3 cloves garlic, crushed
Salt and allspice to taste

Sauté nuts in butter until lightly brown. Add parsley and spices and sauté for one minute. Stuff raw fish with the mixture.

STRING BEAN SALAD

1 pound green string beans
Juice of 1 lemon
3 tablespoons olive oil
2 cloves garlic, crushed
2 to 3 teaspoons salt

Wash tender, fresh green string beans. Remove stems and strings. Cut into 2-inch pieces.

Cook until tender by boiling in plenty of water. Drain. When cool, place in a salad bowl. Dress to taste with lemon juice, olive oil, garlic, and salt.

Makes 4 servings.

_____

MAPLE-WALNUT GRANOLA

4 cups rolled oats
1 cup rice bran
1 cup sesame seeds
½ cup dried cranberries
½ cup dried currants
1 cup chopped walnuts
¼ cup organic canola oil
½ cup maple syrup
¼ cup honey
1 teaspoon vanilla extract

Preheat oven to 250 degrees F. In a large mixing bowl, combine the oats, rice bran, seeds, dried fruit, and nuts. Add the oil and stir evenly.

Pour in maple syrup, honey, and vanilla and mix well until evenly moistened. Mixture should be crumbly and sticky. Spread mixture in a cookie tray, and bake for 90 minutes, stirring every 15 minutes for even toasting until the mixture is golden brown and dry.

Cool well and store in airtight container.

_____

CAROB CHIP COOKIES

⅓ cup organic canola oil
½ cup pure maple syrup
1 teaspoon vanilla extract
1 organic egg
1¾ cups oat or brown rice flour
1 teaspoon baking soda
½ cup carob chips (unsweetened)
Dash allspice (optional)

Oil two baking sheets and preheat oven to 375 degrees F. In a medium-size mixing bowl, combine the oil, maple syrup, and vanilla. Beat the egg and stir into the oil mixture. Gradually stir in flour and baking soda to form a stiff batter. Fold in carob chips and drop the batter onto the baking sheets by the teaspoon. Bake for 10 to 15 minutes, until cookies are lightly browned. Remove from oven and cool.

Makes 3½ to 4 dozen.

KIFTA

2 pounds finely ground lamb meat
1 large onion, finely chopped
2 to 2½ teaspoons salt
1½ teaspoons pepper and allspice
1 cup parsley, finely chopped
½ cup lemon juice

Mix all of the ingredients thoroughly (using a meat grinder, if you have one). Reserve parsley and lemon juice.

To barbecue: Take portions of meat and mold on skewers, making sure it is held firmly.

To broil: Take portions of meat and mold into rolls, lengthwise, 3 inches long. Place on a broiling pan and broil in a preheated oven at 500 degrees F. Broil until brown on one side, then flip to brown the other side.

Serve hot. Sprinkle with lemon juice and garnish with parsley.

For a wealth of additional recipes in every category, check out the blood type–specific cookbooks and recipe database at dadamo .com and 4yourtype.com.

Type O
Supplement Advisory

THE ROLE OF SUPPLEMENTS—be they vitamins, minerals, or herbs—is to add the nutrients that are lacking in your diet and to provide extra protection where you need it. The supplement focus for Type O is

- Supercharging the metabolism
- Balancing the internal biosphere (microbiome)
- Preventing inflammation
- Supporting the thyroid
- Blunting unwarranted stress

The following recommendations emphasize the supplements that help meet these goals and also warn against the supplements that can be counterproductive or dangerous for Type O. The effectiveness of these recommendations relies on your adherence to the Type O diet.

Vitamins

Many Type Os tell me that they feel more energetic when on a high-potency vitamin B complex. You may want to try this for a week or so and see how you feel. A well-designed multivitamin or B complex is safe, and other than possibly experiencing the phenomenon of bright yellow urine, there is little to worry about. (The yellow color is usually just the result of the excess riboflavin in the vitamin being excreted.) If you take a high-potency vitamin B complex, make sure it is free of fillers and binders. Improper binding and compressing can make the pill difficult to absorb in your system. Also avoid using a formula that contains wheat germ.

Type O sometimes requires a vitamin B_{12} supplement, especially if starting the Blood Type Diet after having been a vegan or vegetarian. B_{12} supplements come in a variety of formats. The one you want to avoid is, not surprisingly, the cheapest: cyanocobalamin. Look instead for methylcobalamin, the active form of B_{12}, which does not require transformation into the biologically active form. Methylcobalamin is involved in the synthesis of melatonin, so you might even sleep a bit better at night.

One interesting application of the blood type theory to supplementation involves a supplement called pantethine. Pantethine is actually a form of vitamin B_5, known as pantothenic acid. In fact pantethine is made up of pantothenic acid molecules chained together by a molecule called cysteamine. Studies show that when cysteamine is released from pantethine during digestion it acts to slow down dopamine beta-hydroxylase (DBH), the overactive enzyme in Type O that drains precious dopamine into anxiety-inducing norepinephrine. One added side effect is that supplementing with pantethine also gives you unchained pantothenic acid, which can help support the adrenal glands.

Finally, eat plenty of vitamin B–rich foods.

Minerals

CALCIUM

Although a high-protein diet stimulates unique enzymes in the Type O digestive tract that ramp up calcium absorption, there are situations when you should supplement your diet with calcium. The Type O diet does not include many dairy products, which are some of the best sources of this mineral. Calcium supplementation (600 to 1,100 milligrams elemental calcium) is especially beneficial for Type O children during their growth periods (ages two to five years and nine to sixteen years) and for postmenopausal women. Although the nondairy sources of calcium are not as beneficial, Type O should employ them as mainstays of the diet.

MAGNESIUM

Although a diet of fruits and vegetables usually provides enough magnesium to meet your biological needs, I've found that Type O does well on magnesium supplements. Magnesium tends to optimize the digestive process and may reduce inflammation. If you suffer from migraine headaches or other types of inflammation and pain, you may want to add this to your supplement plan.

IODINE

Type O tends to have unstable thyroid metabolism, which can easily be disturbed by changes in the gut's bacterial population. The wrong types of bacterial flora can activate the immune system to attack them but can also damage the thyroid, a case of harm due to "friendly fire." Iodine is the key element necessary for the production of thyroid hormone. Although iodine supplements are not recommended, adequate amounts of iodine can be found in the Type O diet, especially if you include sea vegetables such as kelp. Not only do these contain small amounts of iodine but they also help optimize the proper balance of gut flora, which keeps the thyroid protected from the inadvertent attentions of the immune system.

Nutraceuticals

DIGESTIVE SUPPORT

Licorice (*Glycyrrhiza glabra*) is helpful for Type O digestion. The high stomach acid typical of Type O can lead to stomach irritations and ulcers. A licorice preparation called deglycyrrhizinated licorice (DGL) can reduce your discomfort and aid healing. It is widely available in health food stores as a pleasant-tasting powder or in the form of lozenges. Unlike most ulcer medicines, DGL actually heals the stomach lining, in addition to protecting it from stomach acids. Avoid crude licorice preparations, because they contain a component of the plant that can cause elevated blood pressure. This component has been removed in DGL. Other remedies to protect your stomach lining and increase resistance to ulcers include slippery elm and marshmallow root, taken as tea or capsules, and ginger rhizome. Clove fruit is a source of eugenol, which has anti-inflammatory and anti-ulcer properties.

PANCREATIC ENZYMES

If you are a Type O who is not used to a high-protein diet, I suggest you take a pancreatic enzyme with large meals for a while, or at least until your system begins to adjust to the more concentrated proteins. Pancreatic enzyme supplements are available at many health food stores and online, usually in a 4× strength.

Stress Support

RHODIOLA HERB

Rhodiola rosea is an herb that has traditional usage as an anti-fatigue agent. It also helps Type O modulate stress more efficiently. It seems to enhance the response of muscle tissue to exercise, help balance neurotransmitters, and may even have a mild antidepressant effect.

Metabolic Support

BLADDERWRACK (*Fucus vesiculosus*)

Bladderwrack (from kelp) is an excellent nutrient for Type O. This herb, actually a seaweed, has some interesting components, including iodine and large amounts of the sugar fucose. As you may recall, fucose is the basic building sugar of the O antigen, and the fucose found in bladderwrack helps protect the intestinal lining of Type O—especially from the ulcer-causing bacteria *H. pylori*, which attaches itself to the fucose lining the stomach. The fucose in bladderwrack acts on *H. pylori* much as dust would on a piece of adhesive tape: clogging the suction cups on the bacteria, preventing it from attaching to the stomach.

I have also found that bladderwrack is very effective as an aid to weight control for Type O—especially for those who suffer thyroid dysfunctions. The fucose in bladderwrack seems to help normalize the sluggish metabolic rate and produce weight loss. (Note, however, that although bladderwrack has a time-honored reputation as an aid to weight loss for Type O, it does not work that way for the other blood types.)

N-ACETYL-GLUCOSAMINE

N-acetyl-glucosamine (NAG) is an amino sugar, found very commonly in nature. Unlike its cousin glucosamine sulfate, which is widely used to promote joint health, NAG works in the digestive tract. Many dietary lectins bind to NAG, so if you are trying to go lectin free or are dealing with gut problems, NAG may be a worthwhile supplement.

Potential Problem Supplements

ST. JOHN'S WORT (*Hypericum* spp.)

A popular herb in health food stores, St. John's wort has a well-regarded reputation for being helpful in mild cases of depression. However, I've noticed that many Type Os feel especially "weird" taking St. John's wort, which may result from the herb interacting with neurotransmitters and stress chemicals that can get out of balance in Type O, such as DBH, monoamine oxidase (MAO), dopamine, and norepinephrine. St. John's wort also can affect how the liver detoxifies certain drugs and environmental chemicals. If you are Type O and using St. John's wort, you may want to consider switching to rhodiola.

HIGH-DOSE VITAMIN C

While the normal doses of vitamin C found in the diet and in rationally designed supplements are probably fine, vitamin C is a known co-factor for the DBH enzyme, which converts dopamine to anxiety-inducing norepinephrine. If you are taking more than 500 milligrams of vitamin C daily and experiencing stressful feelings, high blood pressure, depression or anxiety, you might want to drop the dosage down or take a supplement vacation from vitamin C.

Type O Stress-Exercise Profile

As WE DISCUSSED in Chapter Four, stress is not in itself the problem; it's how your body responds to stress. Each blood type has a distinct, programmed instinct for overcoming stress. With the Blood Type Diet, exercise is really all about personalized stress reduction. As a Type O you want to do whatever you can to increase dopamine (and its accompanying feelings of satisfaction and well-being) and decrease norepinephrine (and its accompanying feelings of anxiety and stress). The ability to reverse the negative effects of stress lives in your blood type. Healthy Type Os are meant to release the built-up hormonal forces through vigorous and intense physical exercise. Your system is literally suited for it. If you are Type O, you have the immediate and physical response of our hunter ancestors. Your blood type carries a patterned alarm response that permits explosions of intense physical energy.

When you encounter stress, your body takes over. As your adrenal glands pump their chemicals into your bloodstream, you become tremendously charged up. Given a physical release at this time, any bad stress you are experiencing may be converted into a positive experience.

Exercise is especially critical to the health of Type O, because the impact of stress is direct and physical. Not only does a regular intense exercise program elevate your spirits, it enables Type O to maintain weight control, emotional balance, and a strong self-image.

Type Os who want to lose weight must participate in highly physical exercise. It blunts their unique form of stress and, in addition to the high-protein diet, builds metabolically active tissue, such as muscle. Each and every increase in metabolically active tissue adds to their metabolic rate.

Type Os who do not express their physical natures with appropriate activity in response to stress are eventually overwhelmed during the exhaustion stage of the stress response. This exhaustion stage is characterized by a variety of psychological manifestations caused by a slower rate of metabolism, such as depression, fatigue, or insomnia. If there is no change, you will leave yourself vulnerable to a number of inflammatory and autoimmune disorders, type 2 diabetes, consistent weight gain, and eventual obesity.

The following exercises are recommended for Type O individuals. Pay special attention to the length of the sessions. To achieve a consistent metabolic effect, you have to get your heart rate up. You can mix any of these exercises, but be sure you do one or several of them at least four times a week for the best results.

EXERCISE	DURATION	FREQUENCY (PER WEEK)
AEROBICS	40–60 min.	3–4x
SWIMMING	30–45 min.	3–4x
JOGGING	30 min.	3–4x
WEIGHT TRAINING	30 min.	3x

TREADMILL	30 min.	3x
STAIR CLIMBING	20–30 min.	3–4x
MARTIAL ARTS	60 min.	2–3x
CONTACT SPORTS	60 min.	2–3x
CALISTHENICS	30–45 min.	3x
CYCLING	30 min.	3x
BRISK WALKING	30–40 min.	5x
DANCING	40–60 min.	3x
IN-LINE OR ROLLER SKATING	30 min.	3–4x

Type O
Exercise Guidelines

THE THREE COMPONENTS of a high-intensity exercise program are the warm-up period, the aerobic exercise period, and the cool-down period. A warm-up is very important to prevent injuries, because it brings blood to the muscles, readying them for exercise, whether it is walking, running, biking, swimming, or playing a sport. A warm-up should include stretching and flexibility moves to prevent tears in the muscles and tendons.

The exercises can be divided into two basic types: isometric exercises, in which stress is created in stationary muscles; and isotonic exercises, such as calisthenics, running, or swimming, which produce muscle tension through a range of movement. Isometric exercises can be used to tone up specific muscles, which can be further strengthened by isotonic exercise. Isometrics may be performed by pushing or pulling an immovable object or by contracting or tightening opposing muscles.

To achieve maximum cardiovascular benefits from aerobic exercise, you must elevate your heart rate to approximately 70 percent of your maximum. Once that elevated rate is achieved during exercise, continue exercising to maintain it for 30 minutes. This regimen should be repeated at least three times each week.

To calculate your heart rate range:

1. Subtract your age from 220. This gives you your maximum heart rate.
2. To calculate the top limit of your target heart rate range, multiply the difference by 70 percent (.70). If you are over 60 years of age or in poor physical condition, multiply the difference by 60 percent (.60).
3. To calculate the bottom limit of your target heart rate range, multiply the difference by 50 percent (.50).

For example, a healthy fifty-year-old woman would subtract 50 from 220 (220 − 50), for a maximum heart rate of 170. To find the top limit of her target heart rate range, multiply 170 by .70. Thus 119 beats per minute is the top heart rate she should strive for. To find the bottom limit of her target heart rate range, multiply 170 by .50. Thus 85 beats per minute is the lowest heart rate she should strive for.

Active, healthy individuals under forty and people under sixty with a low cardiovascular risk can choose their own exercise program from among the recommendations listed.

Remember, your goal is to counter stress with action. For Type O, the best antidote to fatigue and depression is physical work. Think of your metabolism as a fire. You start a fire first by using little pieces of wood called kindling, and then gradually add larger and larger pieces of wood until you have an inferno. If you are too tired to imagine doing aerobics for 45 to 60 minutes, start doing something! As you feel better, add more. At the end, your stress levels will be reduced, your mood will be better, and you'll have renewed energy.

SIX

Blood Type

A

Diet

TYPE A: *The Cultivator*

- REAPS WHAT HE SOWS
- SENSITIVE DIGESTIVE TRACT
- TOLERANT IMMUNE SYSTEM
- ADAPTS WELL TO SETTLED DIETARY AND ENVIRONMENTAL CONDITIONS
- RESPONDS BEST TO STRESS WITH CALMING ACTION
- REQUIRES AGRARIAN DIET TO STAY LEAN AND PRODUCTIVE

The Type A Diet

TYPE A flourishes on plant-based diets—the inheritance of more settled and less warlike farmer ancestors. If you are a Type A currently consuming a diet that includes a lot of meat, you might find it challenging to transition to one that emphasizes soy proteins, grains, and vegetables. Likewise, it might be difficult to eliminate overly processed and refined foods because our civilized diets are increasingly composed of convenient toxins in brightly wrapped packages. But it is particularly important for sensitive Type As to get foods in as natural a state as possible: fresh, pure, organic and primarily vegetarian.

I can't emphasize enough how critical this dietary adjustment can be to the sensitive immune system of Type A. As you will see in Chapters Eleven and Twelve, Type A is biologically predisposed to heart disease, cancer, and diabetes. In other words, these are your risk factors, but they need not be your destiny. If you follow this diet, you can supercharge your immune system and potentially short-circuit the development of life-threatening diseases. A positive aspect of your genetic ancestry is your ability to utilize the best nature has to offer. It will be your challenge to relearn what your blood already knows.

NOTE: Longtime readers will notice a difference in the values of a small number of foods between this edition and the original version of *Eat Right for Your Type*. That is because beginning with the publication of *Live Right for Your Type*, I made a distinction in some foods between secretors and non-secretors. The original version of *Eat Right for Your Type*, which preceded *Live Right for Your Type*, "homogenized" these differences. Like all of my subsequent books, this edition of *Eat Right for Your Type* uses the secretor values as the base values for the A, B, AB, and O blood types.

KEY

‡ Enhances carbohydrate metabolism, helps with
   weight loss

↑ Increases microbiome diversity, discourages microbial
   imbalance

↓ Decreases microbiome diversity, encourages microbial
   imbalance

Meats and Poultry

BLOOD TYPE A	WEEKLY ▪ IF YOUR ANCESTRY IS			
Food	Portion	African	Caucasian	Asian
LEAN RED MEATS	4–6 OZ.	0–1X	0X	0–1X
POULTRY	4–6 OZ.	0–3X	0–3X	1–4X

*The portion recommendations are merely guidelines that can help refine
your diet according to ancestral propensities.*

To receive the greatest benefits, Type A should eliminate all meat.
You do not do well on a Paleo diet. No matter the current trend, I urge
you to look at the Type A diet guidelines with an open mind. This is
a way you can begin reducing Type A risk factors for heart disease and
cancer in your diet. If you're a Type A, you lack some of the digestive
enzymes and stomach acids that would allow you to effectively digest
animal protein.

Having said that, let me acknowledge that if it is new for you, it will
probably take time for you to convert to a totally vegetarian diet. Begin by substituting fish for meat several times a week. When you do
eat poultry, choose lean, chemical- and pesticide-free cuts.

Stay completely away from processed meat products such as ham,
frankfurters, and cold cuts. They contain nitrites, which promote stomach cancer in people with low levels of stomach acid—a Type A trait.

Neutral

Chicken	Grouse	Squab
Chicken liver	Guinea hen	Turkey
Cornish hen	Ostrich	

Avoid

Bear	Goat	Partridge
Beef	Goose	Pheasant
Beef heart	Goose liver	Pork and bacon ↓
Beef liver	Ham ↓	Quail
Beef tongue	Horse	Rabbit
Bone soup	Kangaroo	Squirrel
Buffalo, bison	Lamb	Sweetbreads
Calf liver	Marrow soup	Turtle
Caribou	Moose	Veal
Duck	Mutton	Venison
Duck liver	Opossum	

Seafood

BLOOD TYPE A	WEEKLY ▪ IF YOUR ANCESTRY IS			
Food	*Portion*	*African*	*Caucasian*	*Asian*
ALL RECOMMENDED SEAFOOD	4–6 OZ.	0–3X	1–4X	1–4X

Type A can eat seafood in modest quantities three or four times a week. Many varieties of fish are rich in omega-3 fatty acids, which are protective against Type A's tendencies for cardiovascular disease and cancer. Avoid whitefish, such as sole and flounder, because they contain a lectin that can irritate the Type A digestive tract.

Consider introducing snails into your diet. The edible snail, *Helix aspersa/pomatia*, contains a powerful lectin that may protect against breast cancer, as you will see in Chapter Twelve. This is a positive kind of agglutination; this lectin helps get rid of sick cells.

Seafood should be baked, broiled, or poached to achieve its full nutritional value.

Highly Beneficial

CARP ↑
COD ↑
MACKEREL,
   ATLANTIC ↑
MONKFISH ↑
PERCH ↑
PICKEREL,
   WALLEYE ↑

POLLOCK,
   ATLANTIC ↑
RED SNAPPER ↑ ‡
SALMON,
   ATLANTIC
   (WILD)↑
SALMON,
   CHINOOK ↑

SALMON, SOCKEYE ↑
SARDINE ↑ ‡
SNAIL (ESCARGOT)
TROUT, RAINBOW
   (WILD) ↑
TROUT, SEA ↑
WHITEFISH ↑
WHITING ↑

Neutral

Abalone, sea ear,
   mutton fish
Bass, sea, lake
Bullhead
Butterfish
Chub
Croaker
Cusk
Drum
Halfmoon fish
Mackerel, Spanish
Mahi-mahi
Mullet
Muskellunge
Ocean pout

Orange roughy
Parrotfish
Perch, ocean
Pike
Pilchards
Pompano
Porgy
Rosefish
Sailfish
Sailfish roe
Salmon roe
Scrod
Sea bream
Shark
Smelt

Sturgeon
Sucker
Sunfish,
   pumpkinseed
Swordfish
Tilapia
Trout, steelhead (wild)
Tuna, bluefin
Tuna, skipjack
Tuna, yellowfin
Turbot, European
Weakfish
Yellowtail

Avoid

Anchovy
Barracuda
Bass, blue gill
Bass, striped ↓

Bluefish ↓
Catfish
Caviar
Clam

Conch
Crab
Crayfish
Eel ↓

Flounder
Frog
Grouper
Haddock
Hake
Halibut
Harvest fish
Herring, fresh,
 smoked, pickled

Lobster
Mussels
Octopus
Opaleye fish
Oyster ↓
Salmon,
 smoked (lox)
Scallop
Scup

Shad
Shrimp
Skate
Sole, gray, Dover
Squid, calamari
Tilefish ↓

Dairy and Eggs

BLOOD TYPE A		WEEKLY ▪ IF YOUR ANCESTRY IS		
Food	*Portion*	*African*	*Caucasian*	*Asian*
EGGS	I EGG	I–3X	I–3X	I–3X
CHEESES	2 OZ.	I–3X	2–4X	0
YOGURT	4–6 OZ.	0	I–3X	0–3X
MILK	4–6 OZ.	0	0–4X	0

Type A can tolerate small amounts of fermented dairy products, but should avoid anything made with whole milk and also limit egg consumption to an occasional organically grown egg.

Your Type A choices should be yogurt, kefir, nonfat sour cream, and cultured dairy products. Raw goat's milk is a good substitute for whole milk. And, of course, soy milk and soy cheese are excellent substitutes, and are very good for Type A.

Most commercial dairy products are not digestible for Type A—the sugars in the milk tend to be seen as unfriendly to the gut and they encourage the growth of non-A-friendly bacteria.

If you are a Type A allergy sufferer or are experiencing respiratory problems, be aware that dairy products greatly increase the amount of mucus you secrete. Type A normally produces more mucus than the other blood types, probably because you need the extra protection it provides your somewhat too friendly immune system. However, too much mucus can be harmful because various bacteria tend to live off it. This is another good reason to limit your intake of dairy foods.

Highly Beneficial

PECORINO CHEESE ↑
ROMANIAN URDA ↑

Neutral

Egg, goose
Egg, quail
Egg white, chicken
Egg whole, chicken
Egg whole, duck
Egg yolk, chicken
Farmer cheese

Feta cheese
Ghee, clarified
   butter ↑
Goat cheese
Kefir
Manchego cheese
Milk, goat

Mozzarella cheese,
   all types
Paneer cheese
Quark cheese
Ricotta cheese
Sour cream
Yogurt

Avoid

American
   cheese ↓
Blue cheese
Brie cheese
Butter
Buttermilk
Camembert
   cheese ↓
Casein ↓
Cheddar cheese ↓
Colby cheese ↓
Cottage cheese ↓
Cream cheese ↓
Edam cheese ↓

Emmental, Swiss
   cheese ↓
Gorgonzola
   cheese ↓
Gouda cheese
Gruyère
   cheese ↓
Half-and-half ↓
Ice cream
Jarlsberg cheese
Milk, cow
   (skim or 2%) ↓
Milk, cow
   (whole) ↓

Monterey Jack
   cheese ↓
Muenster cheese ↓
Neufchâtel cheese ↓
Parmesan cheese
Provolone cheese ↓
Romano cheese
Roquefort cheese ↓
Sherbet
Stilton cheese ↓
String cheese ↓
Whey protein ↓

Oils and Fats

BLOOD TYPE A		WEEKLY ▪ IF YOUR ANCESTRY IS		
Food	*Portion*	*African*	*Caucasian*	*Asian*
OILS	1 TABLESPOON	3–8x	2–6x	2–6x

Type A needs very little fat to function well, but a tablespoon of olive oil on salads or steamed vegetables every day will aid in digestion and elimination. As a monounsaturated fat, olive oil also has a positive effect on your heart and may actually reduce cholesterol.

Oils like corn and safflower oil can cause inflammatory reactions on the delicate linings of the Type A blood vessels—quite the opposite effect of the beneficial oils.

Highly Beneficial

APRICOT
  KERNEL OIL
BLACK CURRANT
  SEED OIL ↑ ‡

CAMELINA OIL ↑
FLAXSEED,
  LINSEED OIL ↑ ‡

OLIVE OIL ↑
WALNUT OIL ↑ ‡

Neutral

Almond oil
Avocado oil
Borage seed oil
Canola oil
Chia seed oil
Cod liver oil

Evening
  primrose oil
Hemp seed oil
Macadamia oil
Perilla seed oil
Pumpkin seed oil

Rice bran oil
Safflower oil
Sesame oil
Soybean oil
Sunflower oil
Wheat germ oil

Avoid

Castor oil
Coconut oil
Corn oil ↓

Cottonseed oil
Hazelnut oil
Lard

Margarine
Palm oil
Peanut oil ↓

Nuts and Seeds

BLOOD TYPE A		WEEKLY ▪ IF YOUR ANCESTRY IS		
Food	*Portion*	*African*	*Caucasian*	*Asian*
NUTS AND SEEDS	SMALL HANDFUL	4–6x	2–5x	4–6x
NUT BUTTERS	I TABLESPOON	3–5x	I–4x	2–4x

Many nuts and seeds, such as pumpkin seeds and sunflower seeds, almonds and walnuts, can provide positive supplementation for the Type A diet. Because Type A eats very little animal protein, nuts and seeds supply an important protein component. Walnuts are the most beneficial. They contain proteins and oils that help the cells rid themselves of accumulated debris, a process called autophagy. Pumpkin seeds are also highly beneficial.

If you are Type A and have gallbladder problems, limit yourself to small amounts of nut butters instead of whole nuts.

Highly Beneficial

CHESTNUT,   PEANUT ↑ ‡   PEANUT FLOUR ↑
  CHINESE ↑   PEANUT   PUMPKIN SEED ↑
FLAXSEED ↑   BUTTER ↑   WALNUT ↑ ‡

Neutral

Almond ↑   Chestnut,   Macadamia ↑
Almond butter   European ↑   Pecan ↑
Almond cheese ↑   Chia seed ↑   Pecan butter
Almond milk↑   Filbert, hazelnut   Pine nut,
Beechnut   Hemp seed ↑   pignoli ↑
Butternut ↑   Hickory ↑   Poppy seed ↑
Carob ↑   Litchi/lychee   Safflower seed

Sesame butter, tahini ↑	Sesame seed ↑	Watermelon seed
Sesame flour	Sunflower seed	
	Sunflower butter	

Avoid

| Brazil nut | Cashew butter |
| Cashew | Pistachio |

Beans and Legumes

BLOOD TYPE A	WEEKLY ▪ IF YOUR ANCESTRY IS			
Food	*Portion*	*African*	*Caucasian*	*Asian*
ALL RECOMMENDED BEANS AND LEGUMES	I CUP, DRY	4–7X	3–6X	2–5X

Type A thrives on the vegetable proteins found in beans and legumes. Many beans and legumes provide a nutritious source of protein. Soybeans contain a lectin called genistein that may protect Type A against certain cancers, and one of its main flavones has a truly wonderful, healing effect on the delicate linings of the blood vessels. There is also considerable evidence that genistein stimulates receptors in fat cells called PPARs, which in turn activate fat-busting genes.

Tofu is the staple of the Type A diet. Tofu is a nutritionally complete food that is both filling and inexpensive. Many people in Western societies once had an automatic aversion to tofu, but it is much more common today in markets and restaurants. Try to purchase tofu in its freshest form. Tofu is tasteless; it takes on the flavors of vegetables and spices used in cooking. The best way to prepare it is in a stir-fry with vegetables and flavoring such as garlic, ginger, and soy sauce. Always buy your soy products from manufacturers who certify that they are GMO free.

Be aware, however, that not all beans and legumes are good for you. Some, like kidney, lima, navy, and garbanzo, contain a lectin that can cause a decrease in insulin production, which is often a factor in both obesity and diabetes.

Highly Beneficial

ADZUKI BEAN	NATTO ↑	SOYBEAN CHEESE ‡
BLACK BEAN ↑	PINTO BEAN	SOYBEAN,
BLACK-EYED PEA	PINTO BEAN,	SPROUTED ↑
BROAD BEAN, FAVA	SPROUTED ↑	SOYBEAN,
GREAT	SNAP BEAN	TEMPEH ↑
NORTHERN	SOYBEAN ‡	SOYBEAN, TOFU
BEAN ↑ ‡	SOYBEAN	SOY FLAKES
GREEN BEAN	GRANULES,	SOY MILK
LENTIL,	LECITHIN ‡	SOY MISO
SPROUTED ↑	SOYBEAN	STRING BEAN
LENTIL, ALL	MEAL	
TYPES	SOYBEAN PASTA	

Neutral

Butter bean ↑	Jicama	Northern bean
Cannellini bean	Mung beans,	Pea
Haricot-vert bean ↑	sprouts	White bean

Avoid

Copper bean ↓	Kidney bean ↓	Navy bean ↓
Garbanzo bean,	Lima bean ↓	Tamarind bean
chickpeas ↓		

Grains and Cereals

BLOOD TYPE A		WEEKLY ▪ IF YOUR ANCESTRY IS		
Food	Portion	African	Caucasian	Asian
BREADS, CRACKERS	I SLICE	2–4X	3–5X	2–4X
MUFFINS	I MUFFIN	IX	I–2X	IX
GRAINS	I CUP, DRY	6–10X	5–9X	4–8X
PASTAS	I CUP, DRY	3–5X	4–6X	3–5X

Type A generally does well with grains and cereals, and you can eat these foods one or more times a day. Stay away from processed products, such as frozen meals, prepared noodles with sauces, or packaged rice-and-vegetable combinations. Instead, gain the full nutritional benefits from whole-grain products. Bake your own cakes, prepare your own pasta, or steam your own rice, using the purest ingredients.

Type As trying to lose weight or with a pronounced mucus condition caused by asthma or frequent infections should limit wheat consumption or avoid it altogether, as wheat causes mucus production. You'll have to experiment for yourself to determine how much wheat you can eat.

Be aware that sprouted wheat breads sold commercially often contain small amounts of sprouted wheat and are basically whole wheat breads. Read the ingredient labels. The 100 percent sprouted wheat variety, sometimes called Manna or Essene breads, is acceptable as the wheat lectin is destroyed in the sprouting process.

Highly Beneficial

AMARANTH

ARTICHOKE
  FLOUR, PASTA

BUCKWHEAT,
  KASHA, SOBA

ESSENE, MANNA
  BREAD

FLAXSEED BREAD
  (CONTAINING
  ALLOWABLE
  GRAINS) ↑

LARCH FIBER ↑

LENTIL FLOUR,
  DAHL

MALANGA,
  TANNIA,
  XANTHOSOMA ↑

OAT BRAN

OATMEAL, OAT
  FLOUR, OATS

PAPADUM ↑

SOYBEAN FLOUR ‡

WHEAT, BULGUR

WHEAT, SPROUTED

Neutral

Barley ↑

Barley flour

Black bean flour

Cornflakes

Cornmeal, hominy,
  polenta, all

Cream of rice

Emmer

Fonio ↑

Graham flour

Grits

Job's tears
  (*Coix* spp.) ↑

Kamut

Mastic gum

Millet ↑

Puffed wheat

Quinoa ↑

Rice, basmati

Rice, brown

Rice, puffed,
  rice cakes

Rice, white

Rice, wild ↑

Rice bran ↑

Rice flour, brown

Rice flour, white

Rye ↑

Rye flour ↑

Sorghum ↑

Spelt

Spelt flour, noodles

Sprouted wheat flour

Tapioca, manioc,
  cassava, yucca

Taro, Tahitian, poi,
  dasheen

Wheat, durum,
  semolina, couscous

Wheat, whole grain

White flour

Avoid

Cream of wheat

Familia

Farina

Garbanzo bean
  (chickpea) flour

Grape-Nuts

Lima bean flour

Seven grain

Shredded wheat

Teff

Wheat, bran, germ

Whole wheat flour ↓

Vegetables

BLOOD TYPE A		DAILY ■ IF YOUR ANCESTRY IS		
Food	Portion	African	Caucasian	Asian
VEGETABLES, RAW	I CUP, COOKED	3–6x	2–5x	2–5x
VEGETABLES, COOKED	I CUP, COOKED	I–4x	3–6x	3–6x
SOY PRODUCTS	6–8 OZ.	4–6x	4–6x	5–7x

Vegetables are vital to the Type A diet, providing minerals, enzymes, and antioxidants. Eat your vegetables in as natural a state as possible (raw or steamed) to preserve their full benefits.

Most vegetables are available to Type A, but there are a few caveats: peppers can aggravate the delicate Type A stomach, as do the molds in fermented olives. Type A is also very sensitive to the lectins in domestic potatoes, sweet potatoes, yams, and cabbage. Avoid tomatoes, as their lectins can have a strongly irritating effect on the Type A digestive tract.

Broccoli is highly recommended for its antioxidant benefits. Antioxidants strengthen the immune system and prevent abnormal cell division. Other vegetables that are excellent for Type A are carrots, collard greens, kale, pumpkin, and spinach.

Use plenty of garlic. It's a natural antibiotic and immune system booster, and it's good for your blood. Every blood type benefits from the use of garlic, but perhaps Type A benefits most of all, because your immune system is vulnerable to a number of diseases that garlic ameliorates. Yellow onions are very good immune boosters, too. They contain a powerful antioxidant called quercetin.

Highly Beneficial

ALFALFA SPROUTS
ALOE VERA
ARTICHOKE
BEET GREENS ↑ ‡
BROCCOFLOWER ↑
BROCCOLI ↑ ‡
BROCCOLI RABE,
  RAPINI ‡
BROCCOLI,
  CHINESE
CANISTEL ↑
CARROT ↑
CELERY ↑ ‡
CHICORY
COLLARD
  GREENS ↑ ‡
DANDELION
  GREENS ‡
ESCAROLE ‡

FENNEL
GARLIC
GINGER
GRAPE LEAVES ↑
HORSERADISH ↑
JERUSALEM
  ARTICHOKE
KALE ↑
KOHLRABI
LEEK
LETTUCE,
  ROMAINE
MUSHROOM,
  MAITAKE,
  WHITE
  (COMMON),
  SILVER
  DOLLAR ‡
OKRA

ONION, ALL TYPES
PARSLEY
PARSNIP ↑
PUMPKIN ↑ ‡
SEA VEGETABLE,
  IRISH MOSS
SEA VEGETABLE,
  KELP, KOMBU,
  NORI,
  BLADDERWRACK ↑
SPINACH ↑ ‡
SWISS CHARD ↑ ‡
TOMATILLO ↑
TURNIP
TURNIP GREENS ↑ ‡

Neutral

Arugula
Asparagus
Asparagus pea
Bamboo shoot
Beet
Bok choy,
  pak choi
Broccoli leaves
Brussels sprouts
Cassava
Cauliflower
Celeriac
Chayote, pipinella,
  vegetable pear

Chervil
Chinese kale,
  Kai-lan
Cilantro
Corn, popcorn
Cucumber
Daikon radish
Endive ↑
Fenugreek ↑
Fiddlehead
  fern
Hearts of palm
Jicama ↑
Kelp

Lettuce,
  Bibb, Boston,
  green leaf, iceberg,
  mesclun
Mushroom, abalone,
  black trumpet,
  enoki, oyster,
  portobello, straw,
  tree
Mustard
  greens ↑
Olive, green
Oyster plant,
  salsify ↑

Pimiento
Quorn
Radicchio
Radish sprouts
Radish
Rutabaga

Scallion
Sea vegetables, spirulina
Sea vegetables, wakame
Seaweed

Shallot
Squash
Taro leaves, shoots
Water chestnut, matai
Watercress
Zucchini

Avoid

Cabbage ↓
Capers ↓
Eggplant
Juniper
Mushroom, shiitake ↓
Olive, black, Greek, Spanish ↓

Pepper, cayenne, chili, green, jalapeño, red, yellow
Pickles, all
Potato, blue, red, white, yellow ↓
Rhubarb

Sauerkraut ↓
Sweet potato ↓
Tomato
Yam
Yucca

Fruits

BLOOD TYPE A	DAILY ▪ ALL ANCESTRAL TYPES	
Food	*Portion*	
ALL RECOMMENDED FRUITS	1 FRUIT OR 3–5 OZ.	3–4X

Type A should eat fruits three times a day. Most fruits are allowable, although you should try to emphasize the more alkaline ones, such as berries and plums, which can help balance the grains that are acid forming in your muscle tissues. Melons are also alkaline, but their high mold counts make them hard for Type A to digest. Honeydew melons should be avoided altogether because they have the highest mold counts. Other melons (listed as neutral) can be eaten occasionally.

Type A doesn't do well on tropical fruits, such as mangoes. Although these fruits contain a digestive enzyme that is good for the other blood types, it doesn't work in the Type A digestive tract. Pineapple, on the other hand, is an excellent digestive aid for Type A.

Oranges also should be avoided, as they contain elements that can act like growth factors for undesirable strains of bacteria. This can result in an imbalance of bacteria in the gut, called dysbiosis. Grapefruit, closely related to orange, is an acidic fruit, but it has positive effects on the Type A stomach, exhibiting alkaline tendencies after digestion. Lemons are also excellent for Type A, helping aid digestion and clear mucus from the system.

Because vitamin C is an important antioxidant, especially for stomach cancer prevention, eat vitamin C–rich fruits, such as grapefruit or kiwi.

The banana lectin interferes with Type A digestion. I recommend substituting other high-potassium fruits such as apricots, figs, and allowable melons.

Highly Beneficial

APRICOT ↑	CRANBERRY ↑	LIME ↑
BLACKBERRY ‡	FIG ↑	PAWPAW
BLUEBERRY ‡	GRAPEFRUIT ↑	PINEAPPLE ↑ ‡
BOYSENBERRY	JACK FRUIT	PLUM ‡
CHERRY ‡	LEMON ↑	PRUNE ‡

Neutral

Acai berry	Dewberry	Mamey sapote,
Apple	Durian ↑	mamey apple ↑
Asian pear ↑	Elderberry ↑	Mangosteen
Avocado	Goji, wolfberry	Mulberry
Breadfruit ↑	Gooseberry ↑	Musk melon
Canang melon	Grape	Nectarine
Cantaloupe	Guava ↑	Noni
Casaba melon	Huckleberry	Papaya
Christmas melon	Kiwi	Passion fruit ↑
Crenshaw melon	Kumquat ↑	Peach
Currant	Lingonberry	Pear
Date ↑	Loganberry ↑	Persian melon

Persimmon

Pomegranate

Prickly pear ↑

Quince

Raisin

Raspberry

Sago palm

Spanish melon

Starfruit,
    carambola

Strawberry

Watermelon

Youngberry

Avoid

Banana

Bitter melon

Coconut

Honeydew melon ↓

Loquat ↓

Mango

Orange ↓

Papaya

Plantain ↓

Tangerine ↓

Beverages, Teas and Coffee

BLOOD TYPE A	DAILY ▪ ALL ANCESTRAL TYPES	
Food	*Portion*	
ALL RECOMMENDED JUICES	8 OZ.	4–5X
LEMON AND WATER	8 OZ.	1X (IN MORNING)
WATER	8 OZ.	1–3X

Type A should start every day with a small glass of warm water into which you have squeezed the juice of half a lemon. This will help reduce the mucus that has accumulated overnight in the more sluggish Type A digestive tract and stimulate normal elimination. Lemon and water also possesses slight, but significant anticlotting effects, helping the Type A's naturally more viscous blood to flow smoother.

Alkaline fruit juices, such as black cherry juice concentrate diluted with water, should be consumed in preference to high-sugar juices, which are more acid forming.

Red wine is good for Type A because of its positive cardiovascular effects. A glass of red wine three or four times a week is believed to lower the risk of heart disease for both men and women.

Coffee may actually be good for Type A. Its antioxidants and enzymes are custom-designed for the Type A digestive tract and immune system. Alternate coffee and green tea for the best combination of benefits.

All other beverages should be avoided. They don't suit the digestive system of Type A, nor do they support the immune system.

Pure fresh water, of course, should be consumed freely.

Highly Beneficial

ALFALFA TEA	GINSENG TEA	PINEAPPLE JUICE ↑
ALOE JUICE	GRAPEFRUIT	PRUNE JUICE
APRICOT JUICE	JUICE ↑	ROSE HIPS TEA
BLACKBERRY	GREEN TEA,	SAINT JOHN'S
JUICE	KUKICHA,	WORT TEA
BLUEBERRY JUICE	BANCHA,	SLIPPERY ELM TEA
BURDOCK TEA	GENMAICHA ↑ ‡	VALERIAN TEA
CHAMOMILE TEA	HAWTHORN TEA	VEGETABLE JUICE
CHERRY JUICE	LEMON AND	(FROM HB
COFFEE ↑	WATER ↑	VEGETABLES)
ECHINACEA TEA	LIME JUICE	WINE, RED
FENUGREEK TEA	MILK, SOY ‡	
GINGERROOT TEA	MILK THISTLE TEA	

Neutral

Apple juice, cider	Dandelion tea	Guava juice	Nectarine juice
Beet juice	Dong quai tea	Hops tea	Noni juice
Cabbage juice	Elderberry juice	Horehound tea	Parsley tea
Chickweed tea	Elder tea	Licorice root tea	Pear juice ↑
Coconut water	Gentian tea	Linden tea	Peppermint tea
Coltsfoot tea	Goji berry juice	Milk, almond ↑	Pomegranate juice
Cranberry juice	Goldenseal tea	Milk, rice	Raspberry leaf tea
Cucumber juice	Grape juice	Mulberry tea	
		Mullein tea	

Sage tea	Skullcap tea	Vervain tea	White oak
Sarsaparilla tea	Spearmint tea	Watermelon	bark tea
Senna tea	Strawberry	juice	Wine, white
Shepherd's	leaf tea	White	Yarrow tea
purse tea	Thyme tea	birch tea	Yerba mate tea

Avoid

Beer ↓	Corn silk tea	Seltzer water
Black tea, all	Liquor, distilled ↓	Soda (such as colas
forms	Mango juice	and diet colas)
Cabbage juice	Orange juice ↓	Tangerine juice ↓
Catnip tea	Papaya juice	Tomato juice
Cayenne tea	Red clover tea	Yellow dock tea
Coconut milk	Rhubarb tea	

Herbs and Spices

Type A should view herbs and spices as more than just flavor enhancers. The right combination of herbs and spices can be powerful immune-system boosters. In fact, spices are the original medicines. Many are rich in anti-microbial essential oils, while others are great sources of anti-oxidants, immune-enhancing phytochemicals and fat-burning thermogenic compounds. Try to include your recommended spices in your diet on a regular basis.

Highly Beneficial

DRY MUSTARD	GINGER	PARSLEY ↑
FENNEL	HORSERADISH	TURMERIC
GARLIC		

Neutral

Allspice	Bergamot	Chocolate	Cornstarch
Anise	Caraway	Cilantro	Cream of tartar
Arrowroot	Cardamom	Cinnamon	Cumin
Basil	Chervil	Clove	Curry
Bay leaf	Chives	Coriander	Dill

Dulse	Mustard, dry	Saffron	Tarragon
Guarana	Nutmeg	Sage	Thyme
Kelp	Oregano	Salt, sea salt	Vanilla
Licorice root	Paprika	Savory	
Mace	Peppermint	Senna	
Marjoram	Rosemary	Spearmint	

Avoid

Chili powder
Pepper, black, cayenne, peppercorn, white
Wintergreen

Condiments, Sweeteners, and Additives

Type A should be careful with condiment use. Blackstrap molasses is
a very good source of iron, a mineral that is a bit lacking in the Type A
diet. Vinegar should be avoided because the acids tend to cause stomach
lining irritation and produce dysbiosis in the gut.

Sugar is allowed in the Type A diet, but only in very small amounts.
Use it as you would a condiment, not an energy source. Minimize your
use of white processed sugar. Recent studies have shown that the immune
system is sluggish for several hours after ingesting it.

Highly Beneficial

BARLEY MALT	SOYBEAN SAUCE,
MISO	TAMARI, WHEAT
MOLASSES	FREE
MOLASSES,	
BLACKSTRAP	

Neutral

Agar ↓	Baking soda	Dextrose	Jam, jelly (from
Agave syrup ↑	Brown rice syrup	Fructose	acceptable
Almond extract	Carob syrup	Fruit pectin	fruit)
Apple butter	Cornstarch	Honey	Lecithin
Apple pectin	Corn syrup	Invert sugar	Maple syrup

Mayonnaise, tofu, soy	Rice syrup	Stevia	Vegetable glycerine
Mustard, wheat free, vinegar free ↑	Salad dressing (low fat from acceptable ingredients)	Sugar, brown, white	Yeast, baker's ↑
		Umeboshi plum, vinegar	Yeast, nutritional ↑

Avoid

Acacia (gum arabic)	Ketchup ↓	Sodium carboxy-methyl cellulose ↓
Aspartame	MSG	
Carrageenan ↓	Mayonnaise	Tamarind
Gelatin ↓	Methyl cellulose ↓	Tragacanth gum ↓
Guar gum	Mustard, with vinegar and wheat	Vinegar, all types ↓
High-fructose corn syrup ↓		Worcestershire sauce ↓
High-maltose corn syrup, maltodextrin ↓	Pickle relish ↓ Polysorbate 80 ↓	

Meal Planning for Type A

Asterisk (*) indicates the recipe is provided.

THE FOLLOWING sample menus and recipes will give you an idea of a typical diet beneficial to Type A. They were developed by Dina Khader, MS, RD, CDN, a nutritionist who has used the Blood Type Diets successfully with her patients.

These menus are moderate in calories and balanced for metabolic efficiency in Type A. The average person will be able to maintain weight comfortably and even lose weight by following these suggestions. However, alternative food choices are provided if you prefer lighter fare or wish to limit your caloric intake and still eat a balanced, satisfying diet. (The alternative food is listed directly across from the food it replaces.)

Occasionally you will see an ingredient in a recipe that appears on your avoid list. If it is a very small ingredient (such as a dash of pepper), you may be able to tolerate it, depending on your condition and whether you are strictly adhering to the diet. However, the meal selections and recipes are generally designed to work very well for Type As.

As you become more familiar with the Type A diet recommendations, you'll be able to easily create your own menu plans and adjust favorite recipes to make them Type A friendly.

STANDARD MENU ▪	WEIGHT-CONTROL ALTERNATIVES ▪

SAMPLE MEAL PLAN I

Breakfast

water with lemon (on rising)	cornflakes with soy
oatmeal with soy milk and	milk and maple syrup
maple syrup or molasses	or molasses
grapefruit juice,	
coffee, or herbal tea	

Lunch

Greek salad (chopped lettuce,
   celery, green onions,
   cucumber, with a sprinkling
   of feta cheese, lemon, and
   fresh mint)
apple
1 slice sprouted wheat bread
herbal tea

Midafternoon Snack

2 rice cakes with peanut butter	2 rice cakes with honey
2 plums	
green tea or water	

Dinner

*Tofu-Pesto Lasagna	tofu stir-fry with green
broccoli	beans, leeks, snow peas,
frozen yogurt	and alfalfa sprouts
coffee or herbal tea	
(red wine if desired)	

SAMPLE MEAL PLAN 2

Breakfast

water with lemon (on rising)
*Tofu Omelet   1 poached egg
grapefruit juice   ½ cup low-fat yogurt
coffee or herbal tea   with sliced berries

Lunch

miso soup
mixed green salad
1 slice rye bread
water or herbal tea

Midafternoon Snack

*Carob Chip Cookies   *Tofu Dip with raw
   or yogurt with fruit   vegetables
herbal tea

Dinner

*Turkey-Tofu Meatballs
steamed zucchini
*String Bean Salad
low-fat frozen yogurt
coffee or herbal tea
(red wine if desired)

SAMPLE MEAL PLAN 3

Breakfast

water with lemon (on rising)
*Maple-Walnut Granola with   puffed rice with soy milk
   soy milk
prune, carrot, or vegetable juice
coffee or herbal tea

Lunch

*Black Bean Soup   cold salmon on salad greens
mixed green salad   with lemon juice and
                                        olive oil

Midafternoon Snack

*Apricot Fruit Bread   ½ cup plain yogurt
coffee or herbal tea   with drizzle of honey

Dinner

*Arabian Baked Fish,   *Baked Fish
   made with bass or whitefish
*Spinach Salad
mixed fresh fruit with yogurt
herbal tea
(red wine if desired)

🍽️

Recipes

TOFU-PESTO LASAGNA

*1 pound soft tofu, mashed with
2 tablespoons olive oil
1 cup shredded part-skim mozzarella cheese or part-skim ricotta
1 organic egg (optional)
2 packages frozen, chopped spinach or fresh, cut-up spinach
1 teaspoon salt
1 teaspoon oregano
4 cups pesto sauce (you may use less)
9 rice or spelt lasagna noodles, cooked
1 cup water*

Mix tofu and cheese with egg, spinach, and seasonings. Layer 1 cup sauce in 9 x 13-inch baking dish. Layer noodles, then some of the cheese mixture, then sauce. Repeat, and finish with noodles and sauce on top. Bake in oven at 350 degrees F. for 30 to 45 minutes or until done. Makes 4 to 6 servings.

CAROB CHIP COOKIES

⅓ cup organic canola oil
½ cup pure maple syrup
1 teaspoon vanilla extract
1 organic egg
1¾ cups oat or brown rice flour
1 teaspoon baking soda
½ cup carob chips (unsweetened)
dash allspice (optional)

Oil two baking sheets and preheat oven to 375 degrees F. In a medium-size mixing bowl, combine the oil, maple syrup, and vanilla. Beat the egg and stir into the oil mixture. Gradually stir in flour and baking soda to form a stiff batter. Fold in carob chips and drop the batter onto the baking sheets by the teaspoon. Bake for 10 to 15 minutes until cookies are lightly browned. Remove from oven and cool. Makes 3½ to 4 dozen.

TOFU DIP

1 cup tofu, mashed
1 cup plain nonfat yogurt
1 tablespoon olive oil
juice of 1 lemon
2 tablespoons chopped chives or 1 cup scallions
garlic and salt to season

Combine the tofu, yogurt, olive oil, and lemon juice in a blender and blend at high speed until smooth. Stir in chives or scallions, and seasonings. Remove to a bowl and refrigerate. If mix is too thick to blend well, add a few drops of water.

Serve dip in a glass bowl centered on a platter of fresh vegetables. Makes approximately 3 cups.

TOFU OMELET

1 pound soft tofu, drained and mashed
5–6 tree oyster mushrooms, sliced
½ pound grated red or white radishes
1 teaspoon mirin or sherry for cooking
1 teaspoon tamari or soy sauce
1 tablespoon fresh parsley
1 teaspoon brown rice flour
4 organic eggs, lightly beaten
1 tablespoon canola or extra-virgin olive oil

Combine all the ingredients in a mixing bowl, except for oil. Heat the oil in a large frying pan. Pour in half the mixture and cover the pan. Cook over low heat for approximately 15 minutes until egg is cooked. Remove from pan and keep warm.

Repeat the process and use the remainder of the mixture.

Serves 3 to 4.

TURKEY TOFU MEATBALLS

1 pound ground turkey
1 pound firm tofu
½ cup chestnut flour
1½ cups spelt flour
1 large onion, chopped fine
¼ cup fresh parsley, chopped
2 teaspoons sea salt
4 tablespoons fresh garlic, crushed
allowable seasonings to your preference

Mix well. Refrigerate 1 hour. Roll into small meatballs. To cook, stir-fry in oil until brown and crisp, or bake in the oven at 350 degrees F. for approximately 1 hour.

Makes 4 servings.

STRING BEAN SALAD

1 pound green string beans
juice of 1 lemon
3 tablespoons olive oil
2 cloves garlic, crushed
2 to 3 teaspoons salt

Wash tender, fresh, green string beans. Remove stems and strings. Cut into 2-inch pieces.

Cook until tender by boiling in plenty of water. Drain. When cool, place in a salad bowl. Dress to taste with lemon juice, olive oil, garlic, and salt.

Makes 4 servings.

MAPLE-WALNUT GRANOLA

4 cups rolled oats
1 cup rice bran
1 cup sesame seeds
½ cup dried cranberries
½ cup dried currants
1 cup chopped walnuts
1 teaspoon vanilla extract
¼ cup organic canola oil
¾ cup maple syrup

Preheat oven to 250 degrees F. In a large mixing bowl combine the oats, rice bran, seeds, dried fruit, nuts, and vanilla. Add the oil and stir evenly.

Pour in maple syrup and mix well until mixture is evenly moistened. Mixture should be crumbly and sticky. Spread mixture on a lightly

oiled cookie tray and bake for 90 minutes, stirring every 15 minutes
for even toasting until the mixture is golden brown and dry.
Cool thoroughly and store in airtight container.

BLACK BEAN SOUP

1 pound black beans
2 quarts of water
⅛ cup vegetable broth
⅛ pound diced white onion
⅛ pound green onions plus handful of scallions, for garnish
¼ pound celery
⅛ pound diced leeks
¼ ounce salt
1 ounce cumin
1 cup dried parsley
1 ounce garlic
1 medium bunch of fresh tarragon (chopped)
1 medium bunch of fresh basil (chopped)
1 medium bunch of scallions

Soak beans in water overnight. Pour off the water and rinse. Add 3
quarts of water and bring beans to a boil.
Discard liquid from the beans and add the vegetable broth. Simmer.
Sauté the onion, celery, leeks, seasonings, and garlic together in a pan.
Add this mixture to the beans and continue cooking. Purée ⅛ cup
of this soup for consistency. Add scallions at the end for garnish.
Makes approximately 8 servings.

APRICOT FRUIT BREAD

1¼ cups plain nonfat yogurt
1 organic egg
1 cup apricot conserves (fruit juice sweetened)
2 cups brown rice flour
1 teaspoon ground cinnamon

1 teaspoon ground allspice
1 teaspoon ground nutmeg
1¼ teaspoons baking soda
1 cup chopped, dried, unsulfured apricots
1 cup currants

Grease a standard-size loaf pan and preheat oven to 350 degrees F. In a medium-size bowl, combine the yogurt, egg, and conserves. Add 1 cup of flour and half of the spices plus baking soda. Stir until batter is evenly moist.

Add remaining flour and spices. If consistency feels too thick, you can add a few drops of cold water or vanilla soy milk to mixture. Fold in apricots and currants.

Pour batter into greased loaf pan and bake for 40 to 45 minutes until done. Remove bread from the pan and cool on a wire rack.

ARABIAN BAKED FISH

1 large bass or whitefish (3 to 4 pounds)
dash of salt to taste
¼ cup lemon juice
2 tablespoons olive oil
2 large onions, chopped and sautéed in olive oil
2 to 2½ cups tahini sauce

Wash fish and dry thoroughly. Sprinkle with salt and lemon juice.

Let stand for 30 minutes. Drain fish. Place in baking pan after brushing with oil. Bake in a preheated oven for 30 minutes at 400 degrees F.

Cover with sautéed onions and tahini sauce, and add a dash of salt. Return to oven and bake until fish is easily flaked with a fork (from 30 to 40 minutes).

Serve the fish on a platter and garnish with parsley and lemon wedges. Makes 6 to 8 servings.

TAHINI SAUCE

1 cup organic tahini
juice of 3 lemons
2 cloves of garlic, crushed
2 to 3 teaspoons salt
¼ cup dried, organic parsley flakes or
fresh parsley, chopped finely

In a bowl, mix tahini with lemon juice, garlic, salt, and parsley.
Add enough water to make a thick sauce. Makes approximately 2 cups.

———

BAKED FISH

1 large whitefish (2 or 3 pounds)
or other fish
lemon juice
salt to taste
¼ cup olive oil
1 teaspoon cayenne (optional)
1 teaspoon pepper (optional)
1 teaspoon cumin (optional)

Wash fish. Sprinkle with salt and lemon juice. Add spices if desired.
Let stand for ½ hour. Drain.
Coat fish with oil and place in a baking pan. To prevent fish from drying, wrap with foil, lightly greased with oil. Bake at 350 degrees F.
in a preheated oven for 30 to 40 minutes, or until fish is tender and
easily flaked.
Makes 4 or 5 servings.

WITH STUFFING (OPTIONAL)

⅓ cup pine nuts or shredded almonds
2 tablespoons olive oil
1 cup parsley, chopped
3 cloves garlic, crushed
salt, pepper, and allspice to taste

Sauté nuts in olive oil until lightly browned. Add parsley and spices and
sauté for one minute. Stuff raw fish with the mixture.
Makes 4 to 5 servings.

SPINACH SALAD

2 bunches fresh spinach
1 bunch scallions, chopped
juice of 1 lemon
¼ tablespoon olive oil
salt and pepper to taste (optional)

Wash spinach well. Drain and chop. Sprinkle with salt. After a few minutes, squeeze excess water. Add scallions, lemon juice, oil, salt and
pepper. Serve immediately.
Makes 6 servings.

For a wealth of additional recipes in every category, check out the
blood type–specific cookbooks and recipe database at dadamo
.com and 4yourtype.com.

Type A
Supplement Advisory

THE ROLE OF SUPPLEMENTS—be they vitamins, minerals, or herbs—is
to add the nutrients that are lacking in your diet or to provide extra
protection where you need it. The supplement focus for Type A is

- Toning the immune system
- Supplying cancer-fighting antioxidants
- Balancing the microbiome
- Strengthening the cardiovascular system

The following recommendations emphasize the supplements that
help meet these goals, and warn against the supplements that can be
counterproductive or dangerous for Type A.

Vitamins

Vitamin B$_{12}$

Type A should be alert to vitamin B$_{12}$ deficiency. Not only is the Type A diet somewhat lacking in this nutrient, which is found mostly in animal proteins, but Type A tends to have a hard time absorbing B$_{12}$ because you lack a substance called "intrinsic factor" in the stomach. (Intrinsic factor is produced by the lining of the stomach and it helps B$_{12}$ be absorbed into the blood.) In elderly Type As, vitamin B$_{12}$ deficiency can cause senile dementia and other neurologic impairments. Look for the methylcobalamin form of the vitamin B$_{12}$ supplement. Avoid the cheaper cyanocobalamin form.

Other B Vitamins

Most other B vitamins are adequately contained in the Type A diet. If, however, you suffer from anemia, you may want a small supplement of folic acid. Type A heart patients should ask their doctors about low-dose niacin supplements, as niacin has cholesterol-lowering properties.

Vitamin C

Type A, with higher rates of stomach cancer because of low stomach acid, can benefit from taking additional supplements of vitamin C. Nitrite, a compound that results from the smoking and curing of meats, could be a particular problem for Type A because its cancer-causing potential is greater in people with lower levels of stomach acid. As an antioxidant, vitamin C is known to block this reaction (although you should still avoid smoked and cured foods). However, don't take this to mean that you should take massive amounts. I have found that Type A does not do as well on high doses (1,000 milligrams and up) of vitamin C because it tends to upset the stomach. Taken over the course of a day, two to four capsules of a 250-milligram supplement, preferably derived from rose hips or acerola cherries, should cause no digestive problems.

Vitamin E

There is some evidence that vitamin E serves as a protectant against both cancer and heart disease—two Type A susceptibilities. You may want to take a daily supplement—no more than 400 IU (International Units).

Minerals

CALCIUM

Because the Type A diet includes some dairy products, the need for calcium supplementation is not as acute as for Type O, yet a small amount of additional calcium (300 to 600 milligrams elemental calcium) from middle age onward is advisable. In my experience, Type A does better on particular types of calcium products. The worst source of calcium for Type A is the simplest and most readily available: calcium carbonate (often found in antacids). This form requires the highest amount of stomach acid for absorption. In general, Type As tolerate calcium gluconate, do well on calcium citrate, and do best on a natural calcium derived from the pristine seaweed beds off of northern Ireland, called maerl.

IRON

The Type A diet is naturally low in iron, which is found in the greatest abundance in red meats. Type A women, especially those with heavy menstrual periods, should be especially careful about keeping sufficient iron stores. If you need iron supplementation, do it under a doctor's supervision, so blood tests can monitor your progress.

In general, use as low a dose as possible, and avoid extended periods of supplementation. Try to avoid crude iron preparations such as ferrous sulfate, which can irritate your stomach. Milder forms of supplementation, such as iron citrate or blackstrap molasses, may be used instead. Floradix, a liquid iron and herb supplement, can be found at most health food stores and is highly assimilable by Type A.

ZINC

I have found that a small amount of zinc supplementation (as little as 3 milligrams per day) often makes a big difference in protecting children against infections, especially ear infections. Zinc supplementation is a double-edged sword, however. While small, periodic doses enhance immunity, long-term, higher doses depress it and can interfere with the absorption of other minerals. Be careful with zinc!

Herbs, Phytochemicals, and Probiotics

HAWTHORN

Hawthorn is a great cardiovascular tonic. If you are Type A you should definitely add it to your diet regimen if you or members of your family have a history of heart disease. This phytochemical, with exceptional preventive capacities, is found in the hawthorn tree (*Crataegus oxyacantha*). It has a number of impressive cardiovascular effects. Hawthorn increases the elasticity of the arteries and strengthens the heart, while also lowering blood pressure and exerting a mild solvent-like effect on the plaques in the arteries. Officially approved for pharmaceutical use in Germany, the effects of hawthorn are only now gaining recognition elsewhere. Extracts and tinctures are readily available through naturopathic physicians, health food stores, and pharmacies.

IMMUNE-ENHANCING HERBS

Because the immune system of Type A tends to be open to immune-compromising infections, gentle immune-enhancing herbs, such as purple coneflower (*Echinacea purpurea*), can help ward off colds or flus and may help optimize the immune system's anticancer surveillance. Many people take echinacea in liquid or tablet form. It is widely available. The Chinese herb huang qi (*Astragalus membranaceus*) is also taken as an immune tonic, but is not as easy to find. In both herbs the active ingredients are sugars that act as mitogens that stimulate proliferation of white blood cells, which act in defense of the immune system.

CHONDROITIN SULFATE

Chondroitin sulfate is a constituent of our connective tissue and is often sold as a joint-support supplement (along with glucosamine sulfate). Chondroitin is an interesting molecule that turns out to be made up of a long chain of amino sugars that resemble the Blood Type A antigen. In the stomach these chains are broken down and the liberated A-like sugars are free to attract, trap, and block lectins, working more or less as a decoy.

Calming Herbs

Type A can use mild herbal relaxants, such as chamomile and valerian root, as antistress aids. These herbs are available as teas and should be taken frequently. Valerian has a bit of a pungent odor, which becomes pleasing once you get used to it. There was once a rumor that valerian is so named because it is the natural form of Valium (diazepam), a prescription tranquilizer. This is wrong. Valerian was named for a Roman emperor who had the misfortune to be captured in battle by the Persians. Killed, stuffed, dyed red, and exhibited in a Persian museum, Valerian was fortunate to have had anything named for him. Regardless of the origins of the herb's name, studies show that valerian acts (ever so slightly) on many of the same receptors as do pharmaceutical tranquilizers.

Quercetin

Quercetin is a bioflavonoid found abundantly in vegetables, particularly yellow onions. Quercetin supplements are widely available, usually in capsules of 100 to 500 milligrams. Quercetin is a very powerful antioxidant, many hundreds of times more potent than vitamin E. It can make a powerful addition to Type A cancer-prevention strategies.

Milk Thistle

Like quercetin, milk thistle (*Silybum marianum*) is an effective antioxidant with the additional special property of reaching very high concentrations in the liver and bile ducts. Type A can suffer from disorders of the liver and gallbladder. If your family has any history of liver, pancreas, or gallbladder problems, consider adding a milk thistle supplement to your protocol. Cancer patients who are receiving chemotherapy should use a milk thistle supplement to help protect their liver from damage.

Bromelain (Pineapple Enzymes)

If you are Type A and suffer from bloating or other signs of poor absorption of protein, take a bromelain supplement. This enzyme has a moderate ability to break down dietary proteins, helping the Type A digestive tract assimilate proteins better.

PROBIOTIC SUPPLEMENTS

If the Type A diet is new for you, you may find that adjusting to a vegetarian diet is uncomfortable and produces excessive gas or bloating. A probiotic supplement can counter this effect by supplying the "good" bacteria usually found in the digestive tract.

Supplements to Avoid

BETA-CAROTENE

My father always avoided giving beta-carotene to his Type A patients, saying that he thought it irritated their blood vessels. I questioned his observation, as it had never been documented. Quite to the contrary, the evidence suggested that beta-carotene could prevent artery disease. Yet recently there have been studies suggesting that beta-carotene in high doses may act as a pro-oxidant, speeding up damage to the tissues rather than stopping it. Perhaps my father's observation was correct, at least in the case of Type A. Vitamin A and beta-carotene can be found in seafood and yellow and orange veggies. This caveat is highly individual: There may be times when a vitamin A supplement is needed for short-term benefits. Check with your doctor.

Best Carotene-Rich Foods for Type As

Egg	Broccoli
Spinach	Carrot
Yellow squash	

Type A Stress-Exercise Profile

THE ABILITY to reverse the negative effects of stress lives in your blood type. As we discussed earlier, stress is not in itself a problem; it's how you respond to stress. Each blood type has a distinct, genetically programmed instinct for overcoming stress.

Type A often reacts to stress by mismanaging cortisol, which can cause weight gain, depress the immune system, and interfere with restorative sleep. Even at rest, Type A has higher levels of cortisol than the other blood types. Cortisol-charged bulbs flash in your brain, producing anxiety, irritability, and obsessive tendencies. As the stress signals throb in your immune system, you grow weaker and more tired.

If, however, you adopt a quieting technique, such as yoga or meditation, you can achieve great benefits by countering negative stresses with focus and relaxation. Type A does not respond well to continuous confrontation and needs to consider and practice the art of stillness. If Type A remains in its naturally tense state, stress can produce heart disease and various forms of cancer. Exercises that provide calm and focus are the remedy that pull Type A from the grip of stress.

Tai chi chuan, the slow-motion, ritualistic pattern of Chinese movement, and hatha yoga, the Indian system of yoga commonly practiced in the West, are calming, centering experiences. Moderate isotonic exercises, such as hiking, swimming, and bicycling, are favored for Type As. When I advise calming exercises, it doesn't mean you can't break a sweat. The key is really your mental engagement in your physical activity. For example, heavy competitive sports and exercises will only exhaust your nervous energy, make you tense all over again, and leave your immune system open to illness or disease.

The following exercises are recommended for Type A. Pay special attention to the length of the sessions. To achieve a consistent release of tension and revival of energy, you need to perform one or more of these exercises three or four times a week.

EXERCISE	DURATION	FREQUENCY (PER WEEK)
TAI CHI	30–45 min.	3–5x
HATHA YOGA	30 min.	3–5x
MARTIAL ARTS	60 min.	2–3x
GOLF	60 min.	2–3x
BRISK WALKING	20–40 min.	2–3x
SWIMMING	30 min.	3–4x
DANCE	30–45 min.	2–3x

| AEROBICS
(LOW IMPACT) | 30–45 min. | 2–3x |
| STRETCHING | 15 min. | 3–5x |

Type A
Exercise Guidelines

TAI CHI CHUAN, or tai chi, is an exercise that enhances the flexibility of body movement. The slow, graceful, elegant gestures of tai chi routines seem to mask the full-speed hand and foot blows, blocks, and parries they represent. In China, tai chi is practiced daily by groups who gather in public squares to perform the movements in unison. Tai chi can be a very effective relaxation technique, although it takes concentration and patience to master.

Yoga is also good for the Type A stress pattern. It combines inner rectitude with breath control and postures designed to allow for complete concentration without distraction by worldly concerns. If you learn basic yoga postures, you can create a routine best suited to your lifestyle. Many Type As who have adopted yoga relaxation tell me that they will not leave the house until they do their yoga.

SIMPLE YOGA RELAXATION TECHNIQUES
Yoga begins and ends with relaxation. We contract our muscles constantly, but rarely do we think of doing the opposite—letting go and relaxing. We can feel better and be healthier if we regularly release the tensions left behind within the muscles by the stresses and strains of life.

The best position for relaxation is lying on your back. Arrange your arms and legs so that you are completely comfortable in your hips, shoulders, and back. The goal of deep relaxation is to let your body and mind settle down to soothing calmness, in the same way that an agitated pool of water eventually calms to stillness.

Begin with abdominal breathing. As a baby breathes, her abdomen moves, not her chest. However, many of us grow to unconsciously adopt the unnatural and inefficient habit of restrained chest breathing. One of the aims of yoga is to make you aware of the true center of breathing. Observe the pattern of your breathing. Is your breathing fast, shallow, and irregular or do you tend to hold your breath? Allow your breathing to revert to a more natural pattern—full, deep, regular, and with no constriction. Try to isolate just your lower breathing muscles; see if you can breathe without moving your chest. Breathing exercises are always done smoothly and without any strain. Place one hand on your navel and feel the movement of your breathing. Relax your shoulders.

Start the exercise by breathing out completely. When you inhale, pretend that a heavy weight, such as a large book, is resting on your navel, and that by your inhalation, you are trying to raise this imaginary weight up toward the ceiling.

Then, when you exhale, simply let this imaginary weight press down against your abdomen, helping you exhale. Exhale more air out than you normally would, as if to "squeeze" more air out of your lungs. This will act as a yoga stretch for the diaphragm and further help release tension in this muscle. Bring your abdominal muscles into play here to assist. When you inhale, direct your breath down so deeply that you are lifting an imaginary heavy weight up toward the ceiling. Try to completely co-ordinate and isolate the abdominal breath with no chest or rib movement.

Even if you perform aerobic exercises during the course of your week, try to integrate the relaxing, soothing routines that will help you best manage your Type A stress patterns.

SEVEN

Blood Type

B

Diet

TYPE B: *The Nomad*

- **BALANCED**
- **STRONG IMMUNE SYSTEM**
- **TOLERANT DIGESTIVE SYSTEM**
- **MOST FLEXIBLE DIETARY CHOICES**
- **DAIRY EATER**
- **RESPONDS BEST TO STRESS WITH CREATIVITY**
- **REQUIRES A BALANCE BETWEEN PHYSICAL AND MENTAL ACTIVITY TO STAY LEAN AND SHARP**

The Type B Diet

TYPE O AND TYPE A seem to be polar opposites in many respects, but Type B can best be described as idiosyncratic—with utterly unique and sometimes chameleon-like characteristics. In many ways Type B resembles Type O so much that the two seem related. Then, suddenly, Type B will take on a totally unfamiliar shape—one that is peculiarly its own. You might say that Type B represents a sophisticated refinement in the adaptive journey, an effort to join together divergent peoples and cultures.

On the whole, the sturdy and alert Type Bs are usually able to resist many of the most severe diseases common to modern life, such as heart disease and cancer. Even when you do contract these diseases, you are more likely to survive them. Yet because Type Bs are somewhat offbeat, your system seems more prone to exotic neuro-immune system disorders, such as multiple sclerosis, lupus, and chronic fatigue syndrome (see Chapter Eleven).

In my experience, a Type B who carefully follows the recommended diet can often bypass severe disease and live a long and healthy life.

The Type B diet is balanced and wholesome, including a wide variety of foods. In the words of my father, it represents "the best of the animal and vegetable kingdoms." Think of *B* as standing for "balance"—the balancing forces of A and O.

NOTE: Longtime readers will notice a difference in the values of a small number of foods between this edition and the original version of *Eat Right for Your Type*. That is because beginning with the publication of *Live Right for Your Type*, I made a distinction in some foods between secretors and non-secretors. The original version of *Eat Right for Your Type*, which preceded *Live Right for Your Type*, "homogenized" these differences. Like all of my subsequent books, this edition of *Eat Right for Your Type* uses the secretor values as the base values for the A, B, AB, and O blood types.

KEY

‡ Enhances carbohydrate metabolism, helps with
   weight loss

↑ Increases microbiome diversity, discourages microbial
   imbalance

↓ Decreases microbiome diversity, encourages microbial
   imbalance

Meats and Poultry

BLOOD TYPE B		WEEKLY ▪ IF YOUR ANCESTRY IS		
Food	Portion*	African	Caucasian	Asian
LEAN RED MEATS	4–6 OZ.	3–4X	2–3X	2–3X
POULTRY	4–6 OZ.	0–2X	0–3X	0–2X

*The portion recommendations are merely guidelines that can help refine
your diet according to ancestral propensities.*

Type B can derive benefit from selected meats. If you are fatigued or
suffer from immune deficiencies, you should eat red meat such as lamb,
mutton, or rabbit several times a week, in preference to beef or turkey.

In my experience, one of the most difficult adjustments Type B
must make is giving up chicken. Chicken contains a Blood Type B
agglutinating lectin in its muscle tissue. If you're accustomed to eating
vmore poultry than red meat, you can eat other poultry such as turkey
or pheasant. Although they are similar to chicken in many respects,
neither contains the dangerous lectin.

The news about chicken is troubling to many people because it has
become a fundamental part of many ethnic diets. In addition, people
have been told to eat chicken instead of beef because it is "healthier,"
but here is another case where one dietary guideline does not fit all.

Chicken may be leaner (although not always) than red meat, but that isn't the issue. The issue is the power of an agglutinating lectin to attack your cells and disrupt your digestion. So, even though chicken may be a beloved food, I urge you to begin weaning yourself from it.

Highly Beneficial

GOAT ↑ ‡	MOOSE ↑	RABBIT ↑
LAMB ↑ ‡	MUTTON ↑ ‡	VENISON ↑

Neutral

Beef	Buffalo, bison	Turkey
Beef liver	Calf liver	Veal
Beef tongue	Marrow soup	
Bone soup	Ostrich	
(allowable meats)	Pheasant	

Avoid

Bear	Goose	Pork and bacon ↓
Beef, heart	Goose liver	Quail
Chicken ↓	Grouse	Squab
Chicken liver	Guinea hen	Squirrel
Cornish hen	Ham ↓	Sweetbreads
Duck	Horse	Turtle
Duck liver	Partridge	

Seafood

BLOOD TYPE B	WEEKLY ▪ IF YOUR ANCESTRY IS			
Food	Portion	African	Caucasian	Asian
ALL RECOMMENDED SEAFOOD	4–6 oz.	4–6x	3–5x	3–5x

Type B thrives on seafood, especially deep-ocean fish such as cod and salmon, which are rich in nutritious oils. Whitefish, such as flounder, halibut, and sole, are also excellent sources of high-quality protein for Type B. Avoid all shellfish—crab, lobster, shrimp, mussels, etc. They contain lectins that are disruptive to the Type B system.

Highly Beneficial

CAVIAR	MACKEREL, SPANISH	SALMON, ATLANTIC (WILD) ↑
COD ↑ ‡	MAHI-MAHI ↑	SALMON, CHINOOK ↑
CROAKER ↑	MONKFISH ↑	SALMON, SOCKEYE ↑
FLOUNDER ↑	PERCH, OCEAN ↑	SARDINE ↑ ‡
GROUPER ↑	PICKEREL, WALLEYE ↑	SCALLOP ↑
HADDOCK ↑	PIKE ↑	SHAD ↑ ‡
HAKE ↑	PILCHARDS	SOLE ↑
HALIBUT ↑	PORGY ↑	STURGEON ↑
HARVEST FISH ↑		TUNA, YELLOWFIN
MACKEREL, ATLANTIC ↑ ‡		

Neutral

Abalone, sea ear, mutton fish	Opaleye fish	Squid, calamari
Bluefish	Orange roughy	Sucker
Bullhead	Parrotfish	Sunfish, pumpkinseed
Carp	Perch	Swordfish
Catfish	Pompano	Tilapia
Chub	Red snapper	Tilefish
Cusk	Rosefish	Tuna, bluefin
Drum	Sailfish	Tuna, skipjack
Halfmoon fish	Sailfish roe	Turbot, European
Herring	Scallop ↑	Weakfish
Mullet	Scrod	Whitefish
Muskellunge	Scup	Whiting
Ocean pout	Shark	
	Smelt	

Avoid

Anchovy	Frog	Skate
Barracuda	Herring, pickled	Snail, escargot
Bass, blue gill	Lobster	Sole, gray, Dover
Bass, sea, lake	Mussels	Trout, rainbow
Bass, striped ↓	Octopus	(wild)
Beluga	Oyster ↓	Trout, sea
Butterfish	Pollock, Atlantic	Trout, steelhead
Clam	Salmon roe	(wild)
Conch	Salmon, smoked	Yellowtail
Crab	(lox)	
Crayfish	Sea bream	
Eel ↓	Shrimp	

Dairy and Eggs

BLOOD TYPE B		WEEKLY ▪ IF YOUR ANCESTRY IS		
Food	*Portion*	*African*	*Caucasian*	*Asian*
EGGS	1 EGG	3–4x	3–4x	5–6x
CHEESES	2 OZ.	3–4x	3–5x	2–3x
YOGURT	4–6 OZ.	0–4x	2–4x	1–3x
MILK	4–6 OZ.	0–3x	4–5x	2–3x

Type B is the only blood type that can fully enjoy a variety of dairy foods. That's because the primary sugar in the Type B antigen is galactose, the very same sugar present in milk. Thus, many dairy products, in particular the cultured forms, can act to "fertilize" the Type B digestive tract to encourage the growth of Type B–friendly bacteria. By the way, eggs are fine for Type B; they do not contain the lectin that is found in the muscle tissues of chicken.

However, there are ancestral idiosyncrasies that blur the picture. If you are of Asian descent, you may initially have a problem adapting to dairy foods—not because your system is resistant to them but because your culture typically has been resistant to them. To the Asian mind, dairy products were the food of the barbarian and thus not fit to eat. The stigma remains to this day, although there are large numbers of Type Bs in Asia whose soy-based diet is damaging to their systems. Those of Asian and African descent have been shown to have a lower number of copies of the gene that digests milk. They'll want to adjust their frequencies downward.

What can you do? If you are lactose intolerant, begin using a lactase enzyme preparation, which will make digestion of dairy foods possible. Then, after you have been on your Type B Diet for several weeks, slowly introduce dairy foods, beginning with cultured or soured dairy products, such as yogurt and kefir, which may be tolerated better than fresh milk products, such as ice cream, whole milk, and cream cheese. I've found that lactose-intolerant Type Bs are often able to incorporate dairy foods after they have corrected the overall problems in their diets.

Highly Beneficial

COTTAGE CHEESE ↑ ‡	MILK, COW (SKIM OR 2%)↑	PANEER CHEESE
FARMER CHEESE	MILK, COW (WHOLE) ‡	PECORINO CHEESE ↑
FETA CHEESE ‡	MILK, GOAT ‡	RICOTTA CHEESE ‡
GOAT CHEESE	MOZZARELLA CHEESE, ALL TYPES ‡	ROMANIAN URDA ↑
KEFIR ↑ ‡		YOGURT

Neutral

Brie cheese ↑	Cheddar	Egg whole, chicken
Butter ↑	Colby cheese	Egg yolk, chicken
Buttermilk	Cream cheese	Emmental, Swiss cheese
Camembert cheese	Edam cheese	
Casein	Egg white, chicken	

Ghee, clarified
  butter ↑
Gouda cheese ↑
Gruyère cheese
Half-and-half
Jarlsberg cheese ↑
Manchego cheese

Monterey Jack
  cheese
Muenster cheese
Neufchâtel cheese
Parmesan
  cheese ↑
Provolone cheese

Quark cheese
Sherbet
Sour cream
Stilton cheese
Whey protein

Avoid

American cheese ↓
Blue cheese
Egg, duck
Egg, goose

Egg, quail
Gorgonzola
  cheese ↓
Ice cream

Romano cheese
Roquefort cheese ↓
String cheese ↓

Oils and Fats

BLOOD TYPE B		WEEKLY ▪ IF YOUR ANCESTRY IS		
Food	*Portion*	*African*	*Caucasian*	*Asian*
OILS	1 TABLESPOON	3–5x	4–6x	5–7x

Introduce olive oil into your diet to encourage proper digestion and healthy elimination. Use at least 1 tablespoon every other day. Ghee, an Indian preparation of clarified butter, also can be used in cooking. Avoid sesame, sunflower, and corn oils, which are damaging to the Type B digestive tract.

Highly Beneficial

CAMELINA OIL ↑
OLIVE OIL ↑
RICE BRAN OIL

Neutral

Almond oil	Evening	Macadamia oil
Apricot kernel oil	primrose oil	Perilla seed oil
Black currant	Flaxseed,	Soy oil
seed oil	linseed oil	Sunflower oil
Chia seed oil	Hazelnut oil	Walnut oil
Cod liver oil	Hemp seed oil	Wheat germ oil

Avoid

Avocado oil	Corn oil ↓	Peanut oil ↓
Borage seed oil	Cottonseed oil	Pumpkin seed oil
Canola oil	Lard	Safflower oil ↓
Castor oil	Margarine	Sesame oil ↓
Coconut oil	Palm oil	

Nuts and Seeds

BLOOD TYPE B		WEEKLY ▪ IF YOUR ANCESTRY IS		
Food	*Portion*	*African*	*Caucasian*	*Asian*
NUTS AND SEEDS	6–8 NUTS	3–5X	2–5X	2–3X
NUT BUTTERS	I TABLESPOON	2–3X	2–3X	2–3X

Most nuts and seeds are neutral foods for Type Bs. However, peanuts, sesame seeds, and sunflower seeds, among others, contain lectins that interfere with Type B digestion and may increase inflammation. Walnuts have important neuroprotective effects that make them beneficial.

Highly Beneficial

CHESTNUT, CHINESE ↑
WALNUT ↑ ‡

Neutral

Almond ↑

Almond butter ↑

Almond
  cheese↑

Beechnut

Brazil nut

Butternut ↑

Carob ↑

Chestnut,
  European ↑

Chia seed ↑

Flaxseed ↑

Hemp seed ↑

Hickory ↑

Litchi/lychee

Macadamia ↑

Pecan

Pecan butter↑

Walnut, English

Watermelon seed

Avoid

Cashew

Cashew butter

Filbert, hazelnut

Peanut

Peanut butter

Peanut flour

Pine nut,
  pignoli

Pistachio

Poppy seed

Pumpkin seed

Safflower seed

Sesame butter,
  tahini

Sesame flour

Sesame seed

Sunflower butter

Sunflower seed

Beans and Legumes

BLOOD TYPE B		WEEKLY ■ IF YOUR ANCESTRY IS		
Food	*Portion*	*African*	*Caucasian*	*Asian*
ALL RECOMMENDED BEANS AND LEGUMES	1 CUP, DRY	3–4X	2–3X	4–5X

Type B can eat some beans and legumes, but many beans, such as lentils, garbanzos, pintos, and black-eyed peas, contain lectins that interfere with metabolism, induce dysbiosis, and may increase inflammation.

Highly Beneficial

KIDNEY BEAN

LIMA BEAN

NAVY BEAN

Neutral

Broad bean, fava	Jicama	Soybean pasta ↑
Cannellini bean	Lima bean flour	Soybean, sprouted
Copper bean	Pea	Soybean, tempeh ↑
Great Northern	Snap bean	String bean
bean ↑	Soybean	Tamarind bean ↑
Green bean	Soybean granules,	White bean
Haricot-vert ↑	lecithin	

Avoid

Adzuki bean	Lentil, all types ↓	Soybean cheese ↓
Black bean	Mung beans,	Soybean meal ↓
Black-eyed pea ↓	sprouts ↓	Soybean, tofu ↓
Butter bean↓	Natto ↓	Soy miso
Garbanzo bean,	Pinto bean ↓	Soy tempeh
chickpea ↓	Pinto bean,	
Lentil, sprouted	sprouted	

Grains and Cereals

BLOOD TYPE B		WEEKLY ▪ IF YOUR ANCESTRY IS		
Food	*Portion*	*African*	*Caucasian*	*Asian*
ALL CEREALS	I CUP, DRY	2–3X	2–4X	2–4X
BREADS, CRACKERS	I SLICE	0–IX	0–IX	0–IX
MUFFINS	I MEDIUM	0–IX	0–IX	0–IX
GRAINS	I CUP, DRY	3–4X	3–4X	2–3X
PASTAS	I CUP, DRY	3–4X	3–4X	2–3X

For a Type B individual who is in good balance—that is, following the fundamental tenets of the diet—wheat may not be a problem. However, wheat is generally not tolerated well by Type B. Wheat contains a lectin that attaches to the insulin receptors in the fat cells, prohibiting insulin from attaching. The result is reduced insulin efficiency and failure to stimulate fat "burning."

Type B also should avoid rye, which contains a reactive lectin that can impact the cardiovascular system.

Corn and buckwheat are major factors in Type B weight gain. More than any other food, they contribute to a sluggish metabolism, insulin irregularity, fluid retention, and fatigue.

Try 100 percent sprouted breads, sometimes called Essene or Manna bread. These "live" breads are highly nutritious. Although they are sprouted wheat breads, the problem kernel is destroyed in the sprouting process, and they are perfectly healthful.

Again, for Type B the key is balance. I would, however, advise that you moderate your intake of pasta and rice. You won't need many of these nutrients if you're consuming the meat, seafood, and dairy foods advised.

Eat a variety of grains and cereals. Rice and oats are excellent choices. I also urge you to try spelt, which is highly beneficial for Type B.

Highly Beneficial

ESSENE, MANNA BREAD	MILLET	SPELT
FONIO	MILLET FLOUR	SPELT FLOUR, WHOLE GRAIN, FLOUR, NOODLES
JOB'S TEARS (*COIX* SPP.)	OAT BRAN	
MALANGA, TANNIA, *XANTHOSOMA* ↑	OATMEAL, OAT FLOUR, OATS	
	PUFFED RICE	
	RICE BRAN	
	RICE FLOUR	

Neutral

Barley ↑

Barley flour

Black bean flour

Cream of rice

Emmer

Flaxseed bread
(containing
allowable
grains) ↑

Larch fiber

Lima bean flour

Quinoa ↑

Rice, basmati

Rice, brown

Rice, puffed, cakes

Rice, white

Rice flour, brown

Rice flour, white

Soybean flour

Taro, Tahitian, poi,
dasheen

Wheat, bulgur

Wheat, durum,
semolina,
couscous

White flour

Avoid

Amaranth ↓

Artichoke flour,
pasta ↓

Buckwheat, kasha,
soba ↓

Bulgur wheat flour

Couscous

Cornflakes

Cornmeal, hominy,
polenta, all ↓

Cream of wheat

Durum wheat flour

Garbanzo bean
(chickpea) flour

Gluten flour

Graham flour

Grits

Kamut

Lentil flour, dahl ↓

Mastic gum ↓

Papadum

Puffed wheat

Rice, wild ↓

Rye ↓

Rye flour ↓

Seven grain

Shredded wheat

Sorghum

Tapioca, manioc,
cassava, yucca ↓

Teff

Wheat, bran, germ ↓

Wheat, whole grain ↓

Vegetables

BLOOD TYPE B	DAILY ▪ ALL ANCESTRAL TYPES	
Food	*Portion*	
RAW	I CUP, PREPARED	3–5X
COOKED	I CUP, PREPARED	3–5X

There are many high-quality, nutritious Type B–friendly vegetables—so take full advantage with three to five servings a day. There is only a handful of vegetables that Type B should avoid, but take these guidelines to heart.

Eliminate tomatoes completely from your diet. They contain a lectin that can increase the permeability of the gut, allowing allergens and other elements free entry.

Corn is also off your list, as it contains the insulin- and metabolism-upsetting lectins mentioned before. Also avoid olives because their molds can disrupt your microbiome and trigger allergic reactions.

For the most part, the vegetable world is your kingdom. Unlike other blood types, you can fully enjoy potatoes and yams, cabbage, and mushrooms—and many other delicious foods from nature's bounty.

Highly Beneficial

BEET GREENS ↑ ‡
BEET
BROCCOFLOWER ↑
BROCCOLI ↑ ‡
BRUSSELS SPROUTS
CABBAGE ‡
CANISTEL ↑
CARROT ↑
CAULIFLOWER ‡
COLLARD
  GREENS ↑ ‡
EGGPLANT ↑ ‡
GINGER

GRAPE LEAVES ↑
KALE ↑ ‡
MUSHROOM,
  SHIITAKE ‡
MUSTARD
  GREENS ↑ ‡
PARSLEY
PARSNIP ↑
PEPPERS, BELL,
  CHILI,
  JALAPEÑO ↑
SEA VEGETABLES,
  IRISH MOSS

SEA VEGETABLES,
  KELP, KOMBU,
  NORI, BLADDER-
  WRACK ↑
SEA VEGETABLES,
  SPIRULINA
SEA VEGETABLES,
  WAKAME
SWEET POTATO
TURNIP
  GREENS ↑ ‡
YAM

Neutral

Alfalfa sprouts
Arugula
Asparagus
Asparagus pea
Bamboo shoot
Bok choy, pak choi

Broccoli leaves
Broccoli rabe,
  rapini
Broccoli, Chinese
Capers
Celeriac

Celery
Chayote, pipinella,
  vegetable
  pear
Chervil
Chicory

Chinese kale,
   Kai-lan
Cilantro
Cucumber
Daikon radish
Dandelion greens
Dill
Endive ↑
Escarole
Fennel
Fenugreek ↑
Fiddlehead fern
Garlic
Hearts of palm
Horseradish ↑
Jicama ↑
Kelp
Kohlrabi ↑
Leek

Lettuce, Bibb,
   Boston, green
   leaf, iceberg,
   mesclun,
   romaine
Mushroom,
   abalone, black
   trumpet, enoki,
   maitake, oyster,
   portobello,
   straw, tree,
   white, silver
   dollar
Okra
Onion, all types
Oyster plant,
   salsify ↑
Pickles, all
Pimiento

Potato, blue, white,
   yellow
Radicchio
Rutabaga
Sauerkraut
Scallion
Seaweed
Shallots
Spinach
Squash
Swiss chard
Taro leaves, shoots
Tomatillo
Turnip
Water chestnut,
   matai
Watercress
Zucchini

<u>Avoid</u>

Aloe vera ↓
Artichoke ↓
Cassava ↓
Corn, popcorn ↓
Jerusalem
   artichoke ↓

Olives, black ↓
Olives, green ↓
Pumpkin
Quorn ↓
Radish
   sprouts

Radishes
Rhubarb
Tomato

Fruits

BLOOD TYPE B	DAILY ▪ ALL ANCESTRAL TYPES	
Food	*Portion*	
ALL FRUITS	1 FRUIT OR 3–5 OZ.	3–4X

You'll notice that there are very few fruits a Type B must avoid—and they're pretty uncommon in any case. Most Type Bs won't sorely miss persimmons, pomegranates, or prickly pears in their diets, especially considering the wide range of allowed fruits.

Pineapple can be particularly good for Type B if you're susceptible to bloating—especially if you're not used to eating dairy foods and meats. Bromelain, an enzyme in pineapple, helps with digestion.

On the whole, you can choose your fruits liberally from the following lists.

Try to incorporate at least one or two fruits from the highly beneficial list every day to take advantage of their medicinal qualities for Type B.

Highly Beneficial

BANANA ↑	PAPAYA
CRANBERRY ↑	PAWPAW
GRAPE ↑	PINEAPPLE ↑ ‡
MAMEY SAPOTE,	PLUM
MAMEY APPLE ↑	WATERMELON ‡

Neutral

Acai berry	Crenshaw	Kiwi	Peach
Apple	melon	Kumquat ↑	Pear
Apricot	Currant	Lemon ↑	Persian melon
Asian pear ↑	Date ↑	Lime	Plantain
Blackberry	Dewberry	Lingonberry	Prune
Blueberry	Durian ↑	Loganberry ↑	Quince
Boysenberry↑	Elderberry ↑	Mango	Raspberry
Breadfruit ↑	Fig	Mangosteen	Raisin
Canang melon	Goji, wolfberry	Mulberry	Sago palm
Cantaloupe	Gooseberry ↑	Musk melon	Spanish melon
Casaba	Grapefruit	Nectarine	Strawberry
Cherry	Guava ↑	Noni	Tangerine
Christmas	Honeydew	Orange	Youngberry
melon	Jack fruit	Passion fruit ↑	

Avoid

Avocado	Huckleberry	Pomegranate ↓
Bitter melon	Loquat ↓	Prickly pear
Coconut	Persimmon ↓	Starfruit, carambola

Beverages, Teas and Coffee

BLOOD TYPE B	DAILY ■ ALL ANCESTRAL TYPES	
Food	*Portion*	
ALL RECOMMENDED JUICES	8 oz.	2–3x
WATER	8 oz.	4–7x

Type B does best when you limit beverages to herbal and green teas, water, and juice. Although beverages like coffee, regular tea, and wine do no real harm, the goal of the Blood Type Diet is to maximize your performance, not to keep it in neutral. If you're a caffeinated coffee or tea drinker, try replacing these beverages with green tea, which has caffeine but also provides some antioxidant benefits.

If you'd like a daily juice with built-in immune and nervous-system boosters designed for Type B, try the following beverage first thing every morning. I call it Membrosia:

Mix 1 tablespoon of flaxseed oil, 1 tablespoon of high-quality lecithin granules, and 6 to 8 ounces of fruit juice. Shake and drink. Lecithin is a lipid, found in animals and plants, that contains metabolism- and immune system–enhancing properties. You can find lecithin granules in your local health food store and in some supermarkets.

The Membrosia cocktail provides high levels of choline, serine, and ethanolamine (the phospholipids), which are of great value to Type B. You may be surprised to find that it's rather tasty because the lecithin emulsifies the oil, allowing it to mix with the juice.

Highly Beneficial

CRANBERRY
  JUICE ↑ ‡
GINSENG TEA
GINGERROOT TEA
GRAPE JUICE
GREEN TEA,
  KUKICHA,
  BANCHA,
  GENMAICHA ↑ ‡

LICORICE
  ROOT TEA
MILK, RICE
PAPAYA JUICE
PARSLEY TEA
PINEAPPLE
  JUICE ↑
RASPBERRY
  LEAF TEA

ROSE HIP TEA
SAGE TEA
VEGETABLE JUICE
  (FROM HB
  VEGETABLES)
WATERMELON JUICE

Neutral

Alfalfa tea
Aloe juice
Apple juice, cider
Apricot juice
Beer
Black tea, all forms
Blackberry juice
Blueberry juice
Burdock tea
Carrot juice
Catnip tea
Cayenne tea
Celery juice
Chamomile tea
Cherry juice
Chickweed tea
Coconut water

Coffee
Cucumber juice
Dandelion tea
Dong quai tea
Elderberry juice
Elder tea
Goji berry juice
Grapefruit juice
Hawthorn tea
Horehound tea
Lemon and water
Lime juice
Milk, almond ↑
Mulberry tea
Nectarine juice
Noni juice
Orange juice

Pear juice ↑
Peppermint tea
Prune juice
Saint John's wort tea
Sarsaparilla tea
Slippery elm tea
Spearmint tea
Strawberry leaf tea
Tangerine juice
Thyme tea
Valerian tea
White birch tea
White oak bark tea
Wine, red, white
Yarrow tea
Yellow dock tea
Yerba mate tea

Avoid

Aloe tea
Coconut milk
Coltsfoot tea
Cornsilk tea

Fenugreek tea
Gentian tea
Goldenseal tea
Hops tea

Linden tea
Liquor,
  distilled ↓
Milk, soy ↓

Mullein tea
Pomegranate
  juice
Red clover tea

Rhubarb tea	Shepherd's	Soda (such as	Tomato
Seltzer water	purse tea	cola and diet	juice
Senna tea	Skullcap tea	cola)	

Herbs and Spices

Type B does best with warming herbs and spices, such as ginger, curry, and cayenne pepper. The exceptions are white and black pepper, which increase intestinal permeability (leaky gut).

Highly Beneficial

CAYENNE PEPPER	HORSERADISH
CURRY	LICORICE ROOT
GINGER	PARSLEY ↑

Neutral

Anise	Cilantro	Mustard, dry	Salt, sea salt
Arrowroot	Clove	Nutmeg	Savory
Basil	Coriander	Oregano	Senna
Bay leaf	Cream of tartar	Paprika	Spearmint
Bergamot	Cumin	Pepper, red	Tarragon
Caraway	Dill	flakes	Thyme
Cardamom	Dulse	Peppercorn	Turmeric
Chervil	Fennel	Peppermint	Vanilla
Chili powder	Garlic	Rosemary	Wintergreen
Chives	Mace	Saffron	
Chocolate	Marjoram	Sage	

Avoid

Acacia	Allspice	Cornstarch ↓	Pepper, black,
(gum arabic)	Cinnamon	Guarana	white ↓

Condiments, Sweeteners, and Additives

Condiments are basically either neutral or bad for all types. Type B can handle just about every common condiment except ketchup (tomato lectin), but common nutritional sense would suggest that you limit your intake of foods that provide no real benefit.

Sweeteners, such as white and brown sugar, honey, and molasses, can be consumed, but only as condiments, not as a source of calories. Try to limit your consumption of sweeteners. Needless to say, corn-derived sugars, such as high-fructose corn syrup, are to be avoided. You also may eat small quantities of chocolate, but consider it a condiment, not a main course.

Highly Beneficial

MOLASSES, BLACKSTRAP

Neutral

Agar
Agave syrup ↑
Apple butter
Apple pectin
Baking soda
Carob syrup
Fructose
Fruit pectin
Honey
Jam, jelly (from acceptable fruits)
Lecithin
Maple syrup
Mayonnaise
Molasses
Mustard, wheat free, vinegar free ↑
Mustard, with vinegar and wheat ↑
Pickle relish
Rice syrup
Salad dressing (low fat, from acceptable ingredients)
Soybean sauce, tamari, wheat free
Sugar, brown, white
Vegetable glycerine
Vinegar, all types
Worcestershire sauce
Yeast, baker's ↑
Yeast, nutritional ↑

Avoid

Acacia (gum arabic)
Aspartame
Barley malt ↓
Carrageenan ↓
Cornstarch
Corn syrup
Dextrose ↓
Gelatin ↓
High-fructose corn syrup ↓
High-maltose corn syrup, maltodextrin ↓
Invert sugar
Ketchup ↓
MSG
Mayonnaise, tofu, soy
Miso ↓
Polysorbate 80 ↓
Sodium carboxymethyl cellulose ↓
Stevia ↓
Sucanat
Tragacanth gum ↓
Umeboshi plum, vinegar

Meal Planning for Type B

An asterisk (*) denotes that the recipe is provided.

THE FOLLOWING sample menus and recipes will give you an idea of a typical diet beneficial to Type B. They were developed by Dina Khader, MS, RD, CDN, a nutritionist who has used the Blood Type Diet successfully with her patients.

These menus are moderate in calories and balanced for metabolic efficiency in Type B. The average person will be able to maintain weight comfortably and even lose weight by following these suggestions. However, alternative food choices are provided if you prefer lighter fare or wish to limit your caloric intake and still eat a balanced, satisfying diet. (The alternative food is listed directly across from the food it replaces.)

Occasionally you will see an ingredient in a recipe that appears on your avoid list. If it is a very small ingredient (such as a dash of pepper), you may be able to tolerate it, depending on your condition and whether you are strictly adhering to the diet. However, the meal selections and recipes are generally designed to work very well for Type Bs.

As you become more familiar with the Type B diet recommendations, you'll be able to easily create your own menu plans and adjust favorite recipes to make them Type B friendly.

STANDARD MENU ▪	WEIGHT-CONTROL ALTERNATIVES ▪

SAMPLE MEAL PLAN 1

Breakfast

*Membrosia Cocktail (optional)	
2 slices Essene bread with *Yogurt-Herb Cheese	1 slice Essene bread
poached egg	
green tea	

Lunch
Greek salad: lettuce, cucumber,
   scallions, celery, feta cheese,
   oil, and lemon
banana
iced herbal tea

Midafternoon Snack
*Quinoa Applesauce Cake   1 scoop low-fat cottage
herbal tea   cheese with pear slices

Dinner
*Lamb and Asparagus Stew   broiled lamb chop
*Saffron Brown Rice   asparagus
steamed vegetables (broccoli,
   Chinese cabbage, etc.)
frozen yogurt
(wine if desired)

SAMPLE MEAL PLAN 2

Breakfast
*Membrosia Cocktail
(optional)
rice bran cereal with banana
   and skim milk
grape juice
coffee

Lunch
thin slice of cheese (Swiss or   2 slices turkey breast
   Muenster) and thin slice of   1 slice spelt bread
   turkey breast   mustard only
2 slices spelt bread
mustard or mayonnaise
green salad
herbal tea

Midafternoon Snack
fruit juice–sweetened yogurt
herbal tea

Dinner
*Broiled Fish
steamed vegetables
*Roasted Yams with Rosemary
mixed fresh fruit
herbal tea or coffee
(red or white wine if desired)

SAMPLE MEAL PLAN 3

Breakfast

*Membrosia Cocktail (optional)	
*Maple-Walnut Granola with goat's milk	puffed rice with goat's milk
1 soft-boiled egg	
grapefruit juice	
green tea	

Lunch

*Spinach Salad	
½ cup water-packed tuna with mayonnaise	½ cup plain tuna 1 slice Essene bread
2 rice cakes	
herbal tea	

Midafternoon Snack

*Apricot Fruit Bread	low-fat yogurt with raisins
apple	
coffee or tea	

Dinner
*Scrumptious Fettuccine Alfredo
green salad
frozen yogurt
herbal tea
(red or white wine if desired)

Recipes

YOGURT-HERB CHEESE

2 32-ounce containers of plain nonfat yogurt
2 cloves minced garlic
1 teaspoon thyme
1 teaspoon basil
1 teaspoon oregano
salt and pepper to taste
1 tablespoon olive oil

Spoon yogurt into an old pillowcase or cheesecloth. Tie the cheesecloth with string and allow the yogurt to drip over the kitchen sink
or the bathtub for 4½ to 5 hours.
Remove yogurt from cheesecloth and mix it with all the spices and oil
in a bowl. Cover and chill for 1 to 2 hours before serving. Great
served with raw vegetables.

QUINOA APPLESAUCE CAKE

1¾ cups quinoa flour
1 cup currants or other (allowed) dried fruit
½ cup chopped pecans

½ teaspoon baking soda
½ teaspoon aluminum-free baking powder
½ teaspoon salt
½ teaspoon ground cloves
2 cups unsweetened
organic applesauce
1 large organic egg
1 cup Sucanat sugar or maple sugar
½ cup unsalted, sweet butter

Preheat oven to 350 degrees F. Sprinkle ¼ cup of the flour over the currants and nuts and set aside. Blend the baking soda, powder, salt, and cloves with the remaining quinoa flour.

Add the dried fruit and nut mix and the applesauce. Beat in the egg and mix the sugar and butter in thoroughly.

Spoon into an oiled 8 x 8–inch cake pan and bake for 40 to 45 minutes or until the cake tester inserted in the center comes out clean.

LAMB-ASPARAGUS STEW

1 pound fresh asparagus spears
½ pound free-range lamb meat, cubed
1 medium onion, chopped
3 tablespoons organic, sweet, unsalted butter
1 cup water
salt, pepper to taste
juice of 1 lemon

Cut asparagus spears in 2-inch lengths, discarding tough portion at bottom. Wash and drain.

Sauté meat and onions in butter until light brown. Add water, salt and spices. Cook until tender. Add asparagus. Simmer for 15 minutes or until tender. Add lemon juice.

Makes 2 servings.

SAFFRON BROWN RICE

3 tablespoons extra-virgin olive oil
1 large Spanish onion or red onion
1 teaspoon ground coriander
1 teaspoon nutmeg
2 cardamom pods (use seeds from inside only)
1 teaspoon saffron threads
2 tablespoons rose water (found in Middle Eastern stores)
2 cups brown basmati rice
4 cups filtered water (boiling)

Heat the oil and sauté onion with all spices except saffron for 10 minutes on low heat. In a separate dish crush the saffron threads and add to simmering mixture.

Add half the rose water to the onion mixture. Simmer for another 15 minutes and then add the rice with boiling water. Cook for 35 to 40 minutes.

Just before serving add the rest of the rose water.

Makes 4 servings.

BROILED FISH
(RECIPE BY CHERYL MILLER)

6 tablespoons unsalted butter, ghee, or oil
1 teaspoon hot pepper sauce
1 tablespoon fresh brown garlic
4 slices of your favorite fillet
1 cup puffed rice cereal, crushed
2 tablespoons fresh parsley, chopped

Melt butter, add hot pepper sauce and brown garlic. Pour 4 teaspoons into a glass rectangular baking dish. Arrange fillets, sprinkle with crumbs. Add rest of the butter mixture on top of fillets.

Broil 10 to 15 minutes. Sprinkle with parsley. Serve immediately.
Makes 4 servings.

*My patient and friend Cheryl Miller is a wonderful cook. She supplied this
recipe, and it's just delicious.*

ROASTED YAMS WITH ROSEMARY

5 to 6 medium yams, quartered
¼ cup extra-virgin olive oil
1 tablespoon fresh rosemary or 2 teaspoons dried
dash cayenne or Cajun spice

Blend everything together and put into a Pyrex dish. Bake in the oven
at 350 to 375 degrees F. for 1 hour. This is a wonderful dish to have
with a green salad or roasted vegetables.
Makes 4 servings.

MAPLE-WALNUT GRANOLA

4 cups rolled oats
1 cup rice bran
½ cup dried cranberries
½ cup dried currants
1 cup chopped walnuts
1 teaspoon vanilla extract
¼ cup organic canola oil
¾ cup maple syrup

Preheat oven to 250 degrees F. In a large mixing bowl combine the
oats, rice bran, dried fruit, nuts, and vanilla. Add the oil and stir
evenly. Pour in maple syrup and mix well until evenly moistened.
Mixture should be crumbly and sticky. Spread mixture in a cookie
tray and bake for 90 minutes, stirring every 15 minutes for even
toasting until the mixture is golden brown and dry.
Cool well and store in airtight container.

SPINACH SALAD

2 bunches fresh spinach
dash of salt to taste
1 bunch scallions, chopped
juice of 1 lemon
¼ tablespoon olive oil
pepper to taste

Wash spinach well. Drain and chop. Sprinkle with salt. After a few minutes, squeeze excess water. Add green onions, lemon juice, oil, salt, and pepper. Serve immediately.

Makes 6 servings.

APRICOT FRUIT BREAD

1¼ cups plain nonfat yogurt
1 organic egg
½ cup apricot conserves (fruit juice sweetened)
2 cups brown rice flour
1 teaspoon ground nutmeg
1¼ teaspoons baking soda
1 cup chopped, dried, unsulfured apricots (or any other dried fruit)
½ cup currants

Lightly grease a standard-size loaf pan with butter and preheat oven to 350 degrees F. In a medium-size bowl, combine the yogurt, egg, and conserves. Add 1 cup of flour and half of the spices plus soda. Stir until batter is evenly moist. Add remaining flour and spices. If consistency feels too thick you can add a few drops of cold water to the mixture. Fold in apricots and currants. Pour batter into greased loaf pan and bake for 40 to 45 minutes until done.

Remove bread from the pan and cool on a wire rack.

Makes approximately 8 servings.

SCRUMPTIOUS FETTUCCINE ALFREDO

8 ounces rice or spelt fettuccine/linguine
1 tablespoon extra-virgin olive oil
¾ cup buttermilk
⅓ cup plus 2 tablespoons Parmesan cheese (grated)
¼ cup sliced scallions
2 tablespoons chopped fresh basil or 1 teaspoon dried
¼ teaspoon garlic powder or freshly pressed garlic
¼ teaspoon finely shredded lemon peel

Cook pasta according to package directions to the al dente stage.
Drain; immediately return to pan. Add olive oil; toss to coat the pasta.
In same pan as pasta, add buttermilk, ⅓ cup Parmesan cheese, scal-
lions, basil and garlic. Cook everything together over medium-high
heat until bubbly, stirring constantly.
Decorate with 2 tablespoons Parmesan cheese and fresh basil.
Serve with lemon.
Makes 4 side dishes.

For a wealth of additional recipes in every category, check out the
blood type–specific cookbooks and recipe database at dadamo
.com and 4yourtype.com.

Type B
Supplement Advisory

THE ROLE OF SUPPLEMENTS—be they vitamins, minerals, or herbs—is to
add the nutrients that are lacking in your diet and to provide extra protection where you need it. The supplement focus for Type B is

- Fine-tuning an already balanced diet
- Improving metabolic efficiency
- Strengthening immunity
- Improving brain clarity and focus

Type B is a special (you might say lucky) case. For the most part, you can avoid major diseases by following your Blood Type Diet. Because your diet is so rich in vitamin A, vitamin B, vitamin E, vitamin C, calcium, and iron, there is no need for supplementation of these vitamins and minerals. So enjoy your unique status—but follow your diet!

The following are the few supplements that can benefit Type B individuals.

Minerals

MAGNESIUM

While the other blood types risk calcium deficiency, Type B risks magnesium deficiency. Magnesium is the catalyst for the metabolic machinery in Type B. It's the match head—what makes Type B metabolize carbohydrates more efficiently. Because you are so efficient in assimilating calcium, you risk creating an imbalance between your levels of calcium and magnesium. Should this occur, you find yourself more at risk for viruses (or otherwise lowered immunity), fatigue, depression, and, potentially, nervous disorders. In these instances, perhaps a trial of magnesium supplementation (300 to 500 milligrams) should be considered. Also, many Type B children are plagued with eczema, and magnesium supplementation can often be beneficial. Any form of magnesium is fine, although more patients report a laxative effect with magnesium citrate than with the other forms. An excessive amount of magnesium could, at least theoretically, upset your body's calcium levels, so be sure that you consume high-calcium foods as well, such as cultured dairy products. The key is balance!

Herbs, Phytochemicals, and Probiotics

LICORICE

Licorice (*Glycyrrhiza glabra*) is a plant widely used by herbalists around the world. It has at least four uses: as a treatment for stomach ulcers, as an antiviral agent against the herpes virus, to treat chronic fatigue syndrome, and to combat hypoglycemia. Licorice is a plant to be respected; large doses in the wrong person can cause sodium retention and elevated blood pressure. If you are Type B and suffer from hypoglycemia, a condition in which the blood sugar drops after a meal, drink a cup or two of licorice tea after meals. If you suffer from chronic fatigue syndrome, I recommend that you use licorice preparations, other than deglycyrrhizinated licorice (DGL) and licorice tea, only under the guidance of a physician. Licorice freely used in its supplemental form can be toxic.

MODIFIED CITRUS PECTIN

Modified citrus pectin (MCP) is a special type of pectin, a molecule found in many, if not most, plants. Pectin is widely used in cooking as a thickener. MCP (and pectin in general) is composed of a long chain of a sugar that bears striking resemblance to the Type B antigen. In the stomach, the acids break the chains up, liberating the sugar, which can then act to attract, block, and defuse Type B–specific lectins. This has been extensively studied in regard to blocking lectins from attaching to the tissues of the liver. MCP can be found in some health food stores, from naturopathic physicians, and online.

DIGESTIVE ENZYMES

If you are a Type B who is not used to eating meat or dairy foods, you may experience some initial difficulties adapting to your diet. Take a digestive enzyme with your main meals for a while, and you'll adjust more readily to concentrated proteins. Bromelain, an enzyme found in pineapples, is available in supplemental form.

ADAPTOGENIC HERBS

Adaptogenic herbs increase concentration and memory retention, sometimes a problem for Type Bs who have nervous or viral disorders. The best are Siberian ginseng (*Eleutherococcus senticosus*) and ginkgo biloba, both widely available. Siberian ginseng has been shown in Russian studies to increase the speed and accuracy of teletype operators. Ginkgo biloba is currently the most frequently prescribed drug of any kind in Germany, where more than 5 million people take it daily. Ginkgo increases the microcirculation to the brain, which is why it is often prescribed to the elderly.

LECITHIN. Lecithin, a blood enhancer found principally in soy, allows the cell-surface B antigens to move around more easily and better protect the immune system. Type B should seek this benefit from lecithin granules, not soy itself, as soy doesn't have the concentrated effect. Drinking the Membrosia Cocktail is a good habit to develop, as it allows you to get an excellent modulator for your nervous and immune systems in a rather pleasant way.

Type B Stress-Exercise Profile

TYPE B responds to stress in ways that tend to resemble that of Type A and destresses in ways that resemble Type O. Type B shares the tendency for higher cortisol levels with Type A, but because their levels of the dopamine-busting enzyme DBH are on the low side, they somewhat compensate for this.

As a Type B, you confront stress very well for the most part because you blend more easily into unfamiliar situations. You're less anxious or aggressive than Type O and less physically impacted than Type A. Thus Type B does well with exercises that are neither too aerobically intense nor completely aimed at mental relaxation. The ideal balance for many Type Bs consists of moderate activities that involve other people—such as group hiking, biking excursions, the less aggressive martial arts, tennis, and aerobics classes. You don't do as well when the sport is fiercely competitive—such as squash, football, or basketball.

The most effective exercise schedule for Type B should be three days a week of more intense physical activity and two days a week of relaxation exercises.

EXERCISE	DURATION	FREQUENCY (PER WEEK)
AEROBICS	45–60 min.	3X
TENNIS	45–60 min.	3X
MARTIAL ARTS	30–60 min.	3X

CALISTHENICS	30–45 min.	3x
HIKING	30–60 min.	3x
CYCLING	45–60 min.	3x
SWIMMING	30–45 min.	3x
BRISK WALKING	30–60 min.	3x
JOGGING	30–45 min.	3x
WEIGHT TRAINING	30–45 min.	3x
GOLF	60 min.	2x
TAI CHI	45 min.	2x
HATHA YOGA	45 min.	2x

Type B
Exercise Guidelines

THE THREE COMPONENTS of a high-intensity exercise program are the warm-up period, the aerobic exercise period, and a cool-down period. A warm-up is very important to prevent injuries, because it brings blood to the muscles, readying them for exercise, whether it is walking, running, biking, swimming, or playing a sport. A warm-up should include stretching and flexibility movements to prevent muscle and tendon tears.

The exercises can be divided into two basic types: isometric exercises, in which stress is created against stationary muscles, and isotonic exercises, such as calisthenics, running, or swimming, which produce muscular resistance through a range of movement. Isometric exercises can be used to tone up specific muscles, which can then be further strengthened by isotonic exercise. Isometrics may be performed by pushing or pulling an immovable object or by contracting or tightening opposing muscles.

To achieve maximum cardiovascular benefits from aerobic exercise, you must elevate your heart rate to approximately 70 percent of your maximum. Once that elevated rate is achieved during exercise, continue exercising to maintain that rate for 30 minutes. This regimen should be repeated at least three times each week.

To calculate your maximum heart rate:

1. Subtract your age from 220.
2. Multiply the difference by 70 percent (.70). If you are over sixty years of age, or in poor physical condition, multiply the remainder by 60 percent (.60).
3. Multiply the remainder by 50 percent (.50). For example, a healthy fifty-year-old woman would subtract 50 from 220, for a maximum heart rate of 170. Multiplying 170 by .70 would give her 119 beats per minute, which is the top level she should strive for. Multiplying 170 by .50 would give her the lowest number in her range.

FOR RELAXATION EXERCISES

Tai chi and yoga are the perfect way to balance the more physical activities of your week.

Tai chi chuan, or tai chi, is an exercise that enhances the flexibility of body movement. The slow, graceful, elegant gestures of tai chi seem to mask the full-speed hand and foot blows, blocks, and parries they represent. In China, tai chi is practiced daily by groups who gather in public squares to perform the movements in unison. Tai chi can be a very effective relaxation technique, although it takes concentration and patience to master.

Yoga combines inner rectitude with breath control and postures designed to allow for complete concentration without distraction by worldly concerns. Hatha yoga is the most common form of yoga practiced in the West. If you learn basic yoga postures, you can create a routine best suited to your lifestyle.

Some patients have told me that they are concerned that adopting yoga practices may conflict with their religious beliefs. They fear that the practice of yoga implies that they have adopted Eastern mysticism. I respond, "If you eat Italian food, does that make you Italian?" Meditation and yoga are what you make of them. Visualize and meditate on the subjects that are relevant to you. The postures are neutral; they are just timeless and proven movements.

SIMPLE YOGA RELAXATION TECHNIQUES

Yoga begins and ends with relaxation. We contract our muscles constantly, but rarely do we think of doing the opposite—letting go and relaxing. We can feel better and be healthier if we regularly release the tensions left behind within the muscles by the stresses and strains of life.

The best position for relaxation is lying on your back. Arrange your arms and legs so that you are completely comfortable in your hips, shoulders, and back. The goal of deep relaxation is to let your body and mind settle down to soothing calmness, in the same way that an agitated pool of water eventually calms to stillness.

Begin with abdominal breathing. As a baby breathes, her abdomen moves, not her chest. However, many of us grow to unconsciously adopt the unnatural and inefficient habit of restrained chest breathing. One of the aims of yoga is to make you aware of the true center of breathing. Observe the pattern of your breathing. Is your breathing fast, shallow, and irregular or do you tend to hold your breath? Allow your breathing to revert to a more natural pattern—full, deep, regular, and with no constriction. Try to isolate just your lower breathing muscles; see if you can breathe without moving your chest. Breathing exercises are always done smoothly and without any strain. Place one hand on your navel and feel the movement of your breathing. Relax your shoulders.

Start the exercise by breathing out completely. When you inhale, pretend that a heavy weight, such as a large book, is resting on your navel, and that by your inhalation, you are trying to raise this imaginary weight up toward the ceiling.

Then, when you exhale, simply let this imaginary weight press down against your abdomen, helping you exhale. Exhale more air out than you normally would, as if to "squeeze" more air out of your lungs. This will act as a yoga stretch for the diaphragm and further help release tension in this muscle. Bring your abdominal muscles into play here to assist. When you inhale, direct your breath down so deeply that you are lifting an imaginary heavy weight up toward the ceiling. Try to completely coordinate and isolate the abdominal breath with no chest or rib movement.

EIGHT

Blood Type AB Diet

TYPE AB: *The Enigma*

- MODERN MERGING OF A AND B
- CHAMELEON'S RESPONSE TO
  CHANGING ENVIRONMENTAL
  AND DIETARY CONDITIONS
- SENSITIVE DIGESTIVE TRACT
- OVERLY TOLERANT IMMUNE SYSTEM
- RESPONDS BEST TO STRESS SPIRITUALLY,
  WITH PHYSICAL VERVE AND
  CREATIVE ENERGY
- AN EVOLUTIONARY MYSTERY

The Type AB Diet

BLOOD TYPE AB is rare (2 to 5 percent of the population), and biologically complex. It doesn't fit comfortably into any of the other categories. Multiple antigens make Type AB sometimes A-like, sometimes B-like, and sometimes a fusion of both—kind of a blood type centaur.

This multiplicity of qualities can be positive or negative, depending on the circumstances, so the Type AB diet requires that you read your foods lists very carefully and familiarize yourself with both the Type A and Type B diets to better understand the parameters of your own diet.

Essentially, most foods contraindicated for either Type A or Type B are probably bad for Type AB—although there are some exceptions. Panhemagglutinins, which are lectins capable of agglutinating all of the blood types, seem to be better tolerated by Type AB, perhaps because the lectin reaction is diminished by the double A and B antibodies. Tomatoes are an excellent example. Type A and Type B cannot tolerate the lectins, while Type AB eats tomatoes with no discernible effect.

Type AB is often stronger and more active than the more sedentary Type A. This extra dollop of élan vital may be because Type AB's genetic memory still contains fairly recent remnants of its steppe-dwelling Type B ancestors.

NOTE: Longtime readers will notice a difference in the values of a small number of foods between this edition and the original version of *Eat Right for Your Type*. That is because beginning with the publication of *Live Right for Your Type*, I made a distinction in some foods between secretors and non-secretors. The original version of *Eat Right for Your Type*, which preceded *Live Right for Your Type*, "homogenized" these differences. Like all of my subsequent books, this edition of *Eat Right for Your Type* uses the secretor values as the base values for the A, B, AB, and O blood types.

KEY

‡ Enhances carbohydrate metabolism, helps with weight loss

↑ Increases microbiome diversity, discourages microbial imbalance

↓ Decreases microbiome diversity, encourages microbial imbalance

Meats and Poultry

BLOOD TYPE AB		WEEKLY ■ IF YOUR ANCESTRY IS		
Food	*Portion**	*African*	*Caucasian*	*Asian*
LEAN RED MEATS	4–6 OZ.	1–3X	1–3X	1–3X
POULTRY	4–6 OZ. (MEN)	0–2X	0–2X	0–2X

The portion recommendations are merely guidelines that can help refine your diet according to ancestral propensities.

When it comes to eating meat and poultry, Type AB borrows characteristics from both Type A and Type B. Like Type A, you do not produce enough stomach acid to effectively digest too much animal protein. Yet the key is portion size and frequency. Type AB needs some meat protein, especially the kinds that play to its B-like traits—lamb, mutton, rabbit, and turkey, instead of beef. The lectin in chicken that irritates the blood vessels and digestive tracts of Type B has the same effect on Type AB, so stay away from chicken.

Also avoid all smoked or cured meats. These foods can cause stomach cancer in people with low levels of stomach acid, the trait you share with Type A.

Highly Beneficial

TURKEY ↑ ‡

Neutral

Beef liver	Lamb	Pheasant
Calf liver	Mutton	Rabbit
Goat	Ostrich	

Avoid

Bear	Duck	Partridge
Beef	Duck liver	Pork and bacon ↓
Beef heart	Goose	Quail
Beef tongue	Goose liver	Squab
Bone soup	Grouse	Squirrel
(allowable meats)	Guinea hen	Sweetbreads
Buffalo, bison	Horse	Turtle
Caribou	Kangaroo	Veal
Chicken ↓	Marrow soup	Venison
Chicken liver	Moose	
Cornish hen	Opossum	

Seafood

BLOOD TYPE AB	WEEKLY ▪ IF YOUR ANCESTRY IS			
Food	*Portion*	*African*	*Caucasian*	*Asian*
ALL RECOMMENDED SEAFOOD	4–6 oz.	3–5x	3–5x	4–6x

There is a wide variety of seafoods for Type AB, and it is an excellent source of protein for you. Like Type A, your digestive tract may experience problems from the lectins found in some whitefish, such as sole and flounder. The edible snail, *Helix aspersa/pomatia* (escargot), contains a powerful lectin that may help prevent some cancers that Type AB individuals appear more prone to developing.

Highly Beneficial

COD ↑ ‡	PORGY ↑	SALMON,
GROUPER ↑	RED SNAPPER ↑	SOCKEYE ↑
MACKEREL,	SAILFISH	SARDINE ↑
ATLANTIC ↑ ‡	SAILFISH ROE	SHAD ↑ ‡
MAHI-MAHI ↑	SALMON,	SNAIL, ESCARGOT ↑
MONKFISH ↑	ATLANTIC	STURGEON ↑
PICKEREL,	(WILD) ↑	TUNA, BLUEFIN ↑
WALLEYE ↑	SALMON,	TUNA, SKIPJACK
PIKE ↑	CHINOOK ↑	TUNA, YELLOWFIN

Neutral

Abalone, sea ear, mutton fish	Mackerel, Spanish	Scrod
Bluefish	Mullet	Scup
Bullhead	Muskellunge	Sea bream
Butterfish	Mussel	Shark
Carp	Ocean pout	Smelt
Catfish	Opaleye fish	Squid, calamari
Caviar	Orange roughy	Sucker
Chub	Parrotfish	Sunfish, pumpkinseed
Croaker	Perch	Swordfish
Cusk	Perch, ocean	Tilapia
Drum	Pilchards	Tilefish
Halfmoon fish	Pollock, Atlantic	Weakfish
Harvest fish	Pompano	Whitefish
Herring	Rosefish	
	Scallop	

Avoid

Anchovy	Bass, sea, lake	Clam
Barracuda	Bass, striped ↓	Conch
Bass, blue gill	Beluga	Crab

Crayfish
Eel ↓
Flounder
Frog
Haddock
Hake
Halibut
Herring, pickled, smoked

Lobster
Lox (smoked salmon)
Octopus
Oyster ↓
Salmon roe
Shrimp
Skate
Sole

Trout, rainbow (wild)
Trout, sea
Trout, steelhead (wild)
Whiting
Yellowfish
Yellowtail

Dairy and Eggs

BLOOD TYPE AB		WEEKLY ■ IF YOUR ANCESTRY IS		
Food	*Portion*	*African*	*Caucasian*	*Asian*
EGGS	1 EGG	3–5X	3–4X	2–3X
CHEESES	2 OZ.	2–3X	3–4X	3–4X
YOGURT	4–6 OZ.	2–3X	3–4X	1–3X
MILK	4–6 OZ.	1–6X	3–6X	2–5X

For dairy foods, Type AB can put on the "B" hat, benefiting from dairy foods, especially cultured and soured products—yogurt, kefir, and nonfat sour cream—which are more easily digested and help develop a healthy microbiome.

The primary factor you have to watch out for is excessive mucus production. Like Type A, you already produce a lot of mucus, and you don't need more. Watch for signs of respiratory problems, sinus attacks, or ear infections, which might indicate you should cut back on the dairy foods.

Eggs are a very good source of protein for Type AB. Although they're high in cholesterol and Type AB (like Type A) has some susceptibility to heart conditions, research has shown that the biggest culprits in elevated cholesterol are not cholesterol-containing foods but rather saturated fats.

Highly Beneficial

COTTAGE
CHEESE ↑
EGG WHITE,
CHICKEN ↑
FARMER CHEESE
FETA CHEESE
GOAT CHEESE

KEFIR ↑
MANCHEGO
CHEESE
MILK, GOAT ‡
MOZZARELLA
CHEESE, ALL
TYPES

PECORINO
CHEESE ↑
RICOTTA CHEESE
ROMANIAN URDA ↑
SOUR CREAM ↑
YOGURT

Neutral

Casein
Caviar
Cheddar cheese
Colby cheese
Cream cheese
Edam cheese
Egg, goose
Egg, quail
Egg whole, chicken
Egg yolk, chicken

Emmental, Swiss
cheese
Ghee, clarified
butter ↑
Gouda cheese ↑
Gruyère cheese
Jarlsberg
cheese ↑
Milk, cow
(skim or 2%)

Monterey Jack cheese
Muenster cheese
Neufchâtel cheese
Paneer cheese
Quark cheese
Stilton cheese
String cheese
Swiss cheese
Whey protein

Avoid

American cheese ↓
Blue cheese
Brie cheese
Butter
Buttermilk
Camembert
cheese ↓

Egg, duck
Gorgonzola
cheese ↓
Half-and-half ↓
Ice cream
Milk, cow (whole)
Parmesan cheese

Provolone cheese ↓
Romano cheese
Roquefort cheese ↓
Sherbet

Oils and Fats

BLOOD TYPE AB		WEEKLY ▪ IF YOUR ANCESTRY IS		
Food	*Portion*	*African*	*Caucasian*	*Asian*
OILS	I TABLESPOON	I–5x	4–8x	3–7x

Type AB should use olive oil rather than animal fats, hydrogenated vegetable fats, or other vegetable oils. Olive oil is a monounsaturated fat that is believed to contribute to lower blood cholesterol. You may also use small amounts of ghee, a semifluid clarified butter popular in India, in your cooking. Walnut oil, which can be added to salads, can help promote cell cleansing, especially in the brain and nervous system, a process called autophagy.

Highly Beneficial

APRICOT
  KERNEL OIL
CAMELINA OIL ↑

HEMP SEED OIL
OLIVE OIL ↑ ‡
WALNUT OIL ↑ ‡

Neutral

Almond oil
Black currant
  seed oil
Borage seed oil
Canola oil
Castor oil
Chia seed oil

Cod liver oil
Evening primrose oil
Flaxseed,
  linseed oil
Hazelnut oil
Macadamia oil
Peanut oil

Perilla seed oil
Rice bran oil
Soybean oil
Wheat germ oil

Avoid

Avocado oil
Coconut oil
Corn oil ↓
Cottonseed oil

Lard
Margarine
Palm oil
Pumpkin seed oil

Safflower oil ↓
Sesame oil ↓
Sunflower oil ↓

Nuts and Seeds

BLOOD TYPE AB	WEEKLY ▪ IF YOUR ANCESTRY IS			
Food	*Portion*	*African*	*Caucasian*	*Asian*
NUTS AND SEEDS	6–8 NUTS	2–5X	2–5X	2–3X
NUT BUTTERS	1 TABLESPOON	3–7X	3–7X	2–4X

Nuts and seeds present an unclear picture for Type AB individuals. Choose carefully, eat them in small amounts and consume with caution. Although they can be a good supplementary protein source, seeds are a common source of food lectins, and your double AB antigens afford them ample opportunities for mischief.

Highly Beneficial

CHESTNUT,
  CHINESE ↑
CHESTNUT,
  EUROPEAN ↑
PEANUT ↑ ‡

PEANUT
  BUTTER ↑
PEANUT
  FLOUR ↑
WALNUT ↑ ‡

Neutral

Almond ↑
Almond butter ↑
Almond cheese ↑
Almond milk
Beechnut
Brazil nut ↑
Butternut ↑
Carob ↑

Cashew ↑
Cashew butter
Chia seed ↑
Flaxseed ↑
Hemp seed ↑
Hickory ↑
Litchi/lychee
Macadamia ↑

Pecan ↑
Pecan butter
Pine nut, pignoli ↑
Pistachio ↑
Safflower seed
Watermelon seed

Avoid

Filbert, hazelnut
Poppy seed

Pumpkin seed
Sesame butter, tahini

Sesame flour	Sunflower butter
Sesame seed	Sunflower seed

Beans and Legumes

BLOOD TYPE AB	WEEKLY ■ IF YOUR ANCESTRY IS			
Food	*Portion*	*African*	*Caucasian*	*Asian*
ALL BEANS AND LEGUMES	I CUP, DRY	3–5X	2–3X	4–6X

Beans and legumes are another mixed bag for Type AB. Like seeds, beans are a rich source of food lectins, and like seeds, your double antigen setup gives them twice the opportunity for mayhem. Some of these foods are idiosyncratic to Type AB.

Like Type A, Type AB should make soybean products, like tofu, a regular part of their diet in combination with small amounts of meat and dairy.

Highly Beneficial

LENTIL, GREEN	SOYBEAN	SOYBEAN, TOFU ‡
NATTO ↑	SOYBEAN CHEESE	SOY, MISO
NAVY BEANS	SOYBEAN,	
PINTO BEANS	SPROUTED ↑	
PINTO BEANS,	SOYBEAN,	
SPROUTED ↑	TEMPEH ↑	

Neutral

Cannellini beans	Lentils, all types	Soy cheese
Copper beans	Peas	Soy milk
Great Northern	Snap beans	String beans
beans ↑	Soybean granules,	Tamarind beans ↑
Green beans	lecithin	White beans
Jicama	Soybean meal	
Lentils, sprouted	Soybean pasta ↑	

Avoid

Adzuki beans	Butter beans ↓	Lima beans ↓
Black beans	Garbanzo beans,	Lima bean flour ↓
Black-eyed peas ↓	chickpeas ↓	Mung beans,
Broad beans,	Haricot-vert	sprouts ↓
fava ↓	Kidney beans ↓	

Grains and Cereals

BLOOD TYPE AB	DAILY ▪ IF YOUR ANCESTRY IS			
Food	*Portion*	*African*	*Caucasian*	*Asian*
Breads, crackers	1 slice	0–1x	0–1x	0–1x
Muffins	1 muffin	0–1x	0–1x	0–1x
Grains	1 cup, dry	2–3x	3–4x	3–4x
Pasta	1 cup, dry	2–3x	3–4x	3–4x

Guidelines for Type AB favor both Type A and Type B recommendations. Generally, you do well on grains, even wheat, but need to limit your wheat consumption. Wheat is also not advised if you are trying to lose weight. Type ABs with a pronounced mucus condition, caused by asthma or frequent infections, should also limit wheat consumption.

Limit your intake of wheat germ and bran to once a week. Oatmeal, soy flakes, millet, and soy granules are good Type AB cereals, but you must avoid buckwheat and corn.

Be aware that sprouted wheat breads sold commercially often contain small amounts of sprouted wheat and are basically whole wheat breads. Look for 100 percent sprouted breads (usually called Manna or Essene bread). Read the ingredient labels.

If you're Type AB, you'll benefit from a diet that includes more rice than pasta, although you may have semolina or spinach pasta once or twice a week. Again, avoid corn and buckwheat in favor of oats and rye.

Highly Beneficial

AMARANTH

ESSENE, MANNA
  BREAD

FONIO

JOB'S TEARS,
  (*COIX* SPP.)

MALANGA,
  TANNIA,
  XANTHOSOMA ↑

MILLET

OAT BRAN

OATMEAL, OAT
  FLOUR, OATS

RICE BRAN

RICE FLOUR,
  BROWN

RICE, BASMATI

RICE, BROWN

RICE, PUFFED,
  CAKES

RICE, WHITE

RICE, WILD

RYE

RYE BERRY

RYE FLOUR

SOYBEAN FLOUR ‡

SPELT, WHOLE
  GRAIN

Neutral

Barley ↑

Black bean flour

Cream of rice

Emmer

Flaxseed bread
  (containing
  allowable
  grains) ↑

Graham flour

Larch fiber

Lentil flour, dahl

Mastic gum

Papadum

Puffed wheat

Quinoa ↑

Rice flour, white

Shredded wheat

Spelt flour, noodles

Taro, Tahitian, poi,
  dasheen

Wheat, bran, germ

Wheat, bulgur

Wheat, durum,
  semolina, couscous

Wheat, whole grain
  flour, white flour

Avoid

Artichoke flour,
  pasta ↓

Buckwheat, kasha,
  soba ↓

Cornflakes

Cornmeal, hominy,
  polenta ↓

Garbanzo bean
  (chickpea)
  flour

Grits

Kamut

Lima bean
  flour

Sorghum

Tapioca, manioc,
  cassava, yucca ↓

Teff

Vegetables

BLOOD TYPE AB	DAILY ▪ ALL ANCESTRAL TYPES	
Food	*Portion*	
RAW VEGETABLES	I CUP, PREPARED	3–5X
COOKED OR STEAMED	I CUP, PREPARED	3–5X

Fresh vegetables are an important source of phytochemicals, the natural substances in foods that have a tonic effect in cancer and heart disease prevention. They should be eaten several times a day. Type AB has a wide selection—nearly all the vegetables that are good for either Type A or Type B are good for you as well.

The one interesting exception is the panhemagglutinin in tomatoes, which affects all blood types. Since Type AB has so much blood type material and the lectin isn't specific, you seem able to avoid the ill effects.

Like Type B, you must avoid fresh corn and all corn-based products.

Highly Beneficial

ALFALFA SPROUTS
BEET
BEET GREENS ↑ ‡
BROCCOFLOWER ↑
BROCCOLI ↑ ‡
BROCCOLI,
  CHINESE
CANISTEL ↑
CAULIFLOWER ‡
CELERY ↑ ‡
COLLARD
  GREENS ↑ ‡

CUCUMBER ↑ ‡
DANDELION
  GREENS
EGGPLANT ↑ ‡
GARLIC
GRAPE LEAVES ↑
HEART OF PALM ↑
KALE ↑
MUSHROOMS,
  MAITAKE ‡
MUSTARD
  GREENS ↑ ‡

PARSLEY
PARSNIP ↑
SEA VEGETABLES,
  IRISH MOSS
SEA VEGETABLES,
  SPIRULINA
SWEET POTATO
TURNIP GREENS ↑ ‡
YAM

Neutral

Arugula
Asparagus
Asparagus peas
Bamboo shoot
Bok choy, pak choi
Broccoli leaves
Broccoli rabe, rapini
Brussels sprouts
Cabbage
Carrots
Celeriac
Chayote,
    pipinella,
    vegetable pear
Chervil
Chicory
Chinese kale,
    Kai-lan
Cilantro
Daikon radish
Endive ↑
Escarole
Fennel
Fiddlehead fern
Ginger ↑

Horseradish ↑
Jicama ↑
Kohlrabi ↑
Leeks
Lettuce, green
    leaf, Bibb,
    Boston, iceberg,
    mesclun,
    romaine
Mushroom, black
    trumpet
Mushroom, enoki
Mushroom, oyster
Mushroom,
    portobello
Mushroom, straw
Mushroom, white,
    silver dollar
Okra
Olive, green
Onion, all types
Oyster plant,
    salsify ↑
Pepper, bell
Pimiento

Potato, blue, red,
    yellow, white
    with skin
Pumpkin
Quorn
Radicchio
Rutabaga
Sauerkraut
Scallion
Sea vegetables, kelp,
    kombu, nori,
    bladderwrack ↑
Sea vegetables,
    wakame
Shallot
Spinach
Squash
Swiss chard
Taro leaves, shoots
Tomatillo
Tomato
Turnip
Water chestnut, matai
Watercress
Zucchini

Avoid

Aloe vera ↓
Artichoke ↓
Avocado ↓
Capers ↓
Cassava ↓
Corn, popcorn ↓
Fenugreek ↓

Jerusalem
    artichoke ↓
Mushroom,
    shiitake ↓
Olive, black ↓
Pepper, chili,
    jalapeño

Pickles, all
Radish
Radish, sprouted
Rhubarb

Fruits

BLOOD TYPE AB	DAILY ▪ ALL ANCESTRAL TYPES	
Food	*Portion*	
ALL RECOMMENDED FRUITS	1 FRUIT OR 3–5 OZ.	3–4X

Type AB inherits mostly Type A intolerances and preferences for certain fruits. Emphasize the more alkaline fruits, such as grapes, plums, and berries, which can help balance the grains that are acid forming in your muscle tissues.

Type AB doesn't do particularly well on certain tropical fruits—in particular mangoes and guava—but pineapple is an excellent digestive aid for Type AB.

Oranges also should be avoided, as they can undo some of the good gut rehabilitation that occurs with the diet. Grapefruit is closely related to oranges and is also an acidic fruit, but it has positive effects on the Type AB stomach, exhibiting alkaline tendencies after digestion. Lemons also are excellent for Type AB, aiding digestion and clearing mucus from the system.

Because vitamin C is an important antioxidant, especially for stomach cancer prevention, eat other vitamin C–rich fruits, such as grapefruit or kiwi.

The banana lectin interferes with Type AB digestion. I recommend substituting other high-potassium fruits such as apricots, figs, and certain melons.

Highly Beneficial

CHERRY ‡	JACK FRUIT	PAWPAW
CRANBERRY ↑ ‡	KIWI ↑	PINEAPPLE ↑ ‡
FIG ↑	LEMON ↑	PLUM
GOOSEBERRY ‡	LOGANBERRY ‡	WATERMELON
GRAPEFRUIT ↑	MAMEY SAPOTE,	
GRAPE ↑	MAMEY APPLE ↑	

Neutral

Acai berry	Date ↑	Passion fruit ↑
Apple	Durian ↑	Peach
Apricot	Elderberry ↑	Pear
Asian pear ↑	Goji, wolfberry	Persian melon
Blackberry	Honeydew	Plantain
Blueberry	Kumquat ↑	Prune
Boysenberry↑	Lime	Raisin
Breadfruit ↑	Lingonberry	Raspberry
Canang melon	Mangosteen	Spanish melon
Cantaloupe	Mulberry	Strawberry
Casaba	Musk melon	Tangerine
Christmas melon	Nectarine	Youngberry
Crenshaw melon	Noni	
Currant	Papaya	

Avoid

Avocado	Huckleberry	Prickly pear
Banana	Loquat ↓	Quince
Bitter melon	Mango	Sago palm
Coconut	Orange ↓	Starfruit, carambola
Dewberry	Persimmon ↓	
Guava	Pomegranate ↓	

Beverages, Teas and Coffee

BLOOD TYPE AB	DAILY ▪ ALL ANCESTRAL TYPES	
Food	*Portion*	
ALL RECOMMENDED JUICES	8 oz.	2–3x
WATER	8 oz.	4–7x

Type AB individuals should begin each day by drinking a glass of warm water with the freshly squeezed juice of half a lemon to cleanse the system of mucus accumulated while sleeping. It also has a very mild blood-thinning effect that is desirable for Type AB and aids elimination. Follow with a diluted glass of grapefruit or papaya juice. In general, choose high-alkaline fruit juices such as black cherry, cranberry, or grape.

A glass of red wine three or four times a week can be beneficial for Type AB because of its positive cardiovascular effects. Replace coffee with green tea for the greatest benefit. Green tea has powerful antioxidant qualities, important for Type AB individuals.

Highly Beneficial

ALFALFA TEA	GREEN TEA,	ROSE HIPS TEA
BURDOCK TEA	KUKICHA,	STRAWBERRY
CHAMOMILE TEA	BANCHA,	LEAF TEA
CHERRY JUICE	GENMAICHA ↑ ‡	VEGETABLE JUICE
CRANBERRY	HAWTHORN TEA	(FROM HB
JUICE ↑	LEMON AND	VEGETABLES)
ECHINACEA TEA	WATER ↑	WATERMELON
GINSENG TEA	MILK, RICE	JUICE
GRAPE JUICE	PINEAPPLE JUICE ↑	

Neutral

Apple cider, juice	Elderberry juice	Papaya
Apricot juice	Elder tea	Parsley tea
Beer	Gingerroot tea	Pear juice ↑
Blackberry juice	Goldenseal tea	Peppermint tea
Blueberry juice	Grapefruit juice	Prune juice
Catnip tea	Horehound tea	Raspberry leaf tea
Cayenne tea	Licorice root tea	Sage tea
Chickweed tea	Milk, almond ↑	Saint John's wort tea
Cucumber juice	Milk, soy	Sarsaparilla tea
Club soda	Mulberry tea	Seltzer water
Dandelion tea	Nectarine juice	Slippery elm tea
Dong quai tea	Noni juice	Spearmint tea

Tangerine juice

Thyme tea

Tomato juice

Valerian tea

Vervain tea

White birch tea

White oak bark tea

Wine, red

Wine, white

Yarrow tea

Yellow dock tea

Yerba mate tea

Avoid

Aloe tea

Black tea, all forms

Coconut milk

Coffee

Coltsfoot tea

Corn silk tea

Fenugreek tea

Gentian tea

Guava juice

Hops tea

Linden tea

Liquor, distilled ↓

Mango juice

Mullein tea

Orange juice ↓

Pomegranate juice

Red clover tea

Rhubarb tea

Senna tea

Shepherd's purse tea

Skullcap tea

Soda, cola,
   diet cola, misc.

Herbs and Spices

Spices were the original medicine, so think of them that way. Many herbs and spices are rich in antimicrobial essential oils, while others are great sources of antioxidants, immune-enhancing phytochemicals, and fat-burning thermogenic compounds. Try to work your recommended spices into your diet on a regular basis.

Avoid all pepper and vinegar because they tend to unbalance the absorption machinery of the digestive tract. Instead of vinegar, use lemon juice with oil and herbs to dress vegetables or salads.

And don't be afraid to use generous amounts of garlic. It's a potent tonic and natural antibiotic, especially for Type AB.

Sugar and chocolate are allowed in small amounts. Use them as you would condiments.

Highly Beneficial

CURRY

GARLIC

GINGER

HORSERADISH

OREGANO ↑

PARSLEY ↑

Neutral

Arrowroot	Cinnamon	Licorice root	Savory
Basil	Clove	Mace	Senna
Bay leaf	Coriander	Marjoram	Spearmint
Bergamot	Cream of	Mustard, dry	Tarragon
Caraway	tartar	Nutmeg	Thyme
Cardamom	Cumin	Paprika	Turmeric
Chervil	Dill	Peppermint	Vanilla
Chili powder	Dulse	Rosemary	Wintergreen
Chive	Fennel	Saffron	
Chocolate	Ginger ↑	Sage	
Cilantro	Kelp	Salt, sea salt	

Avoid

Allspice	Guarana	Pepper,
Anise	Pepper, black ↓	red flakes ↓

Condiments, Sweeteners and Additives

Be sure to avoid all pickled condiments, due to their negative effect on the microbiome. Also avoid ketchup, which contains vinegar.

Highly Beneficial

MISO ‡

MOLASSES, BLACKSTRAP

Neutral

Agar	Fruit pectin	Mayonnaise, tofu, soy
Agave syrup ↑	Honey	Molasses
Apple butter	Jams, jelly (with	Mustard, wheat free,
Apple pectin	acceptable	vinegar free ↑
Baking soda	fruits)	Rice syrup
Brown rice syrup	Lecithin	Salad dressing from
Carob syrup	Maple syrup	acceptable
Fructose	Mayonnaise	ingredients

Soybean sauce,	Sugar, brown, white	Vegetable glycerine
tamari, wheat free	Umeboshi plum,	Yeast, baker's ↑
Stevia	vinegar	Yeast, brewer's ↑

Avoid

Acacia	High-fructose	Polysorbate 80 ↓
(gum arabic)	corn syrup ↓	Sodium
Aloe	High-maltose	carboxymethyl
Almond extract	corn syrup,	cellulose ↓
Aspartame	maltodextrin ↓	Soy sauce
Barley malt ↓	Invert sugar	Sucanat
Carob syrup	Ketchup ↓	Tragacanth gum ↓
Carrageenan ↓	Methyl cellulose ↓	Vinegar,
Cornstarch ↓	MSG	all types ↓
Dextrose ↓	Mustard, with vinegar	Worcestershire
Gelatin	and wheat	sauce ↓
Guar gum	Pickle relish ↓	

Meal Planning for Type AB

Asterisk (*) indicates the recipe is provided.

THE FOLLOWING SAMPLE menus and recipes will give you an idea of a typical diet beneficial to Type ABs. They were developed by Dina Khader, MS, RD, CDN, a nutritionist who has used the Blood Type Diet successfully with her patients.

These menus are moderate in calories and balanced for metabolic efficiency in Type AB. The average person will be able to comfortably maintain weight and even lose weight by following these suggestions. However, alternative food choices are provided if you prefer lighter fare or wish to limit your caloric intake and still eat a balanced, satisfying diet. (The alternative food is listed directly across from the food it replaces.)

Occasionally you will see an ingredient in a recipe that appears on your avoid list. If it is a very small ingredient (such as a dash of pepper), you may be able to tolerate it, depending on your condition and whether you are strictly adhering to the diet. However, the meal selections and recipes are generally designed to work very well for Type ABs.

As you become more familiar with the Type AB diet recommendations, you'll be able to easily create your own menu plans and adjust favorite recipes to make them Type AB–friendly.

STANDARD MENU ▪	WEIGHT-CONTROL ALTERNATIVES ▪

SAMPLE MEAL PLAN I

Breakfast

water with lemon (on rising)	
8 ounces diluted grapefruit juice	
2 slices Essene bread	1 slice Essene bread
*Yogurt-Herb Cheese	1 poached egg
coffee	

Lunch

4 ounces sliced turkey breast	
2 slices rye bread	1 slice rye bread or
Caesar salad	2 rye crisps
2 plums	
herbal tea	

Midafternoon Snack

*Tofu Cheesecake	½ cup low-fat yogurt
iced herbal tea	with fruit

Dinner

*Tofu Omelet	
stir-fried vegetables	
mixed fruit salad	
decaffeinated coffee	
(red wine if desired)	

SAMPLE MEAL PLAN 2

Breakfast
water with lemon (on rising)
diluted grapefruit juice
*Maple-Walnut Granola with
   soy milk
coffee

Lunch
*Tabbouleh
bunch of grapes or apple
iced herbal tea

Midafternoon Snack

*Carob Chip Cookies   honeydew melon with a
coffee or herbal tea   scoop of cottage cheese

Dinner
*Baked Rabbit
*String Bean Salad
basmati rice   steamed broccoli and
frozen yogurt   cauliflower
decaffeinated coffee
(red wine if desired)

SAMPLE MEAL PLAN 3

Breakfast
water with lemon (on rising)
diluted grapefruit juice
1 poached egg
2 slices Essene bread with   1 slice Essene bread
   organic almond butter   with low-sugar jam
coffee

Lunch
*Tofu-Sardine Fritters
or   _ tofu-vegetable stir-fry
*Tofu-Pesto Lasagna
mixed green salad
2 plums
herbal tea

Midafternoon Snack
fruit juice–sweetened yogurt

Dinner
broiled salmon with fresh dill
   and lemon
*Saffron Brown Rice   asparagus
*Spinach Salad
decaffeinated coffee
(red wine if desired)

Recibes

YOGURT-HERB CHEESE

2 32-ounce containers of plain nonfat yogurt
2 cloves minced garlic
1 teaspoon thyme
1 teaspoon basil
1 teaspoon oregano
salt and pepper to taste
1 tablespoon olive oil

Spoon yogurt into an old pillowcase or cheesecloth. Tie the cheesecloth with string and allow the yogurt to drip over a kitchen sink or
a bathtub for 4½ to 5 hours.

Remove yogurt from cheesecloth and mix it with all the spices and oil
in a bowl. Cover and chill for 1 to 2 hours before serving. Great
served with raw vegetables.

TOFU CHEESECAKE (BAKED)
(RECIPE BY YVONNE CHAPMAN)

1½ pounds pressed tofu
⅔ cup soy milk
¼ teaspoon salt (optional)
2 teaspoons fresh lemon juice
grated rind of one lemon
1 teaspoon vanilla extract

Blend all ingredients together.

PIE CRUST

¾ cup whole meal flour (or rye flour)
½ cup oatmeal
½ teaspoon salt
½ cup oil
2 tablespoons cold water

Combine ingredients, stir in oil, then water, until mixture holds together. Press over bottom and sides of an 8-inch pie pan. Prick bottom several times with a fork. Fill pie crust with tofu mixture and
bake at 300 degrees F. for 30 to 45 minutes.

Makes approximately 8 servings.

TOFU OMELET

1 pound soft tofu, drained and mashed
5–6 portobello mushrooms, sliced
½ pound grated scallions
1 teaspoon mirin or sherry for cooking
1 teaspoon wheat-free tamari or soy sauce
1 tablespoon fresh parsley, chopped
1 teaspoon brown rice flour
4 organic eggs, lightly beaten
choice of allowable seasonings to taste
2 teaspoons organic extra-virgin olive oil

Combine all the ingredients except for oil. Heat the oil in a large frying pan. Pour in half the mixture and cover the pan. Cook over low heat for approximately 15 minutes until egg is cooked. Remove from pan and keep warm.

Repeat the process and use the remainder of the mixture.
Serves 3 to 4.

MAPLE-WALNUT GRANOLA

4 cups rolled oats
1 cup rice bran
½ cup dried currants
½ cup dried cranberries
1 cup minced walnuts or almonds
1 teaspoon vanilla extract
¼ cup organic canola oil
¾ cup maple syrup

Preheat oven to 250 degrees F. In a large mixing bowl combine the oats, rice bran, dried fruit, nuts, and vanilla. Add the oil and stir evenly. Pour in maple syrup and mix well until evenly moistened. Mixture should be crumbly and sticky. Spread mixture in a cookie tray and bake for 90 minutes, stirring every 15 minutes for even toasting until the mixture is golden brown and dry.

Cool well and store in airtight container.

TABBOULEH

1 cup millet, cooked
1 bunch green onions, chopped
4 bunches parsley, chopped
1 bunch mint, chopped, or 2 tablespoons dried mint
1 large cucumber, peeled and chopped (optional)
⅓ cup olive oil
juice of 3 lemons
1 tablespoon salt

Place millet in a large bowl. Add all chopped vegetables and mix well. Add oil, lemon juice, and salt. Serve over fresh green lettuce. Eat with lettuce leaves, tender grape leaves, or with a fork. Makes a refreshing appetizer or a picnic salad.

Makes 4 servings.

CAROB CHIP COOKIES

⅓ cup organic canola oil
½ cup pure maple syrup
1 teaspoon vanilla extract
1 organic egg
1 teaspoon baking soda
1¾ cups oat or brown rice flour
½ cup carob chips (unsweetened)

Oil two baking sheets and preheat oven to 375 degrees F. In a medium-size mixing bowl, combine the oil, maple syrup and vanilla. Beat the egg and stir into the oil mixture. Gradually stir in soda and flour to form a stiff batter. Fold in carob chips and drop the batter onto

the baking sheets by the teaspoon. Bake for 10 to 15 minutes until cookie is lightly browned. Remove from oven and cool.
Makes 3½ to 4 dozen.

GRILLED RABBIT

2 rabbits
1 cup apple cider vinegar
1 small onion, chopped
2 teaspoons salt
¼ cup water
1 cup rice flour or crushed wheat-free bread crumbs
¼ teaspoon pepper
dash of cinnamon
⅓ cup margarine

Clean dressed rabbits and cut into serving pieces. Marinate meat in vinegar, onion, and salted water for a few hours before cooking. Drain.
Combine flour, salt and spices in a plate. Dip pieces in melted margarine, then in flour or crushed bread crumb mixture until well coated.
Grill in oven at 375 degrees F. for 30 to 40 minutes.
Makes 4 to 6 servings.

STRING BEAN SALAD

1 pound green string beans
juice of 1 lemon
3 tablespoons olive oil
2 cloves garlic, crushed
2 to 3 teaspoons salt

Wash tender, fresh, green string beans. Remove stems and strings. Cut into 2-inch pieces.
Cook until tender by boiling in plenty of water. Drain. When cool, place in a salad bowl. Dress to taste with lemon juice, olive oil, garlic, and salt.
Makes 4 servings.

TOFU SARDINE FRITTERS
(RECIPE BY YVONNE CHAPMAN)

1 can deboned sardines
2 1-inch slices of medium or firm tofu
¼ teaspoon horseradish powder
dash of cider vinegar
olive oil

Mash sardines with a fork until fluffy. Mash tofu into the sardines.
Sprinkle in the horseradish powder. Add a dash of vinegar. Continue
  mixing ingredients until well blended.
Form into small patties. Heat a small amount of olive oil in a heavy
  skillet. Brown both sides of patties, or alternatively brown on a grill.
  This recipe goes well with a salad.
Serves 2.

TOFU-PESTO LASAGNA

1 pound soft tofu, mashed with 2 tablespoons olive oil
1 cup shredded mozzarella cheese (part skim) or part-skim ricotta
1 organic egg (optional)
2 packages frozen, chopped spinach or fresh, cut-up spinach
1 cup water
1 teaspoon salt
1 teaspoon oregano
9 rice or spelt lasagna noodles, cooked
4 cups pesto sauce (you may use less)

Mix tofu and cheese with egg, spinach, water, and seasonings.
Layer 1 cup sauce in 9 x 13 baking dish. Layer noodles, then cheese
  mixture, and then sauce. Repeat and end with noodles and sauce on
  top. Bake in oven at 350 degrees F. for 30 to 45 minutes or until done.

SAFFRON BROWN RICE

3 tablespoons extra-virgin olive oil
1 large Spanish onion or red onion
1 teaspoon ground coriander
1 teaspoon nutmeg
2 cardamom pods (use only seeds from inside)
1 teaspoon saffron threads
2 tablespoons rose water (found in Middle Eastern stores)
2 cups brown basmati rice
4 cups filtered water (boiling)

Heat the oil and sauté onion with all spices for 10 minutes on low heat. In
a separate dish beat the saffron and add to rose water in a small bowl.
To the onion mixture, add 1 tablespoon rose water. Simmer for another 15 minutes and then add the rice with boiling water. Cook for
35 to 40 minutes. Just before serving add the rest of the rose water.
Makes 4 servings.

SPINACH SALAD

2 packages fresh spinach
1 bunch scallions, chopped
juice of 1 lemon
¼ tablespoon olive oil or flaxseed oil
salt and pepper to taste
hot pepper (optional)

Wash spinach well. Drain and chop. Sprinkle with salt. After a few minutes, squeeze excess water. Add scallions, lemon juice, oil, salt and
pepper. Serve immediately.
Makes 6 servings.

For a wealth of additional recipes in every category, check out the
blood type–specific cookbooks and recipe database at dadamo
.com and 4yourtype.com.

Type AB
Supplement Advisory

THE ROLE OF SUPPLEMENTS—be they vitamins, minerals, or herbs—is to add the nutrients that may be lacking in your diet and to provide extra protection where you need it. The supplement focus for Type AB is

- Tuning the immune system
- Supplying cancer-fighting antioxidants
- Blunting stress
- Strengthening the cardiovascular system

Type AB presents a somewhat mixed picture when it comes to supplements. Although you share the vulnerable immune system and disease susceptibilities of Type A, your Type AB diet provides a rich variety of nutrients with which to fight back.

For example, Type AB gets plenty of vitamin A, vitamin B_{12}, niacin, and vitamin E in the diet, receiving a dietary protection against cancer and heart disease. I would suggest further supplementation only if, for some reason, a Type AB individual isn't adhering to the diet. Even iron, which is seriously lacking in the Type A vegetarian diet, is readily available in Type AB foods. There are, however, some supplements that can benefit Type AB.

Vitamins

VITAMIN C
Type AB, with higher rates of stomach cancer because of low stomach acid, can benefit from taking additional supplements of vitamin C. For example, nitrite, a compound that results from the smoking and curing of meats, could be a particular problem for Type AB, because its cancer-causing potential is greater in people with lower levels of stomach acid. As an antioxidant, vitamin C is known to block this reaction (although you should still avoid smoked and cured foods). However, don't take this to mean that you should take massive amounts of the vitamin. I have found that Type AB does not do as well on high doses (1,000 milligrams

and up) of vitamin C because it tends to upset their stomachs. Taken over the course of a day, two to four capsules of a 250-milligram supplement, preferably derived from rose hips or acerola cherries, should cause no digestive problems.

ZINC

I have found that a small amount of zinc supplementation (as little as 5 milligrams per day) often makes a big difference in protecting Type AB children against infections, especially ear infections. Zinc supplementation is a double-edged sword, however. Although small periodic doses enhance immunity, higher doses over the long term can depress it and interfere with the absorption of other minerals. Zinc is widely available as a supplement, but you really shouldn't use it without a physician's advice.

Herbs/Phytochemicals

HAWTHORN

With a tendency toward heart disease, Type AB will want to be serious about protecting your cardiovascular system. Following the Type AB diet will substantially reduce the risk, but if you have family members with heart disease you may want to take your preventive program a step further. A phytochemical with exceptional preventive capacities is found in the hawthorn tree (*Crataegus oxyacantha*). Hawthorn has a number of impressive antioxidant effects. It increases the elasticity of the arteries and strengthens the heart while also lowering blood pressure and exerting a mild solvent-like effect on the plaque in the arteries. Extracts and tinctures are readily available from naturopathic physicians, health food stores, pharmacies and online.

LARCH ARABINOGALACTAN

Arabinogalactan is a sugar molecule found in many plants, but typically extracted from the western larch (*Larix occidentalis*). Arabinogalactan has many positive benefits for Type AB individuals: It helps balance the microbiome by increasing the production of healthy short-chain fatty acids; it acts as a source of soluble fiber; and it is a safe, gentle, and effective immune modulator.

OTHER IMMUNE-ENHANCING HERBS

Because Type AB tends to be vulnerable to viruses and infections, gentle immune-enhancing herbs such as purple coneflower (*Echinacea purpurea*) can help ward off colds or flus and may help optimize the immune system's anti-cancer surveillance. Many people take echinacea in liquid or tablet form. It is widely available. The Chinese herb huang qi (*Astragalus membranaceus*) is also taken as an immune tonic, but is not as easy to find. The active ingredients in both herbs are sugars that act as mitogens to stimulate white blood cell proliferation. The white blood cells, you will remember, defend the immune system.

CALMING HERBS

Type AB will do well to use mild herbal relaxants such as chamomile and valerian root. These herbs are available as teas and should be taken frequently. Valerian has a bit of a pungent odor, which actually becomes pleasing once you get used to it. Another great relaxing herb for Type AB individuals is lemon balm (*Melissa officinalis*), which calms the digestive tract and has been found to improve mood and performance.

QUERCETIN

Quercetin is a bioflavonoid found abundantly in vegetables, particularly yellow onions. Quercetin supplements are widely available in health food stores, pharmacies, and groceries, usually in capsules of 100 to 500 milligrams. Quercetin is a very powerful antioxidant, many hundreds of times more powerful than vitamin E. It makes a beneficial addition to your cancer-prevention strategies.

MILK THISTLE

Like quercetin, milk thistle (*Silybum marianum*) is an effective antioxidant with the additional special property of reaching very high concentrations in the liver and bile ducts. Type AB tends to suffer from digestive disorders, particularly of the liver and gallbladder. If your family has any history of liver, pancreas, or gallbladder problems, add a milk thistle supplement (easily found in most health food stores) to your protocol. Cancer patients who are receiving chemotherapy should use a milk thistle supplement to protect the liver from damage.

Bromelain (Pineapple Enzymes)

If you are Type AB and suffer from bloating or other signs of poor absorption, take a bromelain supplement. This enzyme has a moderate ability to break down dietary proteins, helping the Type AB digestive tract better assimilate them.

Type AB Stress-Exercise Profile

The ability to reverse the negative effects of stress lives in your blood type. As we discussed earlier, stress is not in itself a problem; it's how you respond to stress. Although we've seen again and again that Type AB acts as a marriage between Types A and B, in regard to stress, Type AB appears to share many of the same characteristics of Type O (fight-or-flight), along with a bit of overactive cortisol thrown in for good measure. If, however, you adopt quieting techniques, such as yoga or meditation, you can achieve great benefits by countering negative stresses with focus and relaxation. Type AB does not respond well to continuous confrontation and needs to consider and practice the art of stillness as a calming charm. Concentrate on improving the quality of your sleep. Remove distractions and turn off the TV. Use any of the recommended calming herbs as a tea taken just before bedtime. Exercises that provide calm and focus are the remedy that pulls Type AB from the grip of stress.

Tai chi, the slow-motion, ritualistic pattern of Chinese boxing, and hatha yoga, the timeless Indian stretching system, are calming, centering experiences. Moderate isotonic exercises, such as hiking, swimming, and bicycling, are favored for Type AB. When I advise calming exercises, it doesn't mean you can't break a sweat. The key is really your mental engagement in your physical activity.

The following exercises are recommended for Type AB individuals. Pay special attention to the length of the sessions. To achieve a consistent release of tension and revival of energy, you need to perform one or more of these exercises three or four times a week.

EXERCISE	DURATION	FREQUENCY (PER WEEK)
TAI CHI	30–45 min.	3–5x
HATHA YOGA	30 min.	3–5x
AIKIDO	60 min.	2–3x
GOLF	60 min.	2–3x
CYCLING	60 min.	2–3x
BRISK WALKING	20–40 min.	2–3x
SWIMMING	30 min.	3–4x
DANCE	30–45 min.	2–3x
AEROBICS (LOW IMPACT)	30–45 min.	2–3x
HIKING	45–60 min.	2–3x
STRETCHING	15 min.	every time you exercise

Type AB
Exercise Guidelines

TAI CHI CHUAN, or tai chi, is an exercise that enhances the flexibility of body movement. The slow, graceful, elegant gestures of tai chi routines seem to mask the full-speed hand and foot blows, blocks, and parries they represent. In China, tai chi is practiced daily by groups who gather in public squares to perform the movements in unison. Tai chi can be a very effective relaxation technique, although it takes concentration and patience to master.

Yoga is also good for the Type AB stress pattern. It combines inner rectitude with breath control and postures designed to allow for complete concentration without distraction by worldly concerns. Hatha yoga is the most common form of yoga practiced in the West. If you learn basic yoga postures, you can create a routine best suited to your lifestyle.

Many Type ABs who have adopted yoga relaxation tell me that they will not leave the house until they do their yoga.

SIMPLE YOGA RELAXATION TECHNIQUES

Yoga begins and ends with relaxation. We contract our muscles constantly, but rarely do we think of doing the opposite—letting go and relaxing. We can feel better and be healthier if we regularly release the tensions left behind within the muscles by the stresses and strains of life.

The best position for relaxation is lying on your back. Arrange your arms and legs so that you are completely comfortable in your hips, shoulders, and back. The goal of deep relaxation is to let your body and mind settle down to soothing calmness, in the same way that an agitated pool of water eventually calms to stillness.

Begin with abdominal breathing. As a baby breathes, her abdomen moves, not her chest. However, many of us grow to unconsciously adopt the unnatural and inefficient habit of restrained chest breathing. One of the aims of yoga is to make you aware of the true center of breathing. Observe the pattern of your breathing. Is your breathing fast, shallow, and irregular or do you tend to hold your breath? Allow your breathing to revert to a more natural pattern—full, deep, regular, and with no constriction. Try to isolate just your lower breathing muscles; see if you can breathe without moving your chest. Breathing exercises are always done smoothly and without any strain. Place one hand on your navel and feel the movement of your breathing. Relax your shoulders.

Start the exercise by breathing out completely. When you inhale, pretend that a heavy weight, such as a large book, is resting on your navel and that by your inhalation, you are trying to raise this imaginary weight up toward the ceiling. Then, when you exhale, simply let this imaginary weight press down against your abdomen, helping you exhale. Exhale more air than you normally would, as if to "squeeze" more air out of your lungs. This will act as a yoga stretch for the diaphragm and further help release tension in this muscle. Bring your abdominal muscles into play here to assist. When you inhale, direct your breath down so deeply that you are lifting an imaginary heavy weight up toward the ceiling. Try to completely coordinate and isolate the abdominal breath with no chest or rib movement.

NINE

The 10-Day Blood Type Diet Challenge

*T*HE 10-DAY BLOOD TYPE DIET CHALLENGE IS A FAST AND EASY WAY to test the efficacy of the Blood Type Diet for yourself, while learning how to check for personal markers of success. The 10-day jump-start requires a serious level of dedication. It means focusing on following the exact guidelines to give you a true measure of how the diet works for you.

I recommend as close to 100 percent compliance as possible. Maximum compliance equals maximum effect. That means consuming foods primarily from the highly beneficial lists, supplemented by healthful neutral foods. In my experience, people who start the diet with a high level of compliance quickly reset their biochemistry, boosting metabolism, balancing blood sugar, and repairing past lectin damage. Most people who follow the 10-day challenge with a high degree of compliance can expect the following results:

1. Weight loss between 1 and 5 pounds
2. Decrease in stomach circumference
3. Less bloating after meals
4. Reduced joint pain
5. Greater energy

6. Reduction of digestive distress
7. Improved elimination

Before You Begin . . .

1. Know your blood type and secretor status. (Tests are available at 4yourtype.com.)
2. Clear your cupboards and refrigerator and restock with beneficial foods and supplements.
3. Plan an exercise schedule in advance, based on your physical condition and the specific recommendations in your Blood Type Diet.
4. Join the conversation on social media or check out the dadamo .com or 4yourtype.com websites for support, information, supplements, and inspiration.

The 10-day challenge is divided into two parts:

Days 1-5	Days 6-10
LECTIN DETOX	RESTORATION AND BALANCE

Days 1–5: Lectin Detox

START BY CHOOSING only those foods that are considered highly beneficial for your blood type. By eating highly beneficial foods and taking supplements that are compatible with your blood type, you will be cleansing and detoxifying your body and allowing all your systems to function at their very best. Purchase organic ingredients when possible and stick to buying whole foods, rather than processed foods from a box, bag, or can. And remember, this is not a deprivation diet, so be sure to follow the recommended portion sizes and eat enough food each day.

Start the day with a tall glass of water with a squeeze of fresh lemon juice. Continue drinking water throughout the day. Water promotes cell regeneration and helps cleanse the body. Aim to drink 8 to 10 glasses of water per day.

Avoid being around harsh chemicals and steer clear of chemical cleansers—try vinegar, lemon juice, and baking soda instead. Not only are they better for you; they are better for the environment too.

Supplement your diet with lectin-detoxifying nutrients. Suggestions are included, but you can investigate more options, including blood type–specific products and foods at 4yourtype.com.

Be sure to keep a record of what you eat, your exercise routines, and the supplements you take. Record your reflections on the journey as you begin so that you can track your progress and hold yourself accountable. Make notes about how you feel physically, your energy levels, mood, and whatever else you want to record.

At first, it can be a challenge to focus primarily on highly beneficial foods, but it will give you the purest form of your Blood Type Diet for the first five days. The charts provide a sample detox day for each of the blood types to give you an idea of menus that maximize your Blood Type Diet.

Blood Type O Sample Day: Lectin Detox

Food/Drink	
6:30 a.m.	Water with lemon
7:00 a.m.	Breakfast smoothie: blend together ¼ of a medium pineapple, a handful of blueberries, a splash of pineapple juice, a splash of almond milk, and 2 tablespoons of protein powder
10:00 a.m.	Walnuts, pumpkin seeds, and green tea
12:00	Salmon salad with fresh greens and seaweed, with olive oil and lemon dressing
2:30 p.m.	Plums or dried figs or 1 slice Essene toast with prune butter
6:30 p.m.	Beef and veggie stir-fry, with peppers, onions, broccoli, and leeks; herbal tea

Exercise	Aerobic activity: 45 min.
Supplements	Bladderwrack: 1 (100-milligram) capsule with meals
	N-acetyl glucosamine (NAG): 1 capsule with meals
	Standardized Chinese garlic extract: 1 (400 milligram) capsule, twice daily
	Type O–friendly probiotic (4yourtype.com)
Reflections (example)	"Felt really clear and strong today! Stir-fry I made for the kids was a huge hit—and I loved it too!"

Blood Type A Sample Day: Lectin Detox

Food/Drink	
6:30 a.m.	Water with lemon
7:00 a.m.	Breakfast smoothie: Blend together ¼ of a medium pineapple, a handful of blueberries, a splash of pineapple juice, a splash of soy milk, and 2 tablespoons soy protein powder
10:00 a.m.	2 rice cakes with peanut butter
12:00	Soba noodles with tofu, broccoli, carrots, and garlic
2:30 p.m.	1 cup of lentil soup
6:30 p.m.	Snails, baked salmon, steamed kale, and spinach; herbal tea
Exercise	Tai chi: 45 min.
	Brisk walking: 20–30 min.
Supplements	Chondroitin sulfate: 2 capsules with meals
	Dandelion (Taraxacum officinale): 1 (250-milligram) capsule, twice daily
	Type A–friendly probiotic (4yourtype.com)
Reflections (example)	"Had a tough day at work—very stressful—but tai chi and a walk with my dog really set the tone for a great evening."

Blood Type B Sample Day: Lectin Detox

Food/Drink	
6:30 a.m.	Water with lemon
7:00 a.m.	Breakfast smoothie: Blend together ¼ of a medium pineapple, 1 banana, a splash of pineapple juice, a splash of milk, and 2 tablespoons of protein powder
10:00 a.m.	1 cup of yogurt or cottage cheese and grapes
12:00	Large spinach salad with mushrooms, 1 cup navy bean soup
2:30 p.m.	1 slice toasted Essene bread with melted cheese
6:30 p.m.	Baked sole or halibut, lima beans, and broccoli; herbal tea
Exercise	Swimming: 45 min.
	Yoga class
Supplements	Modified citrus pectin: 1 capsule with each meal
	Type B–friendly probiotic (4yourtype.com)
Reflections (example)	"Got up early to swim at the Y and even though I had to rush to my yoga class, I had a really positive day overall! Capped it off with some delicious new tea!"

Blood Type AB Sample Day: Lectin Detox

Food/Drink	
6:30 a.m.	Water with lemon
7:00 a.m.	Breakfast smoothie: Blend together ¼ of a medium pineapple, 1 kiwi, a splash of pineapple juice, a splash of soy milk, and 2 tablespoons of soy protein powder
10:00 a.m.	1 cup of yogurt with a sprinkling of walnuts
12:00	Tofu stir-fry with mushrooms, carrots, and broccoli on basmati rice

2:30 p.m.	Rice cakes with peanut butter
6:30 p.m.	Lamb chops with steamed greens and baked sweet potato; herbal tea
Exercise	Cycling: 45 min.
Supplements	Larch arabinogalactan: 1 teaspoon, twice daily
	Type AB–friendly probiotic (4yourtype.com)
Reflections (example)	"Took a nice bike ride with my friend and we had so much fun—like kids again! Feeling revitalized!"

Days 6–10: Restoration and Balance

THE RESTORATION and balance stage, which makes up the final five days of the challenge, is less restrictive and allows you to begin to incorporate selected neutral foods into your diet, providing variety. However, continue to favor highly beneficial foods and completely eliminate the avoid foods from your diet.

Sample Day Type O: Restoration and Balance

Food/Drink	
6:30 a.m.	Water with lemon
7:00 a.m.	1 slice Essene toast with almond butter, 1 poached egg, 6 ounces vegetable juice, and green tea
10:00 a.m.	Blueberry-pomegranate juice and almond butter on rye crackers
12:00	A large mixed green salad with shredded chicken, 1 tablespoon olive oil, and lemon; 1 cup of escarole and black-eyed pea soup
2:30 p.m.	Handful of raw walnuts and almonds; herbal tea

6:30 p.m.	Filet of beef with steamed spinach and kale, a baked sweet potato with a pat of butter, and 1 cup pineapple slices; herbal tea
Exercise	Rest day
Supplements	NAG: 1 capsule, with meals
	Type O–friendly probiotic (4yourtype.com)
Reflections (example)	"No exercise today, but I am excited to take my longest jog ever tomorrow at the state park."

Sample Day Type A:
Restoration and Balance

Food/Drink	
6:30 a.m.	Water with lemon
7:00 a.m.	Puffed rice with soy milk and ½ grapefruit; green tea
10:00 a.m.	Apple slices with peanut butter
12:00	1 cup of lentil soup with a large green salad with tofu and lemon–olive oil dressing
2:30 p.m.	1 cup of soy milk or yogurt mixed with blueberries
6:30 p.m.	Baked salmon with steamed broccoli and carrots, and couscous
Exercise	Yoga: 1 hr.
Supplements	Chondroitin sulfate: 1 capsule, with meals
	Type A–friendly probiotic (4yourtype.com)
Reflections (example)	"Tried out a brand-new yoga class today and though it took time for me to catch up, I am really enjoying doing more advanced moves."

Sample Day Type B:
Restoration and Balance

Food/Drink	
6:30 a.m.	Water with lemon
7:00 a.m.	Oatmeal with milk and banana; green tea
10:00 a.m.	Wasa bread with almond butter
12:00	1 cup of navy bean soup; egg salad on a bed of greens
2:30 p.m.	Almonds, walnuts, and 1 plum; herbal tea
6:30 p.m.	Grilled lamb chops with broccoli, rice; licorice tea
Exercise	Tai chi: 45 min.
Supplements	Bromelain digestive enzymes
	Membrosia Cocktail
	Type B–friendly probiotic (4yourtype.com)
	Modified citrus pectin: 1 capsule, with meals
Reflections (example)	"Walked to tai chi today to up that exercise! Had a craving for chocolate cake today. Got through it, and luckily the lamb chops we had for dinner really hit the spot."

Sample Day Type AB:
Restoration and Balance

Food/Drink	
6:30 a.m.	Water with lemon
7:00 a.m.	Oat bran cereal with yogurt and sliced kiwi; green tea
10:00 a.m.	Wasa bread with almond butter
12:00	Open-faced spelt sandwich with sliced turkey and arugula; pineapple slices

2:30 p.m.	2 tablespoons goat cheese and grapes
6:30 p.m.	Baked salmon with mixed peppers, shiitake mushrooms, and basmati rice
Exercise	Add 2 miles extra to daily walk
Supplements	Bromelain digestive enzymes: 1 with meals
	Milk thistle: 1 capsule, twice daily
	Type AB–friendly probiotic (4yourtype.com)
	Larch arabinogalactan: 1 teaspoon twice daily
Reflections (example)	"It was a good day—had fun on my extra-long walk around the lake. Time for some new walking shoes."

Evaluate the Results

- Weight: Before _____ After _____
- Waist circumference: Before _____ After _____

Improvement Scale

On a scale of 1 to 5, with 5 being the greatest result, check the improvements you experienced on the 10-Day Blood Type Diet Challenge.

Sleep	① ② ③ ④ ⑤
Energy	① ② ③ ④ ⑤
Bloating	① ② ③ ④ ⑤
Heartburn	① ② ③ ④ ⑤
Elimination	① ② ③ ④ ⑤
Stress reduction	① ② ③ ④ ⑤
Joint pain	① ② ③ ④ ⑤

Headaches   ① ② ③ ④ ⑤

Mental clarity   ① ② ③ ④ ⑤

Skin condition   ① ② ③ ④ ⑤

Other _____   ① ② ③ ④ ⑤

Other _____   ① ② ③ ④ ⑤

Reflect on Your Results

I HAVE a high level of confidence in the promise that you will see some results in 10 days. While acknowledging that people have individual responses to the diet, it has been my overwhelming experience that the majority of people have noticeable results within this brief period. That usually means some weight loss and also a general improvement in digestive problems, allergy relief, sleep, and energy levels. I suggest you take some time to seriously consider your results—beyond just assigning numbers. List the real-life benefits. Also, if you experienced problems, list those too—they'll help you make adjustments that work for you individually.

Keep in mind that because the Blood Type Diet is designed as an *individualized* plan, there are going to be variations within the confines of your diet. You'll find the Blood Type Diet relatively forgiving—offering lots of choices to suit your preferences.

Next Steps

NOW THAT YOU'RE ON BOARD with 10 days under your belt, keep going by getting comfortable with the full potential of the Blood Type Diet. In addition, check out Appendix F for details about the large online support possibilities and the phone apps, which make it easy to plan, shop, and eat right for your type.

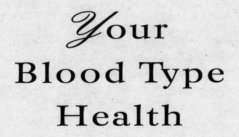

PART III

Your
Blood Type
Health

TEN

Common Health Strategies:

The Blood Type Connection

*B*Y NOW YOU ARE AWARE OF THE STRONG LINK BETWEEN YOUR blood type and your health. I hope you are also beginning to see that you can exert meaningful control, even when you have a susceptibility to a certain condition. Your Blood Type Diet is the cornerstone to a lifetime of health.

In the next three chapters, we will talk in more detail about the specific medical issues that concern everyone and how you can use the Blood Type Diet to make the best choices for your health. We begin with the drugs and treatments that are commonplace in modern life.

Drugs have been used as medicine for thousands of years. When a shaman or witch doctor brewed a potion, that potion had not only medical authority, but spiritual power. Although the infusion was often malodorous and vile, it contained magic, and the patient would gladly drink the bitter brew in hope of a cure.

Not that much has changed.

Today physicians overprescribe overpriced medications, and we overuse them. It's a serious problem. Yet unlike other naturopaths who reject the entire modern pharmacopoeia, I believe we must take a more reasoned and flexible stance. Most medical preparations are designed to be effective for a broad range of the population and should be used to treat the most severe and potentially dangerous conditions.

But we need to keep medication in perspective: All drugs are poisons in one way or another. One genomic database goes so far as to define diseases as "disruptions of the molecular system" and drugs as "anything capable of disrupting the molecular system." So let's get this straight: The basis of drug therapy is to treat a disruption with an additional, highly controlled, further disruption. Not exactly a formula for good health.

The good drugs discovered over the centuries are selective poisons. Many others are broader, less selective poisons. An excellent example of the latter is the diffuse arsenal of drugs used by oncologists for chemotherapy. In the process of destroying cancerous cells, many of these drugs indiscriminately attack healthy cells as well. (It is not my intention to vilify oncologists. This is just the state of the art.)

The good news is that chemotherapy sometimes works. The bad news is that sometimes chemotherapy works but the patient dies of complications related to the treatment. It's a terrible conundrum.

Modern science has presented the medical community with a bewildering array of medications, and all of them are being prescribed by well-meaning physicians worldwide. But have we been careful enough in our use of antibiotics and vaccines? How do you know which medications are best for you, for your family, for your children?

Again, blood type holds the answer.

Over-the-Counter Medications

THERE IS A wide range of over-the-counter (OTC) medications designed for every common ailment—from headaches to aching joints to congestion to indigestion. On the face of it, these seem to be inexpensive, convenient, and effective remedies.

As a naturopathic physician, I try to avoid prescribing OTC medications whenever I can. In most cases, there are natural alternatives that work just as well or better. In addition, there are dangers inherent in using many OTC preparations, including

- Aspirin's blood-thinning properties can be trouble for Type O, who might already have thin blood, although I sometimes recommend it for Types A and AB, especially if they have a history of heart disease or a family history of colon cancer. But even then, aspirin is a mixed bag, as it can mask the symptoms of a serious infection or illness.
- Some antihistamines can raise blood pressure—a particular danger for Types A and AB. They can also cause sleeplessness and exacerbate prostate problems.
- Habitual use of laxatives can actually cause constipation, disrupting the natural process of elimination. They also can be harmful for people with a history of inflammatory bowel disease or a dysregulated microbiome resulting in dysbiosis.
- Cough, throat, and chest remedies often have side effects, including high blood pressure, drowsiness, and dizziness.

Before you take an OTC remedy to treat a headache, cramps, or any other malady, investigate the possible causes of your problem. Often, it relates to your diet or stress. For example, you might ask the following:

- Is my headache a result of stress?
- Is my stomach discomfort caused by eating foods that are indigestible or inflammatory for my blood type?
- Are my sinus problems the result of mucus caused by eating too many mucus-generating foods?
- Is my flu virus the result of immune system weaknesses?
- Is my congestion or bronchitis caused by an overproduction of mucus in my respiratory passages?
- Is my overreliance on commercial laxatives interfering with natural elimination and causing diarrhea?

I urge you to seek medical attention if your symptoms are chronic or particularly severe. Pain, weakness, coughs, fever, congestion, and diarrhea all can be signs of deeper problems. You might cover them up with medications, but you won't be addressing the root cause.

For occasional aches, pains, and irregularities, the following remedies are excellent natural replacements for OTC drugs. They're available in many forms from your local health food store, drugstore or online,
including teas, compresses, liquid tinctures, extracts, powders, and capsules.

To make your own herbal tea, boil water and steep the natural herbs
for about 5 minutes.

Please note the key indicating special considerations for each blood
type.

KEY

●   TYPE O AVOID
■   TYPE A AVOID
▼   TYPE B AVOID
†   TYPE AB AVOID
★   SPECIAL NOTE FOR ALL BLOOD TYPES

HEADACHE

Chamomile   Valerian
Damiana ●   White willow bark (*Salix*)
Feverfew

SINUSITIS

Fenugreek ▼ †   Thyme

ARTHRITIS

Alfalfa ●   Epsom salt bath
Boswellia   Rosemary tea soak
Calcium

EARACHE

Garlic-mullein-olive-oil ear drops

TOOTHACHE

Crushed garlic gum   Oil-of-cloves gum massage

INDIGESTION, HEARTBURN

Bladderwrack   Ginger
Bromelain (from pineapple)   Goldenseal
Gentian ● †   Peppermint

CRAMPS, GAS

Chamomile tea   Peppermint tea
Fennel tea   Probiotic supplement
Ginger   with bifidus factor

NAUSEA

Cayenne ■   Licorice root tea
Ginger

FLU

Echinacea   Larch arabinogalactan
Garlic   Rose hip tea
Goldenseal

FEVER

Catnip ■   Vervain
Feverfew   White willow bark

COUGH

Coltsfoot ● ▼   Linden▼
Horehound

SORE THROAT

Fenugreek tea gargle ▼

Stone root, goldenseal root, and sage tea gargle

CONGESTION

Licorice tea   Nettle

Mullein ▼   Vervain

CONSTIPATION

Aloe vera juice ● ▼ †   Psyllium fiber ★★

Larch tree bark (ARA-6) ★   Slippery elm

DIARRHEA

Blueberries   *L. acidophilus* (yogurt culture)

Elderberries   Raspberry leaf

MENSTRUAL CRAMPS

Jamaican dogwood

★ This is a substance of larch tree bark in a powdered form that is available from my office under the name ARA-6. It has been tested to be an excellent natural immune system booster. Furthermore, a substance in larch tree bark, called butyrate, is a safe and effective natural source of fiber for all blood types. For more information and orders, see Appendix F.

★★ Natural fiber is available in many fruits, vegetables, and grains. Be sure to check your blood type food list before you choose a fiber source.

Vaccines: The Blood Type Sensitivities

VACCINATION is an emotionally charged issue in both the conventional and alternative medical communities. From the more orthodox viewpoint, vaccination represents the first line of defense in preventive medicine. Increasing emphasis is being placed on mandatory universal vaccination by the federal, state, and local levels of government. What are the consequences of such a strategy?

Vaccines have been of unquestioned benefit to humankind, saving millions of lives and preventing needless suffering. In the rare circumstances where there have been problems, the vaccines have sometimes reacted badly in a particularly hypersensitive individual. Our knowledge of the immune system does not yet reveal if vaccines have more profound resonances, possibly lowering some of our innate immunities to cancer. Yet many public health officials and medical scientists behave as though it were somehow unpatriotic to question whether every new vaccine must be injected into the collective national bloodstream.

Meanwhile, the public remains confused. Parents want to know which vaccines, if any, their children should be exposed to. The elderly, the hypersensitive, pregnant women, and others worry about the effects of vaccinations. It shouldn't surprise you that there is no single answer for everyone. Certain reactions to vaccines may have to do with your blood type.

When researchers or doctors speak of the flu, they are being very specific; they mean an infection by the influenza virus. Epidemic influenza is divided into influenza type A and influenza type B. The most common presentation of influenza includes a fever (usually 100 to 103°F. in adults), respiratory symptoms (such as cough, sore throat, runny or stuffy nose), headache, muscle aches, and often extreme fatigue.

In general, we can make the following observations about blood type and influenza A. Blood Types B and AB are much more susceptible to infection during times when new antigenic varieties of influenza virus appear. That's somewhat bad news because this type of influenza A virus change results in widespread flu pandemics. Blood Type O individuals tend to be susceptible to influenza infection when virulent strains are in circulation—so in years when the flu is making people feel really sick, Type O will be hit the hardest. Type As are the lucky ones when it comes to influenza A. They have a generalized susceptibility to the less virulent strains and are less likely to contract the more severe varieties.

Type O Vaccine Sensitivities

With all vaccines, parents of Type O children should be alert to any sign of inflammation, such as fever or joint pain, because the Type O immune system is more prone to these reactions. In general, parents should try to space out immunizations and not pile them up during one or two doctor's visits. Give the immune system sufficient time to adjust to the stimulation. This is analogous to listening to a lecture on geography at the same time you listen to another one on history. You'll probably not remember much of either (or, even worse, get lots of facts wrong). Too much stimulation from multiple vaccines can interfere with the proper education of the immune system.

Recently vaccinated Type O children should be watched carefully for a couple of days to ensure that there are no complications. Don't give them acetaminophen, the most commonly prescribed OTC medication for vaccination-related problems (found in Tylenol). In my experience, Type O children seem to react poorly to this drug. A natural remedy that will work for Type O is an herb called feverfew, derived from the common chrysanthemum flower (*Chrysanthemum parthenium*). It is available at most health food stores in liquid tincture form and can be given to a child every few hours. Four to eight drops of the feverfew tincture in a glass of juice is sufficient to achieve a positive effect.

If you are a pregnant woman with Type O blood, the flu vaccine holds special dangers, especially if the father of your baby is a Type A or Type AB. The flu vaccine could boost the presence of anti-A antibodies in your system, which could attack and damage your fetus. Blood Type O has a relatively effective ability to generate the natural antibody response against influenza A(H1N1) and A(H3N2) viruses. Your antibody response against influenza B is not as dramatic as seen in other blood types if you are Type O. Although most healthy adults do not require a flu shot, there is some evidence that Type O does not seroconvert (build up antibodies) well after a single dose of the flu vaccine and may in fact need two doses to build up proper immunity.

Type A and Type AB Vaccine Sensitivities

Type A and Type AB children typically respond well to vaccines. A full vaccination program—including the whooping cough vaccine—should produce few side effects, although as a rule, I recommend against aggressive scheduling. Type A tends to respond well to the typical flu vaccine, usually seroconverting after one dose. Overall, influenza is probably most problematic year to year for Type ABs. In general, they are more sensitive to infection by both influenza A and B than the other blood types. They are also affected by these viruses earlier and more severely than the other blood types and need to be extra cautious regarding an abrupt change in the influenza A virus as well.

Type B Vaccine Sensitivities

I've observed that Type B children sometimes have severe neurological reactions to vaccinations. Parents should be acutely aware of any signal indicating a complication, be it an alteration in your child's walking or crawling gait or a personality change of some kind. If you intend to vaccinate your Type B child, it is imperative that you make sure he or she is first completely healthy—free of colds, flu, or ear infections. Like Type O, Type B children should use the oral form of the polio vaccine.

Why does Type B tend to react so badly to vaccines? It may be the particular vaccine itself that causes this cross-reaction with either the Type B antigen or with opposing blood type antibodies. Or perhaps it's one of the chemicals used to enhance the vaccine's effectiveness that causes a bad reaction in Type B individuals. It might even be the culture medium used to grow the vaccine. We just don't know yet.

Type B has a reasonable, but not great, ability to generate an antibody response against influenza A(H_1N_1), but has the slowest (it can take three to five months) and weakest ability to generate antibodies against influenza A(H_3N_2) of any blood type. However, Type B has a significant advantage against influenza B virus, responding differently from either Type A or Type O. The Type B immune response happens much earlier and persists longer.

Blood Type B is going to be most severely affected when influenza A(H3N2)—also known as the Hong Kong variety—and its relatives are in circulation. Type B individuals have relatively little difficulty with influenza B but have to be very concerned about an abrupt change in the influenza A strains.

The Pros and Cons of Antibiotic Therapy

WHEN I WAS A YOUNG medical student, I was taught that the drug vancomycin was the official antibiotic of last resort: a drug, like a fire ax, to be kept in a locked glass case with a little hammer to break the glass only in an emergency. Now it is routinely prescribed for common infections, such as Lyme disease. Our misuse of the infection-fighting wonder drugs, from their overprescription for trivial colds and flu to their use in accelerating the growth of livestock, has squandered some of the greatest gifts of modern medicine. The constant misuse of antibiotics is a leading factor in our growing inability to eradicate disease. The overuse of such wonder drugs promotes the development of progressively more resistant pathogens, which require ever stronger antibiotics to treat. If your physician or your child's pediatrician often prescribes antibiotics for simple colds and flu, I have one piece of advice: Find another doctor.

Far more powerful than any of the antibiotics currently being manufactured is the natural prescription of proper diet, proper rest, and stress reduction.

Typically, there is a lag between the time you develop an infection and the time your body's immune system responds. It's like dialing the 911 emergency number; you know they aren't going to be at your door the second they answer your call. Most people don't realize that antibiotics merely allow your body to catch up with the infection by slowing down the rapid growth of pathogenic bacteria. The body and its immune system still have to do the cleanup and resolution.

We race to treat fever with antibiotics, yet fever is generally a good sign. It indicates that your body's metabolic rate has kicked into overdrive, burning out invaders by making the environment as inhospitable to infectious organisms as it possibly can. Continued and heavy use of antibiotics destroys not only the infection but all of the good bacteria in the digestive tract. Many people experience diarrhea, and quite often women become subject to recurring and persistent yeast infections.

Supplements of a friendly digestive bacteria, *L. acidophilus*, may be taken in either tablets or yogurt to restore the proper balance of bacteria in the digestive tract.

Overuse of antibiotics disrupts the microbiome. According to research published in *mBio*, a single course of antibiotics is strong enough to disrupt the normal makeup of microorganisms in the gut for up to a year, leading to resistance. The Centers for Disease Control and Prevention (CDC) has encouraged doctors to limit use of antibiotics, stating that antibiotic-resistant bacteria lead to at least 2 million cases of disease and 23,000 deaths annually in the United States.

There are, of course, times when an appropriate antibiotic is needed and should be used. If you are given an antibiotic, take a supplement of bromelain to ensure that the antibiotic spreads rapidly and penetrates tissue more readily. Pineapples contain this enzyme, so you may drink pineapple juice or take bromelain tablets when you're on a course of antibiotics.

Parents of sick children on antibiotics should set the alarm clock for 3:00 or 4:00 A.M. so they can administer an extra dose during the child's sleep cycle. This ensures a more rapid concentration of the drug to fight the infection.

Once more: If you need antibiotics, take them. If an infection becomes protracted, you certainly should consider using an antibiotic. I just think the body's immune system should be allowed to do what it's been created for—to resist.

Type O Antibiotic Sensitivities

Type O should avoid penicillin-class antibiotics, if another alternative exists. The Type O immune system is more allergically sensitive to this class of drugs. If using sulfa-class drugs, such as Bactrim, make sure that you also take a probiotic supplement.

Try to avoid macrolide-class antibiotics. Erythromycin and the newer macrolides Biaxin and Zithromax can aggravate inflammatory bowel tendencies in Type O. Be especially wary of this problem if you are currently taking blood-thinning medications such as Coumadin or warfarin, as it can increase their effects.

Type A Antibiotic Sensitivities

Carbacephem-class antibiotics seem to work well for Type A. There are very few side effects, although women should take a probiotic to prevent vaginal yeast infections. Most Type As respond well to penicillin-class and sulfa-class antibiotics. These are probably preferable to tetracycline or the newer macrolide-class antibiotics.

If a macrolide-class antibiotic is prescribed for a Type A, erythromycin is preferred over Zithromax or clarithromycin. Both of these antibiotics can cause digestive problems and dysbiosis, and interfere with iron metabolism in the Type A system.

Type AB and Type B Antibiotic Sensitivities

If you are Type AB or Type B, avoid quinolone-class antibiotics, such as Floxin and Cipro, if you can. If you must use them, take them (as Europeans do) in smaller doses than prescribed. Be aware of any sign of a nervous system disorder, such as blurred vision, confusion, dizziness, or insomnia. Discontinue the antibiotic and immediately contact your physician if these symptoms occur.

Antibiotic Therapy at the Dentist

IT IS STANDARD PRACTICE for dentists to use antibiotics as a preventive measure against infection in some patients. Patients with mitral valve prolapse, a heart condition, are almost always given a course of antibiotics to guard against any possibility of bacterial infection and subsequent valve damage. However, a study in the British medical journal *Lancet* found no benefit to a course of antibiotics for the majority of patients before invasive dental procedures.

If you are a non-secretor, you are at much greater risk than a secretor for infections after dental surgery. There are many more instances of streptococcal bacteria causing endocarditis (an inflammation of the lining of the heart muscle) and rheumatic fever in non-secretors because they produce much lower levels of protective antibodies in the mucous membranes of the mouth and throat. Secretors, on the other hand, have higher levels of these IgA antibodies, which trap bacteria and destroy them before they can gain access to the bloodstream.

Non-secretors should consider preventive antibiotic therapy before any invasive dental procedure, from deep cleaning to oral surgery. If you are Type O you may wish to opt out of antibiotic therapy, unless there is deep-rooted infection or the promise of heavy bleeding. Instead, try herbal medications with antistrep activity, such as goldenseal (*Hydrastis canadensis*).

Type A, Type B, and Type AB individuals may wish to discuss alternative therapies with their dentist or physician if they respond poorly to antibiotics.

Many dentists will refuse to treat a patient who declines the prophylactic use of antibiotics. If you are a healthy individual with no prior history of infections, you might want to consider going elsewhere for your dental work.

Surgery: Better Recovery

ANY INVASIVE PROCEDURE is a shock to your system. Never take it lightly, even if it is a minor surgery. Tune up your immune system in advance, no matter what your blood type.

Vitamins A and C have a profound effect on wound healing and minimize the formation of scar tissue. Every blood type can benefit from supplementation before surgery. Start taking vitamins A and C at least four or five days before surgery, and continue for at least a week afterward. All of my patients who have followed this recommendation report that both they and their surgeons were astonished at the rapidity of their recovery.

RECOMMENDED SURGICAL SUPPLEMENTATION PROTOCOL		
Blood Type	*Daily Vitamin C*	*Daily Vitamin A*
TYPE O	2,000 MG	30,000 IU
TYPE A	500 MG	10,000 IU
TYPE AB, TYPE B	1,000 MG	20,000 IU

Type O Surgical Cautions

Type Os often experience greater blood loss than other blood types during and after surgery because of lower levels of serum clotting factors. Make sure that you have plenty of vitamin K in your system before surgery; it is essential to clot formation. Kale, spinach, and collard greens contain ample amounts of this vitamin, although you might want to supplement your diet with liquid chlorophyll. Chlorophyll supplements are available at most health food stores.

Type O individuals can also boost their immune system and metabolism with strong physical activity. If it is realistic for you to pursue this before surgery, exercise will allow your body to deal with the stress of surgery much more effectively and will help you heal more rapidly.

Type B Surgical Cautions

Type B is fortunate, being less likely to experience postsurgical complications. The vitamin A and C protocol given earlier should be followed.

Type Bs who are suffering from a weakened condition may also want to use immune-boosting herbal teas before surgery. Burdock root (*Arctium lappa*) and purple coneflower (*Echinacea purpurea*) are excellent immune boosters. A few cups of tea taken every day over a number of weeks can be a positive stimulant for your immune system.

Type A and Type AB Surgical Cautions

Type A and Type AB individuals are more prone to postsurgical bacterial infections. These infections can become a major stumbling block to recovery and can exacerbate an already difficult situation. I strongly suggest that Type A and Type AB adopt a blood-building, immune system–enhancing protocol of additional vitamin supplementation a week or two before surgery. Vitamin B_{12}, folic acid, and supplemental iron should all be taken daily along with the already suggested levels of vitamins A and C. The concentration of vitamins you need to achieve is difficult to squeeze out of the Type A and Type AB diets, so supplementation is best.

Floradix is a liquid iron and herb source that is both gentle on the digestive tract and highly assimilable. I strongly recommend its use for iron supplementation because iron is usually an irritant to the digestive tracts of Type A and Type AB. Floradix is found in most health food stores.

Avail yourself of the two excellent immune-enhancing herbal teas, burdock root and echinacea. Drink a few cups daily of these herbal teas at least a couple of weeks before surgery.

Relaxation techniques, such as meditation and visualization, can be of tremendous benefit to Type A and Type AB patients, as it has been shown in studies that stress can increase blood thickness (viscosity) in these blood types. Increased viscosity can result in a greater risk of complications, such as postsurgical blood clots. By taking the advice here, you can have a profound influence on your own healing process. Some anesthesiologists will work with patients on visualizations while the patient is under anesthesia. I urge you to ask your doctor about this.

After the Surgery

MARIGOLD (*Calendula succus*) is used to help the wound heal and keep it clean for all blood types. A solution of this homeopathic herb—a form of the marigold flower—is a wonderful healer for all cuts and scrapes in general. The juice has mild antibiotic properties and can be left on after application. Be sure you buy the juice, or succus, and not the calendula tincture, which has a high alcohol content. The tincture will really sting if you try to clean a wound with it.

As your incision heals and after the stitches or staples are removed, a topical vitamin E preparation will minimize scar tissue formation and skin tightening. Many people just snip open a vitamin E capsule and smear it on their skin, but oral supplements aren't formulated for use as skin healers. Use a topical cream or lotion blended for just this purpose.

Listen to Your Blood Type

There are many vitamins and herbal supplements that aid the body in both defending and healing itself. The recommended surgical supplementation is just the minimum you should do to protect and strengthen yourself. Each of the Blood Type Diets contains pertinent information that allows you to make reasoned choices about what you should and should not eat and drink. All of these choices can have a profound effect on your health and the quality of your life. By making knowledgeable choices about what is best for your body, you will be able to dramatically affect the course of your recovery from surgery. This not only grants you greater control over your present circumstances, but enables you to ensure your future health.

Parents whose children are of vaccination age, people who have viral infections, those facing surgery—everyone can achieve benefits from an awareness of the blood type connection. It makes sense. It also solves the puzzle of why some people do very well with conventional treatments, while others suffer complications and pain. I urge you to put yourself in the position of being someone who does well.

ELEVEN

Blood Type:

A Power over Disease

EVERYONE WHO GETS SICK WANTS TO KNOW, WHY ME? EVEN WITH our enormous technological arsenal, we often have no certain answer to that question. It has become clear, however, that there are individuals who are more prone to certain diseases because of their blood type. Perhaps this is the missing link—the way we can understand the cellular causes of disease and devise ways to combat and eliminate it more effectively.

Time and again I've found that people with the most profound long-term results on the Blood Type Diet are those who have suffered from medical conditions. Being sick gives you a barometer of where you are and how to judge results and changes within your body.

Why Some People Are Susceptible . . . and Some Are Not

CAN YOU REMEMBER being young and having a close friend who wanted you to do something that you were reluctant to do? Take a puff of a forbidden cigarette? Sneak a drink of whiskey from your father's liquor cabinet? Did you take that puff? Drink that whiskey? If you did, you exhibited your susceptibility—your lack of resistance—to the suggestion of a friend.

Susceptibility, or lack of resistance, is the basic issue with most disease. The word is derived from the Latin *suscipio*, which means "I take up." Many microbes have the ability to mimic antigens that are considered friendly by the security force of a particular blood type. These clever mimics bypass the security guards and gain entry. Once in the system, they quickly overwhelm it and take control.

Don't you ever wonder why one person stays perfectly healthy while everyone else is falling prey to the latest cold or flu? It is because the healthy person's blood type is not susceptible to those particular invaders.

The Blood Type Connection

THERE ARE MANY causal factors for disease that are clearly influenced by blood type. For instance, Type A individuals with a family history of cardiovascular disease should examine their diets very carefully. Red meats and saturated fats of all kinds are poor choices. The Type A digestive tract has difficulty processing these foods, and the result is higher levels of both triglycerides and cholesterol. The friendly Type A immune system is also more prone to cancer because it has a hard time recognizing foes.

Type O, as I've said, is very sensitive to the agglutinating lectin found in whole wheat. This lectin interacts with the lining of the Type O intestinal tract and produces additional inflammation. If you're Type O and suffer from Crohn's disease, colitis, or irritable bowel syndrome, wheat acts like a poison in your system. Although the Type O immune system is generally hardy, it is also somewhat rigid and limited.

The disease profile of Type B is independent of Type O and Type A by virtue of the idiosyncratic B antigen. Type B tends to be susceptible to slow-moving viral diseases that don't manifest themselves for many years—such as multiple sclerosis and rare neurological ailments, sometimes triggered by the lectins in foods such as chicken and corn.

Type AB has the most complex disease profile because they possess both A-like and B-like antigens. Most of their disease susceptibilities are A-like, so if you had to categorize them you would say they were more A than B. Type AB immune systems have to work a bit harder to make up for the lack of any opposing blood type antibodies.

The blood type connection between good health and disease is a potent tool in our search for the best way to treat the body as it is meant to be treated. Still, I must add a caveat, lest you think that I am proposing a magic formula. There are many factors in every individual life that contribute to disease. It would be overly simplistic and certainly foolish to suggest that blood type is the sole determining factor. If a Type O, a Type A, a Type B, and a Type AB each drank a cup of arsenic, they would all die. By the same token, if four people of different blood types were all heavy smokers, they would all be susceptible to lung cancer. The blood type information is not a panacea but a meaningful refinement that will enable you to function at your peak.

Let's turn to the most common and troubling diseases and conditions for which we can identify a blood type relationship. Some blood type–disease relationships are more clearly defined than others. We are still learning, but every day blood type is revealed as a critical factor—the previously missing link in our quest for health.

CATEGORIES*

- AGING DISEASES
- ALLERGIES
- ASTHMA AND HAY FEVER
- AUTOIMMUNE DISORDERS
- BLOOD DISORDERS
- CARDIOVASCULAR DISEASE
- CHILDHOOD ILLNESSES
- DIABETES
- DIGESTIVE ILLNESSES
- INFECTIONS
- LIVER DISEASE
- SKIN DISORDERS
- WOMEN/REPRODUCTION

Note: Cancer is such a complex topic that I have devoted an entire chapter to it (see Chapter Twelve).

Aging Diseases

All people age, no matter what their blood type. But why do we age—and can we slow down the process? These questions have fascinated us for as long as we can remember. The promise of a Fountain of Youth has appeared in every century. Today, with our sophisticated medical technology and our increased knowledge of the factors that contribute to aging, we are closer to an answer.

But there's another question: Why do individual aging patterns differ so greatly? Why does the 50-year-old runner, lean and seemingly fit, drop dead of a heart attack, while the 89-year-old woman who has never broken a sweat in her life remains hale and hardy? Why do some people develop Alzheimer's disease or dementia, while others do not? At what age does physical deterioration become inevitable?

We understand some pieces of the puzzle. Genetics plays a role; unique variations in chromosomes contribute to susceptibilities that cause deterioration more rapidly in one person than in another.

New studies offer clues to a blood type connection in the instances of declining mental function. These studies have begun to show a definite link between blood type and neurological diseases associated with aging. Researchers at the University of Sheffield in England found that Blood Type O has more gray matter in the brain, offering stronger protection against diseases like Alzheimer's and dementia than the other blood types. In particular, Type O has more gray matter in the posterior area of the cerebellum, and people with Blood Types A, B, and AB have less gray matter in the areas of the brain dealing with memory formation.

In a separate study, published in *Brain and Mental Performance Diagnostics*, researchers found a strong connection between Blood Type AB and memory loss leading to dementia—an 82 percent likelihood over the other blood types. The researchers focused on higher levels of blood clotting factor in Blood Type AB.

We also know that different blood types have special risk factors that can exacerbate medical conditions as you age. For example, Blood Type O is susceptible to inflammatory diseases, which affect the elderly. Blood Type A's tendency toward high cortisol levels is linked to heart disease and lowered immunity. Blood Type B individuals are at risk from slow-moving viruses and neuromuscular problems that can appear and worsen as you age. Blood Type AB's increased blood clotting factors can heighten the risk of strokes from embolism.

A critical link between blood type and aging is the correlation between the agglutinating action of lectins and the biggest physiological association with aging—inflammation. Inflammation has manifestations in virtually all aspects of aging, but we'll look at just two: the brain and the kidneys.

As we age we experience a gradual drop in kidney function so that by the time the average person reaches age 72, his or her kidneys are operating at only 25 percent of their capacity.

Your kidney function is a reflection of the volume of blood that gets cleaned and recirculated into your bloodstream. This filtering system is very delicate—large enough for the various fluid elements of blood to go through but small enough to prevent whole cells from passing through.

Consider the way that lectins can gum up the works. They can induce inflammation and permeability in the gut, which can allow bacteria and allergens access into the lymphatics and circulation. These toxins can then react with the antibodies normally found in the bloodstream and create an immune complex. Immune complexes solidify and float around in the bloodstream, eventually arriving at the kidney where they can clog up the kidney's delicate filtration device, called the glomerulus. Because the kidneys play a central role in the purification of blood, the action of these immune complexes can, over time, upset the delicate process. The process is similar to having a clogged drain. Eventually, the filtration system ceases to function. As more and more deposition occurs, less and less blood is able to be cleaned. It is a slow process, but ultimately deadly. Kidney failure is one of the leading causes of physical deterioration in the elderly.

The second large physiological association with aging occurs in the brain. Here lectins may play an equally destructive role. We know that Alzheimer's disease, the most common form of dementia, is associated with plaques and tangles in the brain. Plaques are dense, mostly insoluble deposits of a peptide called beta-amyloid and cellular material around the neuron. Tangles are bundles of a protein called protein tau, which accumulate inside the cells. The real cause of the onset is unknown, although there is a strong genetic correlation. One factor may be lectins in the diet. Studies have shown that the brain cells of Alzheimer's patients combine a sugar with protein or fat—or "glycosylate"—differently than do normal cells. This can make them more receptive to binding with lectins, and can go on to alter the shapes of many proteins. Lectins that reach the systemic circulation—a part of the cardiovascular system that carries blood to and from the heart—can also stimulate inflammation of the delicate lining of the blood vessels, a process that often causes inflammation of the surrounding tissues.

It is clear to me that by reducing or eliminating the most harmful lectins from your diet, you can maintain healthier kidneys and brain function for a longer period of time. That is one reason some very old people remain mentally sharp and physically active.

A third way that lectins contribute to aging is their effects on our hormonal and assimilation functions. It is well documented that as people age they have more trouble absorbing and metabolizing nutrients. Many, many dietary lectins can act as antinutrients, blocking the proper uptake of other elements in the diet, such as proteins, minerals, and vitamins. That's one reason elderly people often become malnourished, even when they are eating their normal diet. Dietary guidelines usually call for added supplementation for the elderly, but if agglutinating lectins are not overwhelming the system and interfering with hormonal activity, it is likely that elderly people can absorb nutrients as effectively as when they were younger.

I am not proposing that the Blood Type Diet is the Fountain of Youth! It is not a formula for reversing the effects of aging that have already occurred. But you can reduce cellular damage by reducing your lectin intake at any age. Most of all, your Blood Type Diet is designed to be age sparing—enabling you to slow down the process of aging during your entire adult life.

Allergies

Food

In my opinion, no area of alternative medicine is as shot full of humbug as the concept of food allergy. Complex and expensive tests are conducted on practically every patient, resulting in a list of foods to which that person is allergic.

My own patients habitually term any reaction to something they've eaten as a food allergy, although most of the time it is not an allergy they are describing but, rather, a food *intolerance*. If you have a problem with lactose in milk, for example, you are not allergic to it; you lack an enzyme to break it down. You are lactose intolerant, not lactose allergic. This intolerance does not necessarily mean you'll get sick if you drink milk. Type Bs who are lactose intolerant, for example, are often able to gradually introduce small amounts of cultured milk products into their diets. There are also products that add the lactose enzyme to milk products, making them more palatable for the intolerant.

Although the basis of food allergy testing is scientifically valid, sometimes the interpretation is not. Patients have come in with food allergy results that did not show a reaction to foods that they have already had a profound allergic reaction to. Other tests show a food allergy exists, but the patient has eaten the food for years and never had any problems with it. Oftentimes it seems the antibody is being linked to a food protein when in fact it may well be a common protein shared among foods and microbes in the gut.

True food allergies exist, but the effects of a food allergy do not occur in the digestive tract but in the immune system. Your immune system literally creates an antibody to a food. The reaction is swift and harsh—rashes, swelling, cramps, or other specific symptoms that indicate your body is struggling to rid itself of the food it is allergic to.

Food allergies don't just affect the gut. Dietary lectins have been shown to produce immunoglobulin E (IgE), an antibody that triggers allergic reactions, which is why people who follow the Blood Type Diet have a lessening of sinus and asthma symptoms. Each Blood Type Diet is rich in natural antioxidants called flavones, which block specialized cells called basophils from releasing IgE unnecessarily.

Not everything in nature is perfectly cut and dried. Allergic reactions can be genetic, and those genes can be independent of your blood type. Occasionally, I'll come across a person who is allergic to a food that is on his Blood Type Diet. The solution? Simply remove the offending food. The main point is that you have more to fear from the hidden lectins entering your system than you do from food allergies. You may not feel sick when you eat the food, but it is affecting your system nonetheless. Type A should also be aware of excessive mucus production. What may appear to be an allergy is actually the result of eating mucus-producing foods.

ASTHMA AND HAY FEVER

Type Os win the allergy sweepstakes hands down. They are more likely to suffer from asthma. Even hay fever, the bane of so many, appears to be specific to Type O blood. A wide range of pollens contain lectins that stimulate the release of the powerful histamines, and boom! Itching, sneezing, runny nose, wheezing, coughing, watery eyes—all allergy symptoms.

Many food lectins, especially wheat, interact with IgE antibodies found in the blood. These antibodies stimulate basophils to release not only histamines but other powerful chemical allergens called kinins. These can cause severe allergic reactions, such as swelling in throat tissues and constriction in the lungs.

Asthma and hay fever sufferers do best when they follow the diet recommended for their blood type. For example, a Type O who eliminates wheat and corn often finds relief of many symptoms, such as sneezing, respiratory problems, snoring, and persistent digestive disorders.

Type As have a different problem. Instead of environmental reactions, they often develop stress-related asthma as a result of their stress profile, particularly high cortisol levels. When a Type A suffers from excessive production of mucus caused by poor dietary choices, it makes the stress-related asthma worse. In addition, Type As naturally produce copious amounts of mucus, and when they eat foods that are mucus producing (such as uncultured dairy), they'll have more respiratory problems. When Type A is careful to avoid mucus-producing foods, and when the causes of the stress are addressed positively, the asthmatic condition always improves or is eliminated.

By design, Type B appears to be less prone to developing allergies— unless the wrong foods are eaten. For example, chicken and corn lectins may trigger allergies in even the most resistant Type B.

Type ABs seem to have the least problem with allergies, probably because their immune system is the most environmentally friendly. The combination of A-like and B-like antigens gives Type AB a double dose of antigens with which to deal with environmental intrusion.

Autoimmune Disorders

Autoimmune disorders are immune-system breakdowns. Your immune defenses develop what amounts to severe amnesia; they no longer recognize themselves. The result is that they run amok, making autoantibodies, which attack their own tissues. These warlike autoantibodies think they are protecting their turf, but in reality they are destroying their own organs and inciting inflammatory responses. Examples of autoimmune disease are rheumatoid arthritis, lupus nephritis, many forms of kidney disease, and possibly elements of chronic fatigue syndrome (Epstein-Barr virus), multiple sclerosis, and amyotrophic lateral sclerosis (ALS, also known as Lou Gehrig's disease).

ARTHRITIS

My father observed many years ago that Type O tended to develop a gritty sort of arthritis, a chronic deterioration of the bone cartilage. This is the kind of arthritic condition called osteoarthritis, typically found in the elderly. The Type O immune system is environmentally intolerant, and there are many foods—grains and potatoes among them—whose lectins induce inflammatory reactions in the joints. Also, if a Type O individual has had a lifetime of insufficient protein intake, there may be extensive bone demineralization. Remember, Type O needs a reasonable amount of protein and fat in the diet to activate the calcium-absorbing enzyme in the gut.

Type A tends to develop a puffy arthritis, which is the more acute rheumatoid form of the disease—a painful and debilitating breakdown of multiple joints.

In my own practice, most of my patients who suffer from rheumatoid arthritis are Type A. The anomaly of Type A, with its immunological tolerance, developing this form of arthritis may be related to A-specific lectins. Laboratory animals injected with lectins known to react with the A antigen developed inflammation and joint destruction that was indistinguishable from rheumatoid arthritis. Just as likely, there is a stress connection. Some studies show that people with rheumatoid arthritis tend to be more high-strung, more prone to sleep disturbance, and less emotionally hardy. Many of these are the same symptoms of a dysregulated cortisol metabolism, a tendency common in Type A. When Type As have poor coping mechanisms for life stress, the disease progresses more rapidly. This makes some sense in light of what we know about the stress factor and about the risks for Type A. Type A individuals with rheumatoid arthritis should certainly incorporate daily relaxation techniques, as well as calming exercises.

CHRONIC FATIGUE SYNDROME

In recent years, I have treated many people who suffered from the baffling disease called chronic fatigue syndrome (CFS). The primary symptom is great tiredness. Other more advanced symptoms include painful muscles and joints, persistent sore throats, digestive problems, allergies, and chemical sensitivities. The most important thing I've learned from my research and clinical work is that CFS may not be an exclusively autoimmune disease at all, but rather a detoxification issue, caused by poor liver metabolism and the inability to neutralize harmful chemicals. To my reasoning, only this sort of liver problem could produce immunological effects as well as effects characteristic of other systems, such as digestive or musculoskeletal.

I've found that Type O CFS patients in particular do very well on licorice and potassium supplements, in addition to the Blood Type Diet. Licorice has many effects in the body, but in the liver it really shines. The bile ducts, where detoxification occurs, become more efficient, offering greater protection against chemical damage. This preliminary removal of stress to the liver seems to positively influence the adrenals and blood sugar, increasing energy and producing a feeling of well-being. The blood type–specific exercise activities also seem to serve as a valuable guide to help patients return to appropriate forms of physical activity. (Note: Please do not use licorice without a physician's supervision.)

CASE HISTORY: CHRONIC FATIGUE SYNDROME
from Dr. John Prentice, Everett, Washington
KAREN, AGE 44; BLOOD TYPE B

My colleague Dr. John Prentice tried the Blood Type Diet for the first time on a patient with severe CFS. He wasn't totally convinced it would work, but all efforts to help his very sick patient had failed, and he contacted me when he heard of the work I was doing with CFS patients.

Karen was a tough case. She had suffered terrible fatigue for her entire adult life and had needed 12 hours of sleep every night since she was a teenager. She would steal naps when she could. For the past seven years her exhaustion prevented her from holding a job. In addition, her neck, shoulders, and back were constantly in pain, and she suffered debilitating headaches. Recently, Karen had started experiencing terrible anxiety attacks, with heart palpitations so severe she would call 911. It felt as if her circulation was shutting down, along with her whole body.

Karen was a wealthy woman, but most of her inheritance was spent on making the rounds to doctors. She had been to more than 50 doctors, both conventional and alternative, before she came to Dr. Prentice.

Dr. Prentice started Karen on a program of strict adherence to the Type B Diet, supplements, and exercise regimen. Both he and Karen were astonished to see that within only a week she had a tremendous increase in energy. Within a few weeks, most of her symptoms were resolved.

Dr. Prentice tells me that today Karen is a new person. "It's like clockwork," he says. "When she eats 'off' her diet, her body reminds her with severe symptoms, so she sticks with it closely." He shared a letter she had written to him: "I have a whole new life. All my symptoms are practically gone and I hold two jobs, having great energy fourteen hours a day consistently. I believe the diet is key to this tremendous change. I am extremely active and feel like nothing can stop me. Thank you so very much!"

MULTIPLE SCLEROSIS, LOU GEHRIG'S DISEASE

Both multiple sclerosis (MS) and Lou Gehrig's disease (ALS) appear to be more frequent in Blood Type B. It's an example of the Type B tendency to contract unusual slow-growing viral and neurological disorders. The Type B association may explain why many Jewish populations, which have high percentages of Type B individuals, suffer from these diseases more than other groups. Some researchers believe that multiple sclerosis and Lou Gehrig's disease are caused by a virus, contracted in youth, that has a stealthy B-like appearance. The virus cannot be combated by Type Bs since they do not produce anti-B antibodies. The virus grows slowly and produces no symptoms for 20 or more years. From there it activates the more generalized parts of the immune system to produce inflammation and destruction of the myelin sheathing around nerve cells. Another possibility is that because Type B appears to produce nitric oxide easier than Type O and Type A, the reaction to the causative factors (viral, etc.) may be more intense, leading to greater inflammation and nerve cell death. Type ABs are also at risk for MS and ALS because they share many of the same tendencies regarding the production of nitric oxide.

CASE HISTORY: AUTOIMMUNE DISORDER
JOAN, AGE 55; BLOOD TYPE O

Joan, a middle-aged dentist's wife, was a classic example of an individual living with the ravages of autoimmune disorders. She suffered from severe symptoms of chronic fatigue/Epstein-Barr, arthritis, and tremendous discomfort caused by gas and bloating. Joan's digestive system was so disrupted that practically everything she ate caused bouts of diarrhea. By the time she arrived in my office, she had been struggling with these conditions for more than a year. Needless to say, she was terribly weakened and in great pain. She was also very discouraged. Because autoimmune disorders can be hard to pin down, many people (even some physicians) don't believe those who suffer from autoimmune diseases like CFS are really sick. Imagine the humiliation and frustration of feeling deathly ill but having people tell you it's all in your head!

Worse still, Joan's doctors had experimented with a number of drug therapies, including steroids, which made her even sicker and contributed to her bloating. She had also been told to adopt a diet high in grains and vegetables, and to limit or eliminate red meat—exactly the opposite of what this Type O should have been doing.

As severe as Joan's symptoms were, the treatment was fairly simple—a detoxification program, the Type O Diet, and a regimen of nutritional supplements. Within two weeks, Joan experienced significant improvement. By the six-month mark, she was feeling normal again. To this day, Joan's energy level is good, her digestion is healthy, and her arthritis flares up only when she binges on carbs and dairy products.

CASE HISTORY: LUPUS
From Dr. Thomas Kruzel, Gresham, Oregon
MARCIA, AGE 30; BLOOD TYPE A

My colleague Dr. Kruzel was interested in trying the blood type treatments, but he was initially skeptical. It was a case of lupus nephritis that showed him the true value of serotyping for the treatment of disease.

Marcia, a frail young woman suffering from lupus, was carried into Dr. Kruzel's office by her brother after being discharged from the hospital's intensive care unit. She had suffered kidney failure from circulating immune complexes related to her disease. Marcia had been on shunt dialysis for several weeks and was scheduled for renal transplantation within the next six months.

Dr. Kruzel took her history and learned that Marcia's diet was very high in dairy, wheat, and red meat—all dangerous foods for a Type A person in her condition. He placed her on a strict vegetarian diet along with hydrotherapy and homeopathic preparations. Within two weeks, Marcia's condition had improved and her need for dialysis had decreased. Remarkably, within a two-month period, Marcia was taken completely off dialysis and her previously scheduled kidney transplant was canceled.

Blood Disorders

It should come as no surprise that blood-related illnesses, such as anemia and clotting disorders, are blood type specific.

Pernicious Anemia

Type A makes up the greatest number of pernicious anemia sufferers, but the condition has nothing to do with the vegetarian Type A Diet. Pernicious anemia is the result of a vitamin B_{12} deficiency, and Type A has the most difficulty absorbing B_{12} from food. Type AB also has a tendency toward pernicious anemia, although not as great as Type A.

The reason for the deficiency is that the body's use of vitamin B_{12} requires high levels of stomach acid and the presence of intrinsic factor, a chemical produced by the lining of the stomach that is responsible for the vitamin's assimilation. Type A and Type AB have lower levels of intrinsic factor than the other blood types and don't produce as much stomach acid. For this reason, most Type As and Type ABs who suffer from pernicious anemia respond best when vitamin B_{12} is administered by injection. By eliminating the need for the digestive process to assimilate this vital and potent nutrient, it is made available to the body in a more highly concentrated way. This is a case in which dietary solutions alone don't work, although Type A and Type AB are able to absorb Floradix, a liquid iron and herb supplement.

Given a proper diet, Type O and Type B tend not to suffer from anemia; they have high acid contents in their stomachs and sufficient levels of intrinsic factor.

Case History: Anemia
From Dr. Jonathan V. Wright, Kent, Washington
Carol, Age 35; Blood Type O

My colleague Dr. Jonathan Wright successfully used the Blood Type Diet to treat a woman with chronically low blood levels of iron. Carol had tried every available form of iron supplement with no success, and Dr. Wright had tried a number of other treatments also without success. The only thing that worked at all was injectable iron, but that was only a temporary solution. Her iron levels would inevitably drop again.

I had talked to Dr. Wright on an earlier occasion about my work with lectins and blood types, and he called me for more details. He decided to try the Blood Type O Diet for Carol. After eliminating the incompatible lectins, which may have been damaging her red blood cells, and adhering to a high–animal protein diet, Carol improved; her blood iron levels started to rise and the previously ineffective supplementation started to help. Dr. Wright and I agreed that the agglutination of the intestinal tract by the incompatible food lectins prevented the iron from assimilating.

CLOTTING DISORDERS

Type O faces the biggest problems when it comes to blood clotting. Most often, Type O lacks sufficient quantities of the various blood-clotting factors. This can have severe consequences, especially during surgery or in situations where there is blood loss. Type O women, for example, tend to lose significantly more blood after childbirth than women of other blood types.

Type Os with a history of bleeding disorders and stroke should emphasize foods containing chlorophyll to help modify their clotting factors. Chlorophyll is found in almost all green vegetables and also can be taken as a supplement.

In studies, Type A and Type AB individuals tend to predominate with clotting disorders, and their thicker blood can work to their disadvantage in other ways. Thicker blood is more likely to induce inflammation in the arteries—one reason Type A and AB are more prone to cardiovascular diseases. Type A and Type AB women might have problems with heavy clotting during menstrual periods if they don't keep their diets under control. Several diseases have been shown to increase the already high blood viscosity (thickness) in Type A and AB individuals, including cancer, diabetes, peripheral artery disease and stress—another reason to practice targeted stress reduction techniques such as yoga and tai chi.

Type Bs tend not to suffer from clotting disorders or thick blood. As long as they follow the Blood Type B Diet, their balanced systems work efficiently.

Cardiovascular Disease

Cardiovascular disease is epidemic in Western societies, with many factors to blame, including diet, lack of exercise, smoking, and stress.

Is there a connection between your blood type and your susceptibility to cardiovascular disease? When researchers associated with the famous Framingham [Massachusetts] Heart Study examined the connection between blood type and heart disease, they found no clear-cut blood type distinction in terms of who gets heart disease. They did, however, discover a strong connection between blood type and who survives heart disease. The study found that Type O heart patients between the ages of 39 and 72 had a much higher rate of survival than Type A heart patients in the same age group. This was especially true for men between the ages of 50 and 59.

Although the Framingham Heart Study did not explore this subject in real depth, it appears that the same factors involved in surviving heart disease also offer some protection against developing it in the first place. While Type A and Type AB have a higher risk for cardiovascular disease, in general, research and clinical practice also show that the pathway to cardiovascular disease differs depending on your blood type.

High cholesterol is more likely to be a high risk factor for coronary artery disease for Type A and Type AB. Most of the cholesterol in our bodies is produced in our livers, but there is an enzyme called phosphatase manufactured in the small intestine that is responsible for the absorption of dietary fats. High alkaline phosphatase levels, which speed the absorption and metabolism of fats, lead to low serum cholesterol levels. Type O blood normally has the highest natural levels of this enzyme, followed by Type B. Type AB and Type A have lower levels of alkaline phosphatase enzyme. Type A and, to a slightly lesser extent, Type AB have consistently higher levels of serum cholesterol and triglycerides (blood fats) than do Type O and Type B blood. In this case, Type O's "thin" blood, the result of fewer blood clotting factors, is actually protective against plaque deposits.

That is not to say that Blood Types O and B don't have risk factors for cardiovascular disease. Diets high in carbohydrates lead to insulin resistance, obesity, and high triglycerides. Increasing evidence shows that high triglycerides are as great a risk factor for heart disease as high cholesterol. Certain stress profiles, such as the "Type A personality," characterized by excessive anger, anxiety, and aggression, have been associated with a greater incidence of heart disease. As we've discovered, it is rather ironic that such behavior is in fact associated with

Type O blood. Progressive and strenuous exercise is the best way for Type Os to bulletproof themselves against heart disease.

CASE HISTORY: HEART DISEASE
WILMA, AGE 52; BLOOD TYPE O

Wilma was a 52-year-old Lebanese woman with advanced cardiovascular disease. When I first examined her, she had recently come out of the hospital after receiving a balloon angioplasty, a procedure used to treat clogged coronary arteries.

Since Wilma was Type O, I was fairly certain that her problem was mainly dietary.

Wilma had always eaten the traditional Lebanese diet, including lots of grains and fish. However, five years earlier, she began to experience pain in her neck and arms. Heart disease didn't even occur to her! She assumed the pain was arthritis and was stunned when her doctor diagnosed her problem as angina pectoris, pain caused from an inadequate blood and oxygen supply to the heart muscle.

After her angioplasty, Wilma's cardiologist advised her to begin taking a statin to lower cholesterol. A well-read health consumer, Wilma worried about long-term problems with drug therapy, and she wanted to try a natural approach before opting for the drug. That's when she came to me.

Since Wilma was Type O, I suggested that she add lean red meat to her diet. In light of her condition, she was understandably nervous about eating foods that are usually restricted in people with high cholesterol or heart disease. She immediately consulted her cardiologist, who was—no surprise—appalled at the idea. Again, he urged her to take the statin medication. But Wilma was serious about avoiding drug therapy, so she decided to follow the Blood Type O Diet for three months and do a cholesterol check at that time.

Wilma confirmed many of my theories about susceptibility to high cholesterol. Often, through heredity or by other mechanisms, people have high levels of cholesterol in their blood in spite of a severely restricted diet. Usually they have some defect in the manipulation of the internal cholesterol metabolism. My suspicion is that when Type O individuals eat a lot of certain carbohydrates (usually wheat products), it modifies the effectiveness of their insulin, resulting in its becoming more potent and longer lasting. From the increased insulin activity, the body stores more fat in the tissues and elevates the triglyceride stores.

In addition to advising Wilma to increase the percentage of red meat in her diet, I also helped her find substitutes for the large amounts of wheat she was consuming and prescribed an extract of hawthorn (an herb used as a tonic for the heart and arteries) and a low dose of the B vitamin niacin (which helps reduce cholesterol levels).

Wilma was an executive secretary with a stressful job, and she did very little exercise. She was intrigued when I described the relationship between stress and physical activity in people with Type O blood as well as the relationship between stress and heart disease. She had never been a regular exerciser, so hardly knew where to begin. I started her on a walking program to gradually increase her aerobic fitness. After a couple of weeks, Wilma reported that walking was a godsend; she'd never felt better.

Within six months Wilma's cholesterol plummeted, without medication, to 187, where it stabilized. She was elated to have cholesterol in the normal range. It had seemed impossible.

The naturopath intern working in my office was astounded and perplexed. All conventional evidence indicates that people with high cholesterol should avoid red meats, yet Wilma flourished. Blood type was the missing link.

CASE HISTORY: DANGEROUSLY HIGH CHOLESTEROL
JOHN, AGE 23; BLOOD TYPE O

John, a recent college graduate, had a skyrocketing cholesterol level, high triglycerides, and high blood sugar. These were very unusual symptoms for a young man, but as there was a strong family history of heart disease, naturally his parents were alarmed. After extensive workups at Yale by consulting cardiologists, John was told that his genetic predisposition was so overwhelming that even cholesterol-reducing medication would be useless. In effect, John was told that he was destined to develop coronary artery disease—sooner, rather than later.

In the office, John seemed depressed and lethargic. He complained of severe fatigue. "I used to love to work out," he said, "but now I just don't have the energy." John also suffered from frequent sore throats and swollen glands. His past history revealed mononucleosis and two separate incidences of Lyme disease.

John had been following a vegetarian diet prescribed by his cardiologist for some time. He admitted, however, that he was feeling worse on this diet, not better.

After only a few weeks on the Blood Type O Diet, however, the results were amazing. Within five months, John's serum cholesterol, triglycerides, and blood sugar all dropped to normal levels. A repeat blood profile after three months revealed similar results.

If John continues to follow the Blood Type O Diet, exercise regularly, and take nutritional supplements, there is a good chance that he will beat the odds of his genetic inheritance.

Constantly at work within us is the dynamic force of our beating hearts, rhythmically pumping blood through our bodies. The process is normally so smooth that we rarely think much about it. That's why high blood pressure (or hypertension) is called the silent killer. It's possible to have dangerously high blood pressure and be entirely unaware of it.

When blood pressure is taken, two numbers are read. The systolic reading (the number on top) measures the pressure within the arteries as your heart beats out blood. The diastolic reading (the number on the bottom) measures the pressure present within the arteries as your heart rests between beats. Normal systolic pressure is below 120, and normal diastolic pressure is below 80. Elevated blood pressure is any number above 120/80, with high blood pressure (or hypertension) at 140/90.

Depending on the severity and duration, high blood pressure left untreated opens the door to a host of problems, including heart attacks and strokes. Hypertension often occurs in conjunction with heart disease, so Type A and Type AB should be particularly vigilant. Hypertension carries the same risk factors as cardiovascular disease. Smokers, diabetics, postmenopausal women, the obese, the sedentary, and people in stressful positions should pay extra attention to the details of their Blood Type Diet.

CASE HISTORY: HYPERTENSION
BILL, AGE 54; BLOOD TYPE A

Bill was a middle-aged bond trader with high blood pressure. When I first saw him in my office, his blood pressure was an almost explosive 150/105 to 135/95. It didn't take me long to find clues to these numbers in his incredibly stressful life, which included a partnership in a high-powered firm and a host of domestic problems. Against his doctor's urging, Bill had discontinued his blood pressure medication because it made him dizzy and constipated. He wanted to try a more natural therapy, but it had to be done immediately.

I placed Bill on a Blood Type A Diet—a huge adjustment for this burly Italian-American. And I immediately began to address Bill's stress with the exercise regimen designed for Type As. He was initially embarrassed about doing yoga and relaxation exercises, but was soon converted when he saw how much calmer and more positive he felt.

At his first visit, Bill also confided that he had a special problem of a different nature. He and his partners were in the process of negotiating their office health plan, and if his hypertension were detected at his insurance physical, his firm would have to pay a much higher premium. Using the stress-reduction techniques, the Blood Type A Diet, and several botanicals, Bill was able to sail through his insurance physical.

Paradoxically, throughout Bill's treatment his insurance company refused to reimburse him for naturopathic care, claiming that it was not a medical necessity. When presented with his now-lower blood pressure readings, they claimed that his company would still have to pay the higher premiums because his condition was being medically treated! As he tells it, Bill went all the way to the president of the insurance company and said, "Look, you can't have it both ways—refuse to pay for the treatment and then claim that the same treatment is the reason why our premiums must remain high." He got his company's premium reduced that afternoon, and the next day the insurance company president scheduled an appointment at our clinic.

Childhood Illnesses

A large number of the patients who come through my office are children suffering from a host of ailments—from chronic diarrhea to repeated ear infections. Their mothers are usually on the verge of frantic. Some of my most satisfying results have come with children.

Conjunctivitis

Conjunctivitis, commonly called "pink eye," is usually caused by the transmission of the staphylococcus bacteria from one child to another. Type A and Type AB children are more susceptible to conjunctivitis than are Type O or Type B, probably because of their weaker immune systems.

Antibiotic creams or eyedrops are used to treat the condition in the conventional manner. But a soothing and surprising alternative is a freshly cut slice of tomato. (Don't try this with tomato juice!) The freshly cut tomato contains a lectin that can agglutinate and destroy the staphylococcus bacteria. The slight acidity of the tomato appears to resemble closely the acidity of the eye's own secretions. Squeezing the watery juice of a fresh tomato on a gauze pad and applying it to the affected eye is also very soothing.

This is one example of how the same lectins in a food that make it dangerous to eat can be highly beneficial to treat an illness. Later, we'll discuss many other examples of the ways in which lectins play a dual role—good cop, bad cop—in our systems. Especially in the war against cancer.

Diarrhea

Diarrhea can be a disturbing and dangerous condition for children. Not only is it debilitating and terribly uncomfortable but it can lead to severe dehydration, causing weakness and fever.

Most childhood diarrhea is the result of either microbial imbalance or dietary irregularities, and here the Blood Type Diet offers very specific guidelines about which foods trigger digestive problems for each blood type.

Type O children often experience mild to moderate diarrhea, frequently caused by the milder forms of coliform bacteria. This often results from an overreliance on dairy products or an excessive use of grains and carbs due to the child's picky eating habits.

Type A and Type AB children are prone to *Giardia lamblia*, more commonly known as Montezuma's revenge. The giardia parasite mimics the Blood Type A antigen and can evade a proper immune response.

Type B children will often contract diarrhea if they overindulge in wheat products or in reaction to eating chicken and corn. If they are Type B secretors (about 80 percent of all Type Bs), they may have a problem with the norovirus, a very common cause of diarrhea.

If the diarrhea is caused by food-related intolerance or allergy, your child will often exhibit other symptoms, ranging from dark, puffy circles under the eyes to eczema, psoriasis, or asthma.

Unless diarrhea is the result of a more serious condition, such as a parasitic infection, partial intestinal blockage, or inflammation, it usually corrects itself with time. Should your child's stool contain blood or mucus, however, seek immediate medical attention. Acute diarrhea might also be infectious; to protect the rest of your family from contagion, it is best to institute scrupulous standards of cleanliness.

To restore your child's proper balance of fluids during bouts of diarrhea, restrict fruit juice. Instead, feed your child vegetable or meat stocks in soups. One wonderful herb that can be used for all blood types is carob. Not only is carob effective for simple cases of diarrhea but it has a wonderful chocolate-like taste that kids really enjoy.

Ear Infections

Perhaps as many as two-thirds of children under the age of six have chronic ear infections. By chronic, I mean 5, 10, 15, even 20 infections every winter season, one after the other. Most of these children have allergies to both environmental and food-based particles. The best solution is the Blood Type Diet.

The conventional protocol for ear infections is antibiotic therapy, but it obviously fails when there is a chronic infection. If we attack the underlying causes of the problem first instead of trotting out the most currently fashionable nostrum—and by this I mean the ever more sophisticated and newest classes of antibiotics—we have an opportunity to allow the body to mount its own powerful response. For starters, it is helpful to know the blood type susceptibilities.

Children who are Type A and Type AB have greater problems with mucus secretions from improper diet—a factor in ear infections. In Type A children, dairy products are usually the culprit, whereas Type AB may experience sensitivities to corn in addition to milk. In general, these kids are also more likely to have throat and respiratory problems, which can often move into the ears. Because the immune systems of Type A and Type AB children are tolerant of a wider range of bacteria, some of their problems stem from the lack of an aggressive response to the infectious organism. Several studies have shown that ear fluids of children with a history of chronic ear infections lack specific chemicals called complement, which are needed to attack and destroy the bacteria.

Another study shows that a serum lectin called mannose-binding protein is missing in the ear fluids of children with chronic infections. This lectin apparently binds to mannose sugars on the surface of the bacteria and agglutinates them, allowing for their faster removal. Both of these important immune factors eventually develop in their proper amounts, which may help explain why the frequency of ear infections gradually lessens as the child ages. In addition to diet, treating Type A and Type AB children with ear infections almost always involves enhancing their immunity. The simplest way to enhance the immunity of any child is to cut down on their intake of sugar. Numerous studies have shown that sugar depresses the immune system, making the body's white blood cells sluggish and disinclined to attack invading organisms.

Naturopaths have for many years made use of a mild herbal immune stimulant, *Echinacea purpurea*. Originally used by Native Americans, echinacea has the extraordinary properties of being both safe and effective in boosting the body's immunity against bacteria and viruses. Because many of the immune functions that echinacea enhances depend on adequate levels of vitamin C, I often prescribe an extract of vitamin C–rich rose hips. In my experience, echinacea preparations seem to work better for Types A, B, and AB than they do for Type O. I also use an extract of the western larch tree as a sort of super-echinacea. This product, larch arabinogalactan, contains much more concentrated active components than you get with echinacea.

Ear infections are terribly painful for a child, and not too pleasant for the parents either. Most of these infections are a backup of noxious fluids and gases into the middle ear because of an obstructed connecting pipe, the eustachian tube. This tube can become swollen because of allergic reactions, weakness in the tissues surrounding it, or infections.

Many parents have grown frustrated by the increasing inability of antibiotics to work on ear infections. There is a reason for this resistance: A baby's first ear infection is typically treated with a mild antibiotic, such as amoxicillin. With the child's next ear infection, amoxicillin is given again. Eventually, the ever more resistant infection returns, and amoxicillin is no longer effective. The escalation phenomenon—the process of using stronger and stronger drugs and ever more invasive treatments—has begun.

When antibiotics no longer work, and the painful infections continue, a myringotomy is performed. This is a process in which tiny tubes called grommets are surgically implanted through the eardrum to increase the drainage of fluid from the middle ear into the throat.

We are now at the point at which most pediatric medical associations are recommending that simple cases of ear infection not be treated with antibiotics at all; instead, they suggest that patients be given supportive care for the pain and a course of antihistamines to help remove the swelling and pressure, something naturopathic physicians have been doing for decades. When I treat chronic ear infections, I focus on ways to prevent recurrences. It is useless to try to resolve one episode with a quick dose of antibiotics when you know another ear infection is warming up in the bull pen. Almost always, I find a solution in the diet.

I see many children in my practice, representing all blood types. I've found that any child can contract chronic ear infections if he eats foods that react poorly in his system. I have never seen a case where there wasn't an obvious connection with a child's favorite food.

Type O and Type B children seem to develop ear infections less frequently, and when they do occur, they are usually easier to treat. More often than not, a change in diet is sufficient to eliminate the problem.

In Type B children, the culprit is usually a viral infection that then leads to a bacterial infection with haemophilus, to which Type B is unusually susceptible. The dietary fix involves restricting tomatoes, corn, and chicken. The lectins in these foods react with the surface of the digestive tract, causing swelling and mucus secretion, which usually carries over to the ears and throat.

My personal feeling is that ear infections can be prevented in Type O children simply by breast-feeding instead of bottle feeding. Breast-feeding for a period of six months to a year allows a child's immune system and digestive tract time to develop. Type O kids will also avoid ear infections if they are taken off wheat and dairy products. They're unusually sensitive to these foods at an early age, but their immunity is easily augmented by the use of higher value proteins such as fish and lean red meats.

Dietary changes are often difficult in households with children who suffer repeated ear infections. Their misery can tempt the anxious parent to let them eat whatever they wish, thinking that it will comfort them. Many of these kids wind up being picky eaters, eating only a very narrow range of foods, and often the very foods that are provoking their illness!

CASE HISTORY: EAR INFECTION
TONY, AGE 7; BLOOD TYPE B

Tony was a seven-year-old boy who suffered from repeated ear infections. When his mother first brought him to my office, she was frantic. Tony would develop a new ear infection immediately after stopping the antibiotic used to treat his previous infection, at the rate of 10 to 15 per winter season. He'd had grommet treatment twice, to no avail. This was a perfect example of a child on the antibiotic treadmill: escalating levels of antibiotics with fewer results.

My initial questions to Tony's mother were about his diet. She was a bit defensive. "Oh, I don't think that's the problem," she told me. "We eat very well—lots of chicken and fish, fruits and vegetables."

I turned to Tony. "What are your favorite foods?" I asked.

"Chicken nuggets," he replied enthusiastically.

"Do you like corn on the cob?"

"Oh, yes!"

"And therein lies the problem," I said to Tony's mother. "Your son is reactive to chicken and corn."

"He is?" She regarded me doubtfully. "How do you know that?"

"Because he's Blood Type B," I replied. I explained the blood type connection, and although Tony's mother was unconvinced, I suggested she feed Tony the Type B Diet for two or three months to see what would happen.

The rest, as they say, is history. Over the next two years Tony did very well, usually developing a single ear infection per season, as opposed to his previous rate of 10 to 15. These isolated infections were easy to treat either with naturopathic methods or a gentle low-strength antibiotic.

HYPERACTIVITY AND LEARNING DISABILITIES

There is a variety of different causes for attention deficit hyperactivity disorders (ADHDs), and we still need much more information before we can make a conclusive blood type connection. We can, however, gain some insight from our knowledge of how different blood types respond to their environments. For example, my father observed over 35 years of practice that Type O children are happier, healthier, and more alert when they're given the opportunity to exercise to their maximum potential.

A Type O child with ADHD should be encouraged to exercise as much as possible. This might include additional gym classes, team sports, or gymnastics. Type A and Type AB children, on the other hand, seem to benefit from activities that encourage the development of sensory and tactile skills, such as sculpting or artwork, and from basic relaxation techniques, such as deep breathing. Type B children do well with swimming and calisthenics.

One factor that deserves consideration is the influence of stress hormones. Blood Type Os are more prone to high catecholamine levels and dopamine imbalances, which have been associated with hyperactivity.

I recently discovered an interesting connection that might more strongly tie Type O children to ADHD. A Type O child was brought to me who suffered from both ADHD and mild anemia. I placed him on a high-protein diet and gave him supplements of vitamins B_{12} and folic acid, and the anemia cleared up. But his mother also noticed a decided improvement in her child's attention span. I've subsequently treated several Type O ADHD children with low doses of these vitamins and have seen improvements ranging from slight to dramatic.

If your child has ADHD, talk to a nutrition professional about adding supplements of vitamin B_{12} and folic acid, in addition to the Blood Type Diet.

STREP THROAT, MONONUCLEOSIS, AND MUMPS

Because the early symptoms of mononucleosis and the symptoms of strep throat are similar, it is often difficult for parents to differentiate between the two. A child with either illness may exhibit one or more of the following symptoms: sore throat, malaise, fever, chills, headache, swollen glands, or swollen tonsils. A blood test and throat culture will be needed to determine which illness is causing the problem.

Strep throat, caused by the streptococcal organism, is a bacterial infection. It often has the additional symptoms of nasal discharge, cough, earaches, white or yellow patches on the back of the throat, and a rash that starts on the neck and chest and spreads to the abdomen and extremities. Diagnosis of strep throat is based on clinical symptoms and a throat culture. The standard treatment includes antibiotics, bed rest, aspirin, and fluids for aches and fever.

Once again, the focus is on treating the immediate infection, not on solving the larger and more long-term health issues. Especially when your child suffers repeat infections, the standard therapy is ineffective.

In general, Type O and Type B children contract strep throat more often than do Type A and Type AB because of their increased vulnerability to bacterial infections. However, Type O and Type B also recover more easily and completely. Once the strep organism gets into the bloodstream of Type A and Type AB children, it settles in and doesn't want to leave. Thus these children will have repeated infections.

There are naturopathic therapies that can help prevent recurrences. I have found that using a mouth rinse made from the herbs sage and goldenseal is very effective in keeping the throat and tonsils free from strep. Goldenseal contains a component called berberine, which has been well studied for its antistrep activity. The problem with goldenseal is that it has a distinctly bitter, weedy taste, which kids don't exactly relish. It is sometimes easier to purchase an inexpensive atomizer or spray pump bottle and just spray the back of your child's throat a couple of times a day. In addition to the Blood Type Diet, I often use nutritional supplements for immune support, in the form of additional beta-carotene, vitamin C, zinc, and echinacea to help develop the child's resistance.

Type O seems to be more susceptible to the viral infection mononucleosis than Type A, Type B, or Type AB children. Antibiotics are ineffective in the treatment of mononucleosis because it is caused by a virus, not a bacteria. Bed rest while the fever lasts and frequent rest intervals during the one- to three-week recovery period are recommended. Aspirin and adequate fluid intake are encouraged to decrease fever.

Type B children seem to be more at risk for developing severe mumps, a viral infection of the salivary glands under the chin and ears. Like many B-prone illnesses, this one has a neurological connection. If your child is Type B and/or Rh-negative and has the mumps, be alert for signs of neurologic damage, particularly as manifested in hearing problems.

Diabetes

The Blood Type Diet can be effective in the treatment of type 1 diabetes, and in both the treatment and prevention of type 2 diabetes. Type 2 diabetes was once referred to as adult-onset diabetes, but increasingly it is being diagnosed in young people.

Blood Type A and Type B individuals are more prone to type 1 diabetes, caused by a lack of insulin, the hormone manufactured by the pancreas responsible for allowing glucose to enter the cells of the body. The cause of insulin deprivation is the destruction of the beta cells of the pancreas, which are the sole cells capable of producing insulin.

Although there is currently no effective natural treatment alternative for injectable insulin-replacement therapy for type 1 diabetes, one important natural remedy to consider using is quercetin, an antioxidant derived from plants. Quercetin has been shown to help prevent many of the complications stemming from lifelong diabetes, such as cataracts, neuropathy, and cardiovascular problems. Talk with a nutritionist who is skilled in the use of phytochemicals if you plan on using any natural medicine for diabetes; you may have to readjust your insulin dosage.

Several interesting studies show that certain food lectins may actually help the pancreas of diabetics regenerate the insulin-producing beta cells. These include the lectins from fava beans and the standard supermarket silver dollar mushroom. If you are Type A or B, you might want to add fava beans to your diet. If you are Type O or AB, adding silver dollar mushrooms may help.

People with type 2 diabetes typically have high levels of insulin in their bloodstreams, but their tissues lack sensitivity to insulin. This condition develops over time and is usually the result of a poor diet. Type 2 diabetes is often observed in Type Os who have eaten dairy, wheat, and corn products for many years, and in Type As who eat a lot of meat and dairy foods. Type 2 diabetes is associated with being overweight and having high cholesterol, high triglycerides, and elevated blood pressure. In this respect, any blood type can develop type 2 diabetes.

People with type 2 diabetes need to monitor their blood sugar several times a day with glucose strips, and often need to inject insulin. However, it is possible to reduce the symptoms and manage the condition. By sticking to the appropriate Blood Type Diet and exercise regimen, such patients can achieve positive results. A high-potency vitamin B complex can also help counter insulin intolerance. Check with a physician and nutritionist before using any substance to self-treat diabetes. You might have to adjust the dosage of your diabetic medication.

Digestive Illnesses

CELIAC DISEASE

Celiac is a disease of the gastrointestinal tract. Common symptoms include chronic diarrhea, weight loss, iron deficiency and other evidence of nutrient malabsorption. Once virtually unknown, it is now commonly written about in the mainstream press, although as with most "popular" disseminated information, it is often misunderstood.

The disease is thought to be an immune reaction to gluten, or, more specially, gliadin, a protein found in wheat, rye, oats and barley. About four in five people with celiac disease have antibodies to gliadin in their blood.

There is a strong association between being a non-secretor and having celiac disease. Non-secretors are 200 times more likely to have celiac than secretors. One study reported that up to 48 percent of patients with celiac disease were reported to be non-secretors. This would make sense because non-secretors have lower levels of IgA, an antibody produced in the mucosal lining, than secretors.

Lectins have been extensively studied in celiac disease, although the results are mixed and inconclusive. Many people wonder if Type O is more prone to celiac disease because of its aversion to wheat. However, I've found that celiac seems to affect all blood types about equally, though perhaps for different reasons. Part of the reason seems to be that gliadin, the perpetrator here, is different from wheat germ lectin, the major everyday problem for Type O.

That is not to say that gluten doesn't appear to be somewhat lectin-like in its own right. It's just not wheat germ lectin. Yet gluten has been shown to bind to carbohydrate-rich tissues much like a lectin. And much like a lectin, gluten can even be inhibited by a specific sugar, alpha-D-mannose. Curiously, many intestinal influenza viruses bind to alpha-D-mannose as well. In addition to bugs, the lectin from the plant snowdrop (*Galanthus nivalis*), which is used to genetically alter foods, also binds alpha-D-mannose.

CONSTIPATION

Constipation occurs when the stools are unusually hard or a person's bowel patterns have changed and become less frequent. Most chronic constipation is caused by poor bowel habits and irregular meals, with a diet low in bulk and water content. Some other causes are a habitual use of laxatives, a rushed and stressful daily schedule, and travel that requires abrupt adjustments of eating and sleeping patterns. Lack of physical exercise, acute illness, painful rectal conditions, and some medications also may cause constipation.

Every blood type is susceptible to constipation given the circumstances. Constipation is not so much a disease as a warning sign that something is not right with your digestive system. You'll find most of the clues in your diet. Are you eating enough foods in your diet that are high in fiber content? Are you drinking enough fluids—in particular, water and juices? Are you exercising regularly?

Many people simply take a laxative when they're constipated, but that doesn't solve the natural systemic causes of constipation. The long-term solution is in the diet. However, Type A, Type B, and Type AB individuals can supplement their diets with fibrous unprocessed bran. Type O, in addition to eating plenty of the fibrous fruits and vegetables, can take a supplement of butyrate, a natural bulk-forming agent, as a substitute for bran, which is not advised for them.

CROHN'S DISEASE AND COLITIS

Crohn's disease and colitis are depleting, enervating diseases that add the elements of uncertainty, pain, blood loss, and suffering to the process of elimination. There are an enormous number of genes linked to these inflammatory bowel conditions, virtually all of which alter the immune response in the gut. Many food lectins can cause digestive irritation by attaching to the mucous membranes of the digestive tract. As many of the food lectins are blood type specific, it is possible for each blood type to develop the same problem from different foods. Also, these types of disorders are characterized by a process called aberrant glycosylation, a situation in which the cells do not properly attach particular sugars to proteins. These sugars provide instructions on how the protein must properly fold to give it the shape needed for it to function. Mis-folded proteins trigger a stress alarm system in the cell, which then attempts to refold the protein correctly. If it cannot do this, the cell sends out signals that cause it to commit suicide, a process known as apoptosis.

Apoptosis is the cellular equivalent of taking one for the team, for if the cell had lived it might have passed on its dysfunction to many more generations of daughter cells. However, if there are many cells committing apoptosis you can have massive amounts of tissue destruction, such as seen with inflammatory bowel disease. Lectins can sometimes cause aberrant glycosylation, but more often they prolong and exaggerate its effects. In these cases other genes may be the cause of inflammatory bowel disease, but a consistent diet of avoids for your blood type will amplify and prolong it.

In Type A and Type AB, Crohn's disease and colitis often involve a major stress component. If you have Type A or Type AB blood and suffer from inflammatory bowel disease, pay careful attention to your stress patterns and refer to the discussion of stress in your Blood Type Diet.

Type O tends to develop the more ulcerative form of colitis that causes bleeding with elimination. This is probably due to the lack of adequate clotting factors in the blood or the more pronounced response to common grain lectins. Type A, Type AB, and Type B tend to develop more of a mucous colitis, which is not as bloody. In either case, follow the diet for your blood type. You will be able to avoid many of the food lectins that can aggravate the condition, and you may find your symptoms easing.

CASE HISTORY: IRRITABLE BOWEL SYNDROME
VIRGINIA, AGE 26; BLOOD TYPE O

I first examined Virginia, a 26-year-old woman with chronic bowel trouble, after she had received extensive treatment from a variety of conventional gastroenterologists. Her problems included chronic irritable bowel syndrome with painful constipation alternating with an unpredictable, almost explosive diarrhea that made it difficult for her to leave the house. She also suffered from fatigue and low-grade chronic anemia. Her previous doctors conducted an enormous amount of costly testing and could suggest only antispasmodic drugs and a daily dose of fiber. Food allergy testing was inconclusive. Virginia was a vegetarian who followed a strict macrobiotic diet, and I immediately detected the foods in her diet that were causing her suffering. The absence of meat was a primary factor. She also was unable to properly digest the grains and pasta she was eating on a regular basis.

Since Virginia was Type O, I suggested a high-protein diet, including lean red meats, fish, and poultry, and fresh fruits and vegetables. Because the digestive tract of Type O does not tolerate most grains very well, I suggested that she avoid whole wheat altogether and severely limit her consumption of other grains.

Initially, Virginia was resistant to the idea of making these dietary changes. She was a vegetarian, and she believed that her current diet was truly healthful. I urged her to look again, asking, "How has this diet helped you, Virginia? You seem to be pretty sick."

Eventually, I convinced her to try it my way for a limited period of time. In eight weeks Virginia returned looking hale and hardy, with a ruddy complexion. She boasted that her bowel problems were 90 percent better. Blood tests showed a complete resolution of her anemia, and she said her energy levels were almost back to normal. A second follow-up visit one month later resulted in Virginia being discharged from my care, completely free of bowel problems.

CASE HISTORY: CROHN'S DISEASE
YEHUDA, AGE 50; BLOOD TYPE O

I first saw Yehuda, a middle-aged Jewish man, for active Crohn's disease. By that point he had already had several bowel surgeries to remove sections that were obstructing his small intestine. I put Yehuda on a wheat-free diet, with an emphasis on lean meats and boiled vegetables. I also gave him a high-powered extract of licorice and a fatty acid supplement called butyrate.

Yehuda's compliance was exemplary, a testament to the concerns both he and his family had for his health. For example, his wife, the daughter of a baker, baked him a special wheat-free bread. Yehuda took his supplements, including the licorice, very seriously, as he took everything else.

From the start, Yehuda consistently improved. He never required additional surgery, even though his gastroenterologist had earlier said it was inevitable. His father-in-law is now the largest manufacturer of wheat-free breads in his religious community.

CASE HISTORY: CROHN'S DISEASE
SARAH, AGE 35; BLOOD TYPE B

Sarah was a 35-year-old woman of eastern European ancestry who came to my office for treatment of Crohn's disease. She had already had several surgeries to remove scarred tissue from the bowel, was anemic, and suffered from chronic diarrhea.

I prescribed a basic Type B Diet, instructing Sarah to refrain from eating chicken and other lectin-containing foods. I also used supplemental licorice and fatty acids as part of her protocol.

Sarah was very cooperative. Within four months, most of her digestive symptoms, including the diarrhea, were eliminated. Because she wanted to have more children, Sarah had surgery to remove scar tissue from her bowel that had attached to her uterus. Her surgeon told her that there was no sign of active Crohn's disease anywhere in her abdominal cavity.

FOOD POISONING

Anyone can get food poisoning, but certain blood types are naturally more susceptible because of their tendency toward a weakened immune system. In particular, Type A and Type AB individuals are more likely to fall prey to salmonella food poisoning, which is usually the result of leaving food uncovered and unrefrigerated for long periods of time. Furthermore, the bacteria will be harder for Type A and Type AB to get rid of once they've found a home in their systems.

Type B is more likely to be severely affected by consuming food contaminated with the shigella organism, a bacteria found on plants that causes dysentery.

GASTRITIS

Many people confuse gastritis with ulcers, but it is exactly the opposite. Ulcers are produced by hyperacidity, more common for Type O and Type B. Gastritis is caused by very low stomach acid content, more common for Type A and Type AB. Gastritis occurs when the stomach acid gets so low that it no longer functions as a microbial barrier. Without adequate levels of acid, microbes will live in the stomach and cause serious inflammation.

The best course of action that Type A and Type AB can take is to stress the more acidic food choices in the Blood Type Diet.

STOMACH AND DUODENAL ULCERS

It has been known since the early 1950s that peptic ulcer of the stomach is more common in Blood Type O individuals, with the highest occurrence in Type O non-secretors. Type O also has a higher rate of bleeding and perforation, which was not shown to be different between secretors and non-secretors. One reason is that Type O has higher stomach acid levels and an ulcer-producing enzyme called pepsinogen.

Scientific research has uncovered another reason Type O is prone to ulcers. That is, people with Type O blood are a favorite target for the bacteria now known to cause ulcers. This bacteria, *Helicobacter pylori*, was found to be able to attach itself to the Type O antigen lining the stomach and then work its way into the lining. As we've seen, the Type O antigen is the sugar fucose. Researchers found an inhibitor in breast milk, which apparently blocked the attachment of the bacteria to the stomach surface. No doubt this inhibitor is one of the many fucose sugars found in human breast milk.

The common seaweed bladderwrack is an inhibitor of *H. pylori*. The content of fucose in bladderwrack is so great that it factors into its Latin name—*Fucus vesiculosus*. If you are Type O and suffer from ulcers or want to prevent them, using bladderwrack will make the ulcer-causing bacteria *H. pylori* slide off your stomach lining.

CASE HISTORY: CHRONIC STOMACH ULCERS
PETER, AGE 34; BLOOD TYPE O

Peter had suffered from stomach ulcers since he was a child and had used every conventional ulcer medication available, with little result. I began by prescribing the basic high-protein Blood Type O Diet, stressing that he avoid the whole wheat products that had always been a major part of his diet. I also prescribed a supplement of bladderwrack and a combination medicine of licorice and bismuth.

Within six weeks Peter had made considerable progress. On a follow-up visit to his gastroenterologist, he was scoped and heard the encouraging news that 60 percent of his stomach lining now appeared normal. A second examination a year later showed complete resolution of Peter's stomach ulcers.

Infections

As we discussed earlier, many bacteria prefer specific blood types; in fact, one study showed that over 50 percent of 282 bacteria carried antigens of one blood type or another. It has been observed that viral infections in general seem to be more frequent in Type Os because they do not possess any antigens. These infections are less frequent and milder in Type A, Type B, and Type AB.

HIV/AIDS

While AIDS was once fatal, advances in medicine have made it possible for people to live with HIV. Today, over 1.1 million Americans and 3.3 million people worldwide live long, normal lives with the disease, thanks in large part to new advances in drug therapy. The current state-of-the-art treatment is an antiretroviral drug cocktail, given in one pill a day, which can be started as soon as a person is diagnosed with HIV.

Research is inconclusive about the connection between blood type and susceptibility to HIV; however, one compelling paper published in the journal *Blood* suggested that transmission of HIV is modified by ABO blood type. Comparing transmission to bad transfusion reactions, scientists proposed that it is harder for Blood Type O individuals to contract HIV infection from people of other blood types because they carry both anti-A and anti-B antigens in their blood. On the other hand, Type AB, with no opposing blood type antigens, would more easily contract HIV from other blood types. Much more research needs to be done on this. Having said that, let's look at how the information in this book can be used to help people hold their own against the virus.

If you are HIV positive or have AIDS, modify your diet to encompass the suggestions that are specific to your blood type. For example, if you are Type O, begin to increase the amount of animal proteins in your diet and develop a physical training program. Following the blood type program will help fully mobilize and optimize your immune functions by stressing the highest-value foods for your particular needs. Be careful to limit your fat intake, choosing lean cuts of meat, because bowel parasites, common in people with AIDS, interfere with fat digestion and lead to diarrhea. Also avoid foods such as wheat that contain lectins that could further compromise your immune system and bloodstream.

Because many of the opportunistic infections associated with AIDS cause nausea, diarrhea, and mouth sores, AIDS is often a wasting disease. Type A will need to work a little harder to consume enough calories because many Type A foods are calorically low. Rigorously eliminate any foods, such as meat or dairy, that can cause digestive problems. Your immune system is already naturally sensitive; don't give harmful lectins a chance to get in and weaken you further. Meanwhile, increase your portions of good Type A foods, such as tofu and seafood.

Type B should avoid the obvious problem foods, such as chicken, corn, and buckwheat. But you should also eliminate nuts, which are hard to digest, and reduce the amount of wheat products in your diet. If you are lactose intolerant, avoid dairy foods; even if you're not, dairy can be a digestive irritant for immunocompromised Type B individuals. This is a case in which the disease contraindicates a favored food.

Type AB should limit intake of lectin-rich beans and legumes, and eliminate nuts. Your primary protein source should be fish, and there is a wide variety available to Type AB. Occasional servings of meat and dairy are okay, but watch the fat, and limit your wheat consumption. A lectin isolated from bananas showed amazing ability to deactivate the AIDS virus. Type O and B individuals may want to take advantage of this little-known information.

In general, whatever your blood type, you want to avoid lectins that could damage the cells of your immune system and digestive tract. These cells cannot be easily replaced, the way they are in a healthy body. This cell-sparing aspect of the Blood Type Diet makes it invaluable to the person with AIDS who has anemia or low T-helper cells.

BRONCHITIS AND PNEUMONIA

In general, Type A and Type AB have more bronchial infections than Type O and Type B. This may result from improper diets that produce excessive mucus in the respiratory passages. This mucus facilitates the growth of blood type–mimicking bacteria, such as the A-like pneumococcus bacteria in Type A and Type AB individuals and the B-like haemophilus bacteria in Type B and Type AB individuals. (Because Type AB has both A-like and B-like characteristics, the risk is double.)

The Blood Type Diet seems to substantially reduce the incidences of bronchitis and pneumonia for all blood types. However, we are just beginning to discover some other blood type connections that are not so easily remedied. For example, it appears that Type A children born to Type A fathers and Type O mothers die more frequently of bronchopneumonia in early life. It is thought that some form of sensitization occurs at birth between the Type A infant and the mother's anti-A antibodies that inhibits the infant's ability to fight the pneumococcus bacteria. There are no solid data yet to confirm the reason for this occurrence, but information of this kind can spark research interest in a potential vaccine. We'll have to gather much more data before we can make a valid scientific conclusion.

CANDIDIASIS (Common Yeast Infection)

The *Candida* organism appears to use its own lectins to attach to cells by binding to the sugar fucose. Fucose is the antigen of Type O, and it is perhaps not surprising that studies have shown that Type O carries more candida than the other blood types. Perhaps because of this, Type O tends to develop more of an allergic-type hypersensitivity to the candidiasis organism, especially when eating too many grains. This has been the basis of a theory called the yeast syndrome and a variety of candida diets. These diets stress high protein intake and the avoidance of grains, but they tend to be generalized across blood types, when it is only Type O who appears to have this yeast sensitivity. Type A and Type AB individuals tend to develop more yeast infections after antibiotic usage. Type B appears less prone to this organism, as long as they follow the Blood Type B Diet. If you are a Type B who has a history of candidiasis, cut down on your wheat consumption.

As noted earlier, being a non-secretor dramatically increases your susceptibility for candidiasis.

CHOLERA

According to the CDC, between 3 and 5 million cases of cholera are reported around the world every year. This infection is characterized by extreme diarrhea and severe fluid and mineral depletion. Cholera is known to be blood-type dependent, with the worst cases seen in Blood Type O. After a severe outbreak in Peru, a report in the UK medical journal the *Lancet* attributed it to the high incidence of Type O in the Peruvian population. Historically, the susceptibility of Type O to cholera was probably responsible for the decimation of the populations of many of the ancient cities, leaving as survivors the more cholera-resistant Type A.

COMMON COLD AND FLU

There are hundreds of different strains of cold virus, and it would be impossible to see blood type specificity in all of them. However, studies of British military recruits showed a slightly lower overall incidence of cold viruses in recruits who were Type A, which is consistent with our findings that Blood Type A was developed to resist these common viruses. Viruses also have less impact on Type AB. The A antigen, carried by both Type A and Type AB individuals, blocks the attachment of various strains of flu to the membranes of the throat and respiratory passages.

Influenza, a more serious virus, shows surprising variations in severity between the blood types. (This was discussed earlier in the section on vaccines.)

The symptoms of a common cold and the flu are miserable, but they are actually a sign that your immune system is trying hard to fight off the offending virus. While your immune system is doing its job, there are measures you can take that will make coexistence on the battlefield more comfortable:

1. Maintain general good health with adequate rest and exercise, along with learning to cope with the stresses of life. Stress is a major factor in the depletion of immune system resources. This may protect you from frequent infections and may even shorten the duration of the colds and flus you do get.
2. Follow the basic dietary protocol for your blood type. It will optimize your immune response and help shorten the course of your cold or flu.
3. Take vitamin C (250 to 500 milligrams), or increase the sources of vitamin C in your diet. Many people feel that taking small doses of the herb echinacea helps prevent colds or at least helps shorten their duration.
4. Ensure adequate hydration and increase the humidity in your room with a vaporizer or humidifier to prevent a dry throat and nasal tissue.

5. If your throat is sore, gargle with salt water. One half teaspoon of ordinary table salt and a tall glass of comfortably warm water provides a soothing and cleansing rinse. Another good gargle, especially if you are prone to tonsillitis, is a tea of equal parts goldenseal (*Hydrastis canadensis*) root and sage. Gargle with this mixture every few hours.

6. If your nose is runny or stuffy, use an antihistamine to reduce the reaction of tissues to the infecting virus and relieve nasal congestion. Be especially careful with ephedrine-containing antihistamines, such as those found in many popular antihistamines. These can raise blood pressure, keep you awake at night, and complicate prostate problems in men.

7. Antibiotics are not effective against viruses, so if someone offers you leftover antibiotics or if you have some around the house, don't take them.

Plague, Typhoid, Smallpox, and Malaria

Known during the Middle Ages as the black death, the plague is a bacterial infection carried largely by rodents. Blood Type O is more susceptible to plague. Although plague is rare in industrialized societies, it continues to be a problem in the developing world. A recent report by the World Health Organization warned that we may be facing a crisis in the appearance of plague and other infectious diseases as a result of the overuse of antibiotics and other medicines as well as of human settlement of previously uninhabited areas, international travel, and poverty. The fact that Western societies rarely encounter these diseases should not make us feel immune to their social, economic, cultural, and human cost. Occasionally an outbreak does occur in developed countries. In fact, as the world gets "smaller," and people travel more easily, plague could be a problem for any location.

Smallpox has been officially eradicated through extensive worldwide immunization, although its course has probably influenced world history to a largely unappreciated degree. Blood Type A is especially susceptible to smallpox.

Typhoid, a common infection in areas of diminished hygiene or in times of war, usually infects the blood and the digestive tract. Type O is most susceptible to typhoid infection. Typhoid also shows a connection to the Rh blood groups, being found more frequently in Rh-negative individuals.

Malaria is an unfamiliar disease to many in the Western world, yet its global impact is tremendous. According to the World Health Organization, more than half the world's population is at risk for malaria, although aggressive preventative measures have substantially reduced the incidence. It is claimed that the anopheles mosquito, which carries malaria, tends to bite Type B and Type O individuals in preference to Type A and Type AB individuals, whereas the common mosquito seems to prefer Type O secretors (83.3 percent) and Type A secretors (46.5 percent).

POLIO AND VIRAL MENINGITIS

Polio, a viral infection of the nervous system, shows a higher frequency in Type B, which is more susceptible to virally sparked nervous system disorders. Polio was epidemic and caused most cases of juvenile paralysis before the development of the Salk and Sabin vaccines. Eradicated in most of the world, polio is still seen in Afghanistan and Pakistan.

Viral meningitis, an increasingly frequent and serious infection of the nervous system, is significantly more common in Type O than in other blood types, probably because of the Type O weakness against aggressive infections. Be alert to symptoms of fatigue, high fever, and a characteristic of meningitis called nuchal rigidity, a stiffness in the muscles of the neck.

SINUS INFECTIONS

Type O and Type B individuals are more prone to chronic sinus infections. Very often, their physicians will prescribe an almost continuous supply of antibiotics, which banish the problem temporarily. The sinus infections inevitably return, however, prompting the use of more antibiotics and, finally, surgery.

I have found that the herb collinsonia (stoneroot), which is used to treat swelling problems, such as varicose veins, also helps sinusitis—perhaps because chronic sinusitis is a sort of hemorrhoid or varicose vein of the head. When I prescribe this herb to my patients with chronic sinusitis, the results are often astounding. Many of these patients no longer need antibiotics to treat their infections because the collinsonia removes the cause of the problem, which is swelling of the sinus tissue. If you have sinus problems, you may wish to try this herb, which you can order online or find in health food stores in liquid form. A typical dose is 20 to 25 drops in warm water taken orally two or three times daily. No need to worry about toxicity; this is a safe herb.

Occasionally a Type A or Type AB will develop sinusitis, although this is almost always the result of a highly mucus-forming diet. Sinusitis in Type A usually responds well to diet changes alone.

PARASITES (Amoebic Dysentery, Giardia, Tapeworm, and Ascaris)

Given enough of a head start, parasites can live fairly well in anyone's digestive tract. By and large, however, they seem to have a special preference for Type A and Type AB digestive tracts, usually mimicking the Type A blood antigen to avoid detection. For example, the common amoeba parasite shows a preference for Type A and Type AB individuals. In addition, it appears that Type A and Type AB are more prone to complications should amoebic cysts lodge in the liver. Type As and Type ABs with amoebic dysentery should adopt strong measures to deal with the infection before it has a chance to migrate farther into their bodies.

Type A and Type AB individuals are also sitting ducks for a common water contaminant, the parasite *Giardia lamblia*, cause of the condition famously known as Montezuma's revenge. This clever parasite mimics the appearance of Type A, which allows it entry into the Type A and Type AB immune systems and then quickly into the intestines. Type A and Type AB travelers should equip themselves with the herb goldenseal or Pepto-Bismol to help stave off infection. Type As and Type ABs who drink well water should also be on the alert for the giardia parasite.

Many of the parasitic worms, such as the tapeworm and the ascaris parasite, have a resemblance to Type A and Type B and are found in greater frequency in people with these blood types. Because Type AB carries a double A-like, B-like characteristic, Type AB is particularly susceptible.

I have used an herb called Chinese wormwood (*Artemisia annua*) to treat parasites with notable success. Ask your naturopathic physician about this herb.

TUBERCULOSIS AND SARCOIDOSIS

Once considered almost completely eradicated from Western industrialized society, tuberculosis has now become more common. This is largely due to the high incidence of the disease among people with AIDS and the homeless. An opportunistic infection, tuberculosis thrives in immune systems weakened by poor hygiene and chronic disease. Tuberculosis of the lungs (pulmonary tuberculosis) is more common in Type O, whereas tuberculosis in other parts of the body shows a higher frequency in Type A.

Sarcoidosis, or sarcoid, is an inflammatory condition of the lungs and connective tissue that may actually be a form of immune reaction to tuberculosis. It was once thought to be much more common in African-Americans versus the general population, but in recent times it is being diagnosed more frequently in the white population, especially in women. It shows a higher frequency in Type A over Type O. Rh-negative individuals seem to be more susceptible to both tuberculosis and sarcoidosis.

URINARY TRACT INFECTIONS

There is good evidence that if you are Type B or Type AB, you are more susceptible to recurrent bladder infections (cystitis), especially if you are a non-secretor. That's because the most common bacteria-producing infections, such as *E. coli*, pseudomonas, and klebsiella, possess a B-like appearance, and Type B and Type AB produce no anti-B antibodies.

Type B also has higher rates of kidney infections, such as pyelonephritis. This is especially true of Type B non-secretors. If you are Type B and suffer from recurrent urinary problems, try to drink one or two glasses of a mixture of cranberry and pineapple juice every day.

Liver Disease

ALCOHOLIC-RELATED LIVER DISEASE

Alcoholism affects many bodily systems, but perhaps its most dramatic impact is on the liver. The 20 percent of the population who are non-secretors seem to be the most prone to alcoholism, but their susceptibility has little to do with secretor status. In an unfortunate and possibly random cellular twist, the gene that determines whether you're a non-secretor is located on the same part of the DNA as the gene for alcoholism. My patients who type as non-secretors often have an extensive family history of alcoholism.

Oddly enough, it is also non-secretors who seem to derive the most benefit to their hearts from a moderate intake of alcohol. A Danish study showing non-secretors to be at higher risk for ischemic heart disease (a lack of blood flow into the arteries) theorized that a moderate consumption of alcohol altered the rate of insulin flow, slowing the accumulation of fats in the blood vessels. This conflicting message is hard to decipher.

The answer is probably that decisions about the role of alcohol should be made on an individual basis and with consideration of your blood type. Due to the effects of alcohol on the digestive and immune systems, none of the Blood Type Diets allows hard liquor.

It is also clear that alcoholism has a major stress component. A Japanese research team discovered that a greater number of Type A than Type O or Type B received treatment for alcoholism. It is thought that Type A may have a predilection for seeking relaxation from stress by the ingestion of inhibition-releasing chemicals. It is certainly well documented that humans have a long history of using intoxicants for pleasure, for pain, for transport to other realms, and for medicine.

Only about 3 percent of the alcohol you consume passes through your body and is excreted. The rest is metabolized by the liver and processed in the stomach and small intestines. Over time, with heavy and regular consumption, the liver begins to deteriorate. The end result can be cirrhosis of the liver, severe malnutrition from malabsorption of foods, and ultimately death.

GALLSTONES, CIRRHOSIS, AND JAUNDICE

Of course, not all liver disease is linked to alcohol. Infections, allergies, and metabolic disorders all can cause liver damage. For example, jaundice, or yellowing of the skin, is often seen in people with hepatitis, and gallstones have been linked to obesity. Cirrhosis can be caused by infections, diseases of the bile ducts, or other illnesses that affect the liver.

For reasons we do not fully understand, Type A, Type B, and Type AB tend to have higher levels of gallstones, diseases of the bile ducts, jaundice, and cirrhosis of the liver than Type O, with Type A having the highest levels. Type A is also reported to be more susceptible to pancreatic tumors.

LIVER FLUKES AND OTHER TROPICAL INFECTIONS

Common tropical infections of the liver causing fibrosis or scarring appear to a marked degree more frequently in Type A and to a lesser extent in Type B and Type AB individuals. Type O, which may have developed anti-A and anti-B antibodies as an early protection against these parasites, is relatively immune to them.

My office has successfully treated many cases of liver disease using many of the herbal compounds discussed in Chapter Ten. In many cases, the patients who develop liver disease are Type A or Type B and non-secretors.

CASE HISTORY: LIVER DISEASE
GERARD, AGE 38; BLOOD TYPE B

Gerard was a 38-year-old man with a history of sclerosing cholangitis, an inflammatory condition of the liver's bile ducts, causing scarring. Usually this condition leads to the necessity of a liver transplant. When I first saw Gerard in July 1994, he was jaundiced and had horrible pruritus (itching) from deposits of bilirubin, a bile pigment, in his skin. Because of this condition, his cholesterol was also elevated (325). Gerard's serum bile acids were over 2,000 (normal is under 100), he had a bilirubin level of 4.1 (normal is under 1), and all his liver enzymes were sharply elevated, indicating extensive damage to his liver tissue. Gerard was a pretty sharp guy, who knew what his chances were, and frankly, he was preparing to die.

I started Gerard on the basic Blood Type B Diet and a botanical protocol of liver-specific antioxidants. These are antioxidants that preferentially deposit in the liver instead of in other organs. Gerard did very well in the intervening year, having only one flare-up of his itching and jaundice.

Recently Gerard underwent surgery to remove his gallbladder. After the surgeon examined his liver and major bile ducts, she told him that they looked normal, although the tissue around his bile ducts was a little thinner than usual.

CASE HISTORY: CIRRHOSIS
ESTEL, AGE 67; BLOOD TYPE A

Estel was a 67-year-old woman who first came to my office for an inflammatory condition of the liver called primary biliary cirrhosis, which results in destruction of the liver. Most cases eventually go on to a liver transplant.

Estel admitted that she was once a heavy drinker, but no longer. Her condition was probably linked to lifelong alcohol consumption. Although she may not have even been an alcoholic in the strictest sense, her three or four drinks a day, every day, for 40 years resulted in cirrhosis.

Estel's liver enzymes were markedly elevated. The alkaline phosphatase, for example, was in the high 800s. Normal is under 60. Because she was a Type A non-secretor, I immediately put her on the Blood Type A Diet and a protocol of liver-specific antioxidants. Estel began to show results almost immediately, and her condition continued to improve. A year after her first visit, Estel's alkaline phosphatase had dropped to 500.

Although her liver has shown no signs of further deterioration since that time, Estel developed swelling of the veins around her esophagus, a common condition in people with liver disease, which was controlled successfully.

CASE HISTORY: LIVER DETERIORATION
SANDRA, AGE 70; BLOOD TYPE A

Sandra arrived in my office suffering from a difficult-to-determine liver condition. All of her liver enzymes were elevated, and she also had a condition called ascites, an extensive amount of fluid being retained in her abdomen. Ascites is common in many cases of advanced liver failure. Sandra's internist was not treating her liver deterioration, probably expecting her to eventually require a transplant. He was prescribing diuretics to help remove the fluid from her abdomen, but the diuretics were causing her to lose large amounts of potassium, which probably accounted for her overwhelming fatigue.

I prescribed the Type A Diet with liver-specific botanicals. Within four months, all evidence of Sandra's fluid retention disappeared, and her liver enzymes returned to normal. Sandra was initially quite anemic, with a hematocrit of 27.1 (normal for a woman is over 38). Within a year her hematocrit had risen to 40.8, and she continued to be asymptomatic.

Skin Disorders

To date, there is little blood type–specific information available on skin disorders. We do know, however, that conditions such as dermatitis and psoriasis usually result from allergic chemicals acting within the blood. It is worth noting again that many of the common food lectins specific for one blood type or another can interact with the blood and digestive tissues, causing the liberation of histamines and other inflammatory chemicals. For example, it is well-known that psoriasis is aggravated/caused by excessive levels of growth factors called polyamines.

Polyamines result from the action of the gut bacteria or are made in the liver, where they are used as growth stimulants, especially in young children. Polyamines also make cancer cells grow. Certain dietary lectins stimulate the production of polyamines. Studies also show a stress component to psoriasis.

Allergic skin reactions to chemicals or abrasives show the highest incidences in Type A and Type AB individuals. Psoriasis is found more frequently in Type O. My own experience is that many Type Os who develop psoriasis are eating diets too high in grains or dairy products.

CASE HISTORY: PSORIASIS
From Dr. Anne Marie Lambert, Honolulu, Hawaii
MARIEL, AGE 66; BLOOD TYPE O

My colleague Dr. Lambert used the blood type protocol to treat a complicated case of psoriasis in an older woman. Mariel's symptoms included severe shortness of breath, difficulty walking, with limited range of motion in all joints, psoriasis lesions covering 70 percent of her skin surface, and burning pain throughout her body, especially in her muscles and joints. Her medical history was a catalog of constant medical problems: vaginal/bladder/bowel repairs, appendectomy, hysterectomy, ovarian cysts, psoriasis, hospitalization for pneumonia, psoriatic arthritis, and osteoporosis.

Mariel told Dr. Lambert that her typical diet was high in dairy, wheat, corn, nuts, and processed foods, with a high sugar and fat content. She said that she craved sweets, nuts, and bananas. This was a terrible diet for almost anyone, but it was anathema to someone of Mariel's blood type.

Dr. Lambert immediately started Mariel on a moderated Blood Type O Diet, which initially excluded red meat and nuts, plus vitamins and minerals. Within two months, there was a marked decrease in the swelling of Mariel's joints and improved breathing, and her psoriatic lesions were healing. By June, Mariel's psoriasis covered only 20 percent of her body, and the lesions were nearly healed. There was a marked improvement in her breathing, her pain had lessened by half, and the range of motion in her joints continued to improve. A month later, Mariel's psoriasis was no longer evident, there was only slight swelling in the joint spaces, and her breathing was no longer labored.

At a follow-up visit to Dr. Lambert seven months after her first visit, Mariel's breathing had improved, and she had no new lesions on her skin.

Mariel had been to numerous medical professionals since she became ill. She had tried all types of conventional and alternative therapies, including food plans specifically designed for psoriatic arthritis and asthma. Although those diets were well intended, none of them was specifically tailored to ensure compatibility with Mariel's blood. The Blood Type O Diet was able to provide nutrition without causing health problems from foods that were incompatible with Mariel's blood. With the exception of some minor pain relief from Chinese herbs, none of the other treatments had been successful. Mariel considered her progress a miracle!

Women/Reproduction

Pregnancy and Infertility

Many of the disorders related to pregnancy result from some form of blood type incompatibility—either between the mother and the fetus or between the mother and the father. Increasingly, we are learning that blood type incompatibility may be a critical factor in infertility. ABO incompatible couples (a Type A male fertilizing a Type O female) are a frequent occurrence in miscarriages, especially very early in the gestational term. One study of 288 miscarriages showed that there was an excess of Blood Type A and Type B in otherwise normal fetuses. It has been concluded that an ABO incompatibility between mother and fetus is likely to be a cause of early miscarriages, but almost exclusively in chromosomally normal fetuses.

A study of 102 infertile couples showed that 87 percent were blood type incompatible. The same study also found that in 7 couples with markedly delayed fertility, the 9 children that did result were all Blood Type O and hence would have been compatible with the mother. The authors suggested that the infertility was due to the presence of antibodies in the secretions of the mother's genitalia or incompatible sperm from the father.

Blood type incompatibility can also lead to infertility. Opposing blood type antibodies can be induced by foods that contain opposing blood type antigens. It is not unreasonable to conclude that the many case histories of previously infertile women conceiving and producing healthy offspring by simply eating correctly for their blood type are the result of the lowering of these opposing blood group antibodies. How? By avoiding continued consumption of the problematic foods that introduced them.

TOXEMIA OF PREGNANCY

As early as 1905 it was proposed that some form of blood type sensitization resulted in pregnancy toxemia—a poisoning of the blood that can occur in late pregnancy and cause grave illness and even death. In a later study, an excess of Type O women was found to suffer from toxemia, resulting possibly from a reaction to a Type A or Type B fetus.

BIRTH DEFECTS

Blood type incompatibility, which may occur between a Type O mother and a Type A father, has been implicated in several common birth defects, including hydatidiform mole, choriocarcinoma, spina bifida, and anencephaly. Several studies imply that these disorders appear to be caused by maternal ABO incompatibility with fetal nervous and blood tissue.

HEMOLYTIC DISEASE OF THE NEWBORN

Hemolytic (blood-destroying) disease of the newborn is the primary condition related to the positive/negative aspect of your blood. It is a condition that afflicts only the offspring of Rh-negative women, so if you are O, A, B, or AB positive, it doesn't concern you.

Some 70 years ago, researchers discovered that Rh-negative women who were missing an antigen and who were carrying Rh-positive babies had a unique situation. The Rh-positive babies carried the Rh antigen on their blood cells. Unlike with the major blood type system, in which the antibodies to other blood types develop from birth, Rh-negative people do not make an antibody to the Rh antigen unless they are first sensitized. This sensitization usually occurs when blood is exchanged between the mother and infant during birth, so the mother's immune system does not have enough time to react to the first baby, and that baby suffers no consequences. However, should a subsequent conception result in another Rh-positive baby, the mother, now sensitized, will produce antibodies to the baby's blood type, potentially causing birth defects and even infant death. Fortunately, there is a vaccine for this condition, which is given to Rh-negative women after the birth of their first child, and after every subsequent birth. It shouldn't arise as a problem, but it's best to know your Rh status so you can be certain that the vaccine is administered.

INFERTILITY AND HABITUAL MISCARRIAGE

For more than 50 years, scientists have been studying the reasons childlessness seems more common among Type A, Type B, and Type AB women than in Type O women. Many researchers have suggested that infertility and habitual abortion may be the result of antibodies in a woman's vaginal secretions reacting with blood type antigens on the man's sperm. A 1975 study of 288 miscarried fetuses showed a preponderance of Type A, Type B, and Type AB blood, which may have been the result of incompatibility with Type O mothers and their anti-A and anti-B antibodies.

A study looking at a large sample of families showed that the rate of miscarriages was highest when the mother and father were ABO incompatible, such as with a Type O mother and a Type A father. For both white and African-American women of Type O or Type A blood, incompatible Type B fetuses were more frequently found among miscarriages.

The blood group link to infertility is not yet fully established. In my own practice, I find that there are many reasons for fertility problems, including food allergies, poor diet, obesity, and stress.

CASE HISTORY: REPEATED MISCARRIAGE
LANA, AGE 42; BLOOD TYPE A

Lana came to my office after a long history of repeated miscarriages. She told me she'd heard about me from someone she had been talking with in the waiting room of her fertility doctor's office. Lana was desperate. In the previous 10 years she'd had over 20 miscarriages, and she was just about to give up on trying to start a family. I suggested that she try the Blood Type A Diet. For the next year, Lana followed the Blood Type Diet assiduously, while also taking several botanical preparations to strengthen the muscular tone of her uterus. At the end of the year, she became pregnant. She was thrilled, but also very nervous.

Now, in addition to her previous miscarriages, Lana was worried about her age and the possibility of Down syndrome. Her obstetrician recommended amniocentesis, which is common for women over age 40, but I advised against it because the procedure carries a risk of miscarriage. After talking with her husband, Lana decided to forgo the amniocentesis, accepting the possibility of a birth defect. Happily, she delivered a perfectly healthy baby boy.

I saw Lana years later for a problem unrelated to pregnancy. Next to her sat three small kids. "Yours?" I asked. "Yes," she replied. "How did you get them?" I queried. "Oh," she coyly replied. "We had business troubles, and I could not afford a visit for quite a while. So I just redid everything you taught me from the first visit."

CASE HISTORY: INFERTILITY
NIEVES, AGE 44: BLOOD TYPE B

Nieves, a 44-year-old South American massage therapist, first came to see me for a variety of digestive problems. Within one year of beginning the Type B Diet, most of her digestive complaints were resolved.

One day Nieves shyly announced to me that she was pregnant. Although she had not told me before, she now said that she and her husband had tried for many years to conceive a child, but had finally given up hope. She believed that the Type B Diet was responsible for restoring her fertility. When Nieves delivered a healthy baby girl, she named her Nasha, meaning "gift from God."

SEX RATIOS
In both European and non-European populations, the rate of male offspring is higher in Type O babies born to Type O mothers. This is also true if both the baby and mother are Type B. The opposite is true of Type A babies born to Type A mothers, where female offspring are more frequent.

MENOPAUSE AND MENSTRUAL PROBLEMS
Menopause affects every midlife woman regardless of her blood type. A decrease in estrogen and progesterone, the two basic female hormones, causes profound mental and physical problems for many women, including hot flashes, loss of libido, depression, hair loss, and skin changes.

The decline in female hormones also creates a risk for cardiovascular disease, as it appears that estrogen provides protection to the heart and lowers cholesterol levels. Osteoporosis, a thinning of the bones that leads to frailty and even death, is another outcome of estrogen deficiency. With our newfound understanding of the risks associated with hormone depletion, many doctors prescribe hormone-replacement therapy, involving high doses of estrogen and sometimes progesterone. Many women are concerned about conventional estrogen-replacement therapy because some studies show a greater risk of breast cancer in women who use these hormones, primarily when there is a family history of breast cancer. The question of whether to take these synthetic hormones is a dilemma.

Knowing your blood type may help you resolve the conflict and decide which approach is best for your own personal needs.

If you are Type O or Type B and entering menopause, begin to exercise in a manner recommended for your blood type, and in a way appropriate to your current fitness and lifestyle. Eat a high-protein diet. Conventional estrogen replacement generally works reasonably well for Type O and Type B women, unless you have high risk factors for breast cancer.

If you are Type A or Type AB, you should avoid using conventional estrogen replacement, because of your unusually high susceptibility to breast cancer (see Chapter Twelve). Instead, use the newly available phytoestrogens, which are estrogen- and progesterone-like preparations derived from plants, principally soybeans, alfalfa, and yams. Many of these preparations are available as a cream that can be applied to the skin several times a day. Plant phytoestrogens are typically high in the estrogen fraction called estriol, whereas chemical estrogens are based on estradiol. The medical literature conclusively shows that supplementation with estriol inhibits the occurrence of breast cancer.

Phytoestrogens lack the potency of the chemical estrogens, but they are definitely effective against many of the troubling symptoms of menopause, including hot flashes and vaginal dryness. Because they are only weak estrogens, they will not suppress any estrogen production by the body, unlike the chemical estrogen. For the woman who is not taking any estrogen supplementation because of a family history of breast cancer, phytoestrogens are a godsend. Talk to your gynecologist about using these preparations. If you have no special risk factors for breast cancer, the stronger chemical estrogen is more effective for reducing heart disease and osteoporosis, in addition to the symptoms of menopause.

It is interesting that in Japan, where the typical diet is high in phytoestrogens, there is no precise Japanese word for menopause. Undoubtedly the widespread use of soy products, which contain the phytoestrogens genistein and daidzein, serves to modulate the severe symptoms of menopause.

CASE HISTORY: MENSTRUAL PROBLEMS
PATTY, AGE 45; BLOOD TYPE O

Patty was a 45-year-old African-American woman with a variety of problems, including arthritis, high blood pressure, and severe premenstrual syndrome with heavy bleeding. She came to my office accompanied by her husband. At the time, she was being treated with one drug or another for her ailments. I learned that Patty had been consuming a basically vegetarian diet, so it was no surprise that she was also anemic. I recommended that she begin exercising and adopt the Type O high-protein diet, and I prescribed a course of botanical medicines.

Within two months, Patty made an astounding turnabout. Arthritis: cured. Hypertension: under control. PMS: last two periods, all symptoms gone. Menstrual flow: normal.

New associations between blood type and common diseases are being studied every year. The idea that many diseases show a strong propensity for one blood type over another is gaining acceptance in scientific circles. I regularly report these associations on my website, www.dadamo.com.

Knowing your chances, assessing your risk factors, and understanding the situation give you more ways to take positive action against forces that may often leave you feeling without control.

Now let's look at cancer. Cancer is such a major cause of death and disease—and has such a clear-cut blood type connection—that I'm devoting an entire chapter to its discussion.

TWELVE

Blood Type
and Cancer:

The Fight to Heal

J EXPERIENCE A PARTICULAR SURGE OF PASSION WHENEVER I EXAM-
ine the healing connection between blood type and cancer. My mother
died of breast cancer, and her experience was agonizing.

My mother was a wonderful woman, whose simple Spanish values
guarded us all against any pretense or pomp. Mom was an anomaly in
our family—a Type A who ate what she chose to eat. She had the no-
torious Catalan strong will. In her house (my parents were divorced),
she served a basic Mediterranean diet of meats and salads and some
processed foods. In spite of my father's blood type work, there wasn't
a soybean or a legume in sight when we stayed with Mother.

Anyone who has seen a family member or friend engage in a valiant
but ultimately fruitless struggle against cancer knows that there is nothing quite so heartbreaking. Watching my mother as she went from mastectomy to chemotherapy to brief remission to recurrence, I could almost
visualize the armies of invisible invaders, stealing their way into her
healthy tissues and gaining a strong foothold before sweeping away her
immune system, like barbarians waging a surprise attack. In the end,
nothing could be done to stop them. They won.

In the years since my mother's death, I have found myself return-
ing again and again to the mysteries of cancer. I have often wondered

whether my mother might have been spared had she adhered to a Type A Diet, or whether she was somehow genetically preselected to fight and lose this battle. I have dedicated myself to finding those answers on her behalf. You might say I have a Catalan-style vendetta against breast cancer, above all other cancers.

Does cancer find an inherently more fertile ground to grow and develop in the body of one blood type than in another? The answer is a definite yes.

There is undeniable evidence that persons with Type A or Type AB blood have an overall higher rate of cancer and poorer odds of survival than Type O and Type B.

Actually, as early as the 1940s, the American Medical Association stated that Type AB had the greatest rate of cancer of all the blood types, but the news didn't make headlines, probably because Type ABs constitute such a low percentage of the population. Statistically, their high numbers didn't cause the same kind of alarm as the information about the more common Type A. But from a personal standpoint, that's surely of little comfort to the individuals with Type AB blood. Researchers may treat cancer like a numbers game; I prefer to treat it as a personal crisis in the life of a single individual.

Type O and Type B show lower incidences of cancer, but we don't yet have enough information to say exactly why that is. There are important clues, however, in the antigen and antibody activity of the different blood types that we can explore.

Having said that, the blood type–cancer connection is highly complex and in many ways mysterious. Be clear that being Type AB or Type A doesn't mean it's certain or even likely that you personally are going to get cancer, any more than being Type O or Type B means you'll absolutely be spared. There are many causes of cancer, and we are still haunted by the mystery of why some people with no seeming risk factors contract the disease.

Increasingly, blood type has emerged as a vital factor, but it is only one piece of the puzzle. There are many causes of cancer—chemical carcinogens, radiation, and other genetic factors, to name a few. These factors are largely independent of blood type, and as such would not produce enough of a difference in the population to be able to be predicted by blood type alone. For example, cigarette smoking could easily mask or weaken a blood type association because it is a powerful enough carcinogen to cause cancer all by itself—regardless of your inherent susceptibility or lack of it.

There is an enormous amount of scientific research on the molecular relationship between blood type and cancer. Research, however, has practically ignored the question of whether a person with one blood type or another has a better chance of surviving particular cancers.

Who lives and who dies? Who survives and who doesn't? This, in my opinion, is the great missing link in the research on cancer and blood type. The real blood type–cancer connection resides in the rates of resolution rather than in the rates of occurrence among the different blood types, and that connection may be the glue of lectins.

The Cancer-Lectin Connection

SHAKESPEARE once wrote, "There is some soul of goodness in things evil." In some instances, like chemotherapy treatments to fight cancer, it is expedient and even beneficial to use a poison. In relation to cancer, lectins can serve a positive purpose. They can be used to agglutinate cancerous cells, thus acting as a catalyst for the immune system—a wake-up call to get busy and protect the good cells.

How does this happen? Under normal circumstances, the production of surface sugars by a cell is highly specific and controlled. Not in a cancer cell. Because the genetic material is scrambled, cancer cells lose control over the production of their surface sugars and usually manufacture them in greater amounts than a normal cell would. Cancer cells are more liable than normal cells to tangle up if they come in contact with the appropriate lectin.

In 1963, Joseph Aub, a researcher at Massachusetts General Hospital, discovered by chance that there were many surface differences between normal cells and cancer cells, an idea that was thought at the time to be so strange as, in the words of one biographer, "to border on lunacy."

Aub believed that these differences enabled cancer cells to multiply when normal cells would not, detach from their primary site, and spread throughout the body. He originally worked with enzymes, attempting to digest certain portions of the cancer cell's surface to see if there were any differences.

Then, as with many medical discoveries, luck intervened. Of all the enzymes he used, only one, derived from wheat germ, showed any effect, agglutinating the cancer cells. When he replaced this enzyme with an identical one from hog pancreas, again, nothing happened. Obviously, something in the wheat germ other than the enzyme Aub was looking at was agglutinating the cancer cells. As a matter of fact, when he heated the wheat germ extract and destroyed the enzyme, it continued to destroy cancer cells. Aub and his colleagues soon found that the wheat germ enzyme was contaminated with a small protein that was responsible for the agglutinating activity. Aub had discovered a lectin in wheat germ that agglutinated the cancer cells.

Malignant cancerous cells are as much as 100 times more sensitive to the agglutinating effects of lectins than are normal cells. If two slides

The Lectin-Cancer Connection

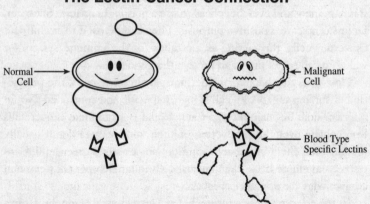

Why lectins agglutinate cancer cells. The cells depicted on the left side of the drawing represent nonmalignant cells. Because the production of surface sugars is controlled by intact genetic material, normal cell walls have surface sugars arranged in an orderly pattern. Malignant cells, however, have many more surface sugars because their genetic material is flawed, resulting in the malignant cell producing uncontrolled amounts of these sugars. If a blood type–specific food lectin is added to a suspension of normal and malignant cells, it will interact more aggressively with the "fuzzier" malignant cells than with the "smoother" normal cells.

are prepared, one containing normal cells and the other malignant, an equal dose of the appropriate lectin will convert the slide with malignant cells into a huge entangled clump, whereas the slide of normal cells will show little, if any, change.

When malignant cells become agglutinated into huge tangles of hundreds, thousands, or millions of cancer cells, the immune system becomes reactivated. Now the antibodies can target the clumps of cancer cells, identifying them for destruction. This search-and-destroy mission is usually carried out by powerful scavenger cells found in the liver.

If you were to go into a medical database and key in lectins and cancer, the printer would probably be working overtime for days. Lectins are extensively used to study the molecular biology of cancer because they make excellent probes, helping identify unique antigens, called markers, on the surface of the cancer cells. Beyond this, their use is limited, which is a shame because they are so ubiquitous in common foods. By identifying the blood type of a person with a particular cancer and by using the appropriate lectins derived from the Blood Type Diet, a powerful new tool can be used by any cancer patient to improve the odds of survival.

Enter the Blood Type

AN ENORMOUS amount of cell division occurs in the course of one's lifetime. Given these odds, it is amazing that more cancer doesn't occur. This is probably because the immune system has a special ability to detect and eliminate the vast majority of mutations that take place on a day-to-day basis. Cancer probably results from a breakdown in this surveillance, the successful cancer cell tricking the immune system into impotency by mimicking normal cells. As we have already seen, the blood types possess unique powers of surveillance, depending on the shape and form of the intruder.

A number of tumor antigens (tumor markers) show blood type antigen characteristics. Many of them are A-like, which explains the predominance of Type A and Type AB with cancer. However, that's not the whole story.

This gives you a rough idea of how blood types, agglutinating lectins, and cancer interact together. The obvious next question is, what does it mean? And if you are personally worried about cancer, what does this mean for you?

The work goes on. The more we learn, the more we live. Let me tell you what I've discovered about the cancers themselves and then about what steps you can take.

Breast Cancer

A NUMBER OF YEARS AGO, while taking histories on new patients, I began to notice that many women who had suffered from breast cancer at some time in their distant pasts and had fully recovered were Type O or Type B. Their rate of recovery was especially impressive because most of them told me that their treatment had not been very aggressive— usually no more than surgical excision, only rarely including radiation or chemotherapy.

How could this be? The statistics on breast cancer show that, even with the most aggressive treatment, only 19 to 25 percent of the women survive 5 to 10 years after the diagnosis. Yet these women had survived for a much longer time with only minimal therapy. Was it possible that being Type O or Type B helped protect them against the spread of the disease or a recurrence?

Over the years, I also began to notice a distinct tendency in Type A women with breast cancer—and also in Type AB women, although I haven't seen many with that rare blood type—to suffer from a more aggressive malignancy and a lower survival rate, even when biopsies taken from the lymph nodes showed that they were free of cancer. Through my own clinical experiences and study of scientific literature, I concluded that there is a major connection between surviving breast cancer and your blood type.

In 1991, a study appeared in the *Lancet*, an English medical journal, that may have provided part of the answer. Researchers reported that it appeared possible to predict whether a breast cancer would spread to the lymph nodes by virtue of its characteristics when treated with a strain containing a lectin from the edible snail, *Helix aspersa/pomatia*. They reported a strong association between the uptake of the snail lectin and the subsequent development of metastasis to the lymph nodes. In other words, antigens on the surface of the primary breast cancer cells were changing, and this change was allowing the cancer to spread into the lymph nodes. Now, here comes the punch line: The lectin of *Helix aspersa/pomatia* is highly specific—to Blood Type A.

The researchers studying breast cancer discovered that as the cancer cells changed, they made themselves more A-like. This allowed them to bypass all of the body's defenses and rage unimpeded into the defenseless lymph.

Did my Type O patients survive because they were Type O? Did my Type B patients survive because they were Type B? It certainly looked that way.

And there is a confirmation in our scientific understanding of cancer. Many tumor cells have unique antigens, or markers, on their surfaces. For instance, breast cancer patients often show high levels of cancer antigen 15-3 (CA15-3), a marker for breast cancer; ovarian cancer patients often have high levels of CA125; and prostate cancer patients may have an elevated prostate-specific antigen (PSA). These antigens, called tumor markers, are often used to track the progress of the disease and effectiveness of treatment. Many tumor markers possess blood type activity. Sometimes the tumor markers are incomplete or corrupted blood type antigens, which in a normal cell would have gone on to form a part of a person's blood type system.

It is not surprising that many of these tumor markers have A-like qualities, which allow them easy access to the Type A and Type AB systems. There they are welcomed as self—the ultimate molecular Trojan horse. Obviously, the A-like intruders would be more easily detected and eliminated if they were to slip into a Type O or Type B system.

Many breast cancer markers are surprisingly A-like. That's the answer to my question about the differing rates of recurrence on the part of my patients. Although my Type O and Type B patients developed breast cancer, their anti-A antigens were better able to fight it off, rounding up the early cancer cells and destroying them. My Type A and Type AB patients, however, couldn't fight the cancer as well because their systems couldn't see their opponents. Everywhere they turned, the cells looked just like them—and they were unable to detect the mutated cancer cells beneath their clever masks.

CASE HISTORY: PREVENTING BREAST CANCER
ANNE, AGE 47; BLOOD TYPE A

Anne came to the office for a general wellness visit, without any real physical complaints. But while I was doing her medical history, I learned that Anne's family had a high incidence of breast cancer on both her mother's and father's sides, and the mortality rate among those who had the disease was very high.

Anne knew about her genetic risk factors, but she was surprised to learn that her Type A blood presented an additional risk factor. "I don't suppose it makes any difference, though," she said. "Either I'm going to get breast cancer or I'm not. There's nothing I can really do about it."

I advised Anne that there were several measures she could take. First, because of her family history, she needed to be hypervigilant about suspicious breast lumps, perform frequent breast self-examinations, and make sure to get routine mammograms.

"When was your last mammogram?" I asked. Anne sheepishly told me that her last mammogram had been seven years before. It turned out that Anne was strongly disinclined to avail herself of any conventional medical techniques. She had educated herself about herbs and vitamins and often used them to treat herself effectively. But when it came to more intrusive medical treatments, she shied away. However, she did promise to schedule a mammogram.

Anne's mammogram was clean, and she began a concentrated program of cancer avoidance. The Blood Type A Diet was an easy transition for Anne because she already ate a primarily vegetarian diet. I fine-tuned the diet with anti-cancer foods, especially increasing the amount of soy and adding specific naturopathic herbs. Anne began to study yoga. She told me that for the first time in her adult life, she wasn't constantly worrying about cancer.

A year later, Anne had a second mammogram. This time a suspicious mark was detected in her left breast. A biopsy showed it to be a precancerous condition known as neoplasia. Essentially, neoplasia is the presence of mutated cells. It's not cancer, but it can become cancer if the cells continue to deteriorate and multiply. During the biopsy, Anne's doctor completely removed the precancerous tissue.

Over the years, there have been no new growths detected, although we watch Anne very carefully. She continues to follow the Blood Type A Diet religiously and says she has never felt healthier.

Of all the functions a physician can perform, none is more elegant and valuable than successful prediction and intervention. I was glad Anne came to me when she did, and that she took all the right steps.

Immunotherapy

Breast cancer continues to be baffling and too often deadly, but there are some signs that blood type may represent a key to the cure. Immunotherapy is the most promising area of study in fighting all cancers, including breast cancer. There are currently a multitude of clinical trials examining the efficacy of vaccine treatment for cancer. It's a promising direction. One of the early pioneers of this approach used blood type as his basis in creating a vaccine.

The late Georg Springer, a research scientist with the Bligh Cancer Center at the University of Chicago School of Medicine, investigated the effects of a vaccine whose basis is a molecule called the T antigen. Since the 1950s, Springer had been one of the most important investigators in the role of blood type in disease. His contributions to the field were phenomenal, and his work on the T antigen was most promising.

The T antigen is a common tumor marker (pancarcinoma antigen) found in many cancers, especially breast cancer. It shares some similarity with the antigen against Blood Type A. Healthy, cancer-free people carry antibodies against the T antigen, so it is never seen in them. In fact anti-T antibodies are one of the few antibodies that you carry against yourself, although it has been shown that if you are Blood Type A you manufacture less of the antibody than the other blood types. The structure of the T antigen was discovered in the early 1960s by Gerhard Uhlenbruck at the University of Cologne using the lectin from peanuts.

Springer believed that a vaccine composed of the T antigen and several helper molecules called adjuvants could jolt and then reawaken the suppressed immune systems of cancer patients, helping them attack and destroy the cancerous cells. Springer and his colleagues used a vaccine derived from the T antigen, hot-rodded with another common vaccine against typhoid, as a long-term treatment against the recurrence of advanced breast cancer. Although the study group was small—fewer than 25 women—the results are impressive. All of the 11 breast cancer patients who had severely advanced disease (stage III and stage IV) survived for more than five years—remarkable in what is considered end-stage cancer—and 6 of those patients survived more than 10 years. These results are nothing short of miraculous.

Springer's work on blood type systems and cancer convinced me that the natural evolution of our understanding of blood types will eventually provide not just information on risk factors, but also a cure for every manifestation of the disease. Unfortunately Springer's work languished after his death, but I'm happy to report that there has been a considerable surge in research interest in the T antigen in recent years.

There are other ways that blood type may influence the course and outcome of breast cancer. One mechanism involves a molecule called vascular endothelial growth factor (VEGF), which is involved in the development of our vascular network, a process known as angiogenesis. Some evidence suggests that there may be a direct interaction between the Blood Type A antigen and the receptor for VEGF that perhaps could lead to increased production of blood vessels, a process that can help the spread of cancer cells. There is even noncancer evidence of this link: VEGF is responsible for the growth of large birthmarks called port wine stains (hemangiomas), whose occurrence is also known to be more common in Type A individuals.

Other Forms of Cancer

THE PATHOLOGY of cancer—wild marauders out for a night on the town—is fundamentally the same in all variations, but differences related both to cause and to blood type exist. The A-like or B-like tumor markers exert remarkable control over the way the body's immune system reacts to the cancer's invasion and growth.

Again, almost all cancers show a preference for Type A and Type AB individuals, although there are occasional forms that are B-like, such as female reproductive and bladder cancers. Type O seems to be far more resistant to developing almost any cancer. I believe the intolerant and hostile Type O system, with its more simple fucose sugars, has an easier time tossing off the A-like or B-like cancer cells and developing anti-A or anti-B antibodies.

Again, we unfortunately know little about the full implications of the blood type link in cancers other than breast cancer. However, they most likely follow a similar course. Let's examine some of the most common forms of cancer.

BRAIN TUMORS. Most cancers of the brain and nervous system, such as glioma multiforme and astrocytoma, show a preference for Type A and Type AB individuals. Their tumor markers are A-like.

FEMALE REPRODUCTIVE CANCERS. Cancers of the female reproductive system (uterine, cervical, ovarian, and labial) show a preference for Type A and Type AB. However, there is also a numerically high number of Type B women who suffer from these cancers. This implies there are different tumor markers created, depending on the circumstances. Ovarian cysts and uterine fibroids, which are usually benign but may be a sign of susceptibility to cancer, generate copious amounts of Type A and Type B antigens.

COLON CANCER. Blood type is not the strongest determinant for the various forms of colon cancer. The real risk factors for the conditions that lead to colon cancer are related to diet, lifestyle, and temperament. Ulcerative colitis, Crohn's disease, and irritable bowel syndrome left unmitigated eventually leave the system depleted and open to cancer. A high-fat diet, combined with smoking and alcohol consumption, create the ideal environment for digestive cancers. The risk is greater if you have a family history of colon cancer. That said, Type A and Type AB individuals are at higher risk.

MOUTH AND UPPER DIGESTIVE CANCERS. Cancers of the lip, tongue, gums, and cheek; tumors of the salivary gland; and esophageal cancer are all strongly linked to Type A and Type AB blood. Most of these cancers are self-generated, in that the risks can be minimized if you abstain from tobacco, moderate your alcohol consumption, and watch your diet.

STOMACH AND ESOPHAGEAL CANCER. Stomach cancer is attracted to low levels of stomach acid, a Type A and Type AB trait. In well over 63,000 cases of stomach cancer studied, Type A and Type AB were predominant. Stomach cancer is epidemic in China, Japan, and Korea because the typical diet is rich in smoked, pickled, and fermented foods. These Asian dietary staples seem to counter any of the good that soybeans might do, perhaps because they are packed with carcinogenic nitrates. Asian Type Bs, who have higher levels of stomach acid, aren't as prone to stomach cancer, even if they eat some of the same foods.

PANCREATIC, LIVER, GALLBLADDER, AND BILE DUCT CANCERS. Cancers of the pancreas, liver, and gallbladder are rare in Type O, with its hardy digestive systems. A study by the Dana-Farber Cancer Institute showed that people with Blood Types A, B, and AB were more likely to develop pancreatic cancer than Type Os. Type A and Type AB are at most risk; Type B has some susceptibility, especially when consuming certain nuts and seeds that are unsuitable.

Several of the earlier therapies for these cancers included large portions of fresh liver from sheep, horse, and buffalo. They seemed to help, but no one knew why. It was later discovered that the livers of these animals contained lectins that slowed the growth and spread of pancreatic, liver, gallbladder, and bile duct cancers.

CASE HISTORY: LIVER CANCER
CATHY, AGE 49; BLOOD TYPE A

Cathy first sought medical attention for a suspicious growth in her abdomen, which turned out to be an aggressive form of liver cancer. She was treated at Harvard's Deaconess Hospital in Boston, Massachusetts, and eventually received a liver transplant. She was referred to me two years later.

In the subsequent two years, most of my focus was on using naturopathic techniques to replace the immunosuppressing antirejection drugs needed to help her keep her transplanted liver. Cathy's condition improved to the point that she was able to stop her drug therapy.

However, after two years of this protocol, Cathy was experiencing some shortness of breath, and at her checkup at Harvard, doctors noticed suspicious lesions on a chest X-ray. These turned out to be cancer.

Cathy and her physicians were on the horns of a dilemma. Her lungs were so heavily laced with cancer, surgery was out of the question ("It would be like picking cherries," said her surgeon), and her liver transplant ruled out chemotherapy.

We went to work, using the basic Type A–lectin cancer diet and other immune-enhancing botanicals. I also recommended a preparation made from shark cartilage for Cathy to take orally and use as an enema.

In an amazing series of correspondences, Cathy's surgical team at Harvard kept me up-to-date on her progress, including informing me that the lesions in Cathy's lungs had shrunk and looked more like scar tissue. Subsequent letters confirmed these findings. In time even the scar tissue began to disappear.

Cathy was stunned and overjoyed. "When they told me that the cancer seemed to be going into remission, I felt as if I had won the lottery," she said happily. Cathy went on to live three symptom-free years. Unfortunately, her cancer finally returned, and she later died.

The case is especially interesting for two reasons: First, throughout this time Cathy received no treatment other than naturopathic. Second, her team at Harvard was open-minded about and supportive of her using a naturopathic doctor. Perhaps what we have seen here is a tiny glimpse of the future: all medical systems working together for the betterment of the patient.

By the way, the total cost of Cathy's naturopathic therapy was less than $1,500, as opposed to the tens of thousands she might have spent on conventional treatment.

LYMPHOMAS, LEUKEMIAS, AND HODGKIN'S DISEASE. Type O may be predisposed to lymphomas, leukemias, and Hodgkin's disease.

Although these diseases of the blood and lymph preferentially afflict Type O, they may not be true cancers at all, but rather viral infections that have run amok. This would make some sense in light of what we know about Type Os; they're actually pretty good at fighting most cancers, but the Type O antigen is not well designed for fighting viruses.

LUNG CANCER. Lung cancer is truly nonspecific. It is one of the few cancers that has no particular blood type connection. Lung cancer is most commonly caused by cigarette smoking. Yes, lung cancer is caused by many other things as well. There are people who have never smoked who will die of lung cancer as you are reading this sentence. But we all know that smoking is the overwhelming cause of lung cancer. Tobacco is such a powerful carcinogen in its own right that it bypasses anything so obvious and so ordered as predilection.

PROSTATE CANCER. There appears to be a higher level of prostate cancer in secretors. My own experience has been that a greater number of Type A and Type AB men suffer from prostate cancer than do Type O or Type B men. A Type A or Type AB secretor is at the highest risk.

SKIN AND BONE CANCERS. Type A and Type AB individuals are at greatest risk for malignant melanoma, the deadliest form of skin cancer, although Type O and Type B are not immune. Bone cancers seem to show a consistent preference for Type B, although there is some risk for Type A and Type AB individuals.

URINARY TRACT, KIDNEY, AND BLADDER CANCERS. Bladder cancer in both men and women occurs most often in Type A and Type B individuals. Type ABs, who have the double whammy of both A and B characteristics, are probably at the greatest risk of all. Far more than Type A, Type B individuals who suffer from recurrent bladder and kidney infections should be especially careful with the management of this problem, as it inevitably leads to more serious diseases. One puzzling connection that is yet to be unraveled: Wheat germ agglutinin, the lectin that can act favorably against both lobular and intraductal breast cancers, paradoxically accelerates the growth of bladder cancer cells.

Fighting Back

CANCER ALWAYS seems to present a discouraging picture. I imagine that if you are Type A or Type AB, you may be thinking grim thoughts. Remember, though, that susceptibility is a single factor among many. I believe that knowing your predilection for cancer and understanding the workings of your specific blood type gives you more opportunity than you would otherwise have to fight back. The following strategies provide a way to make a difference for yourself, especially if you are Type A or Type AB. In particular, many of the foods suggested are tailored for these blood types. Current research has focused primarily on the A-like markers for breast cancer, and little investigation has been conducted regarding the B-like cancers. Unfortunately, this means that while the cancer-fighting foods suggested here may be very effective for Type A and Type AB, they won't necessarily help Type B or Type O. In fact, most of these foods (peanuts, soy, lentils, and wheat germ) cause other problems for the latter two blood types.

Continued research will one day give us a deeper understanding of the cancer-diet connection for all the blood types. In the meantime, here are some special recommendations for people with Type A and AB.

YOU LIVE AS YOU EAT

People with Type A blood have digestive tracts that find it difficult to break down animal fats and proteins. Type A and Type AB should adhere to a diet high in fiber and low in animal products.

There are specific foods that must be given extra consideration as cancer preventives.

SOYBEANS . . . AGAIN

Between 3 and 11 percent of every cake of tofu is composed of soybean agglutinins. Soybean agglutinins are able to selectively identify early mutated cells producing the Type A antigen and sweep them from the system, leaving normal Type A cells alone. Although soy foods are a rich source, only a minute amount is needed for agglutination.

The soybean agglutinin especially discriminates when it comes to breast cancer cells; it is so specific that it's been used to remove cancerous cells from harvested bone marrow. In experimental work breast cancer patients had their bone marrow removed and were then bombarded with high levels of chemotherapy and radiation. These oncology tools would normally destroy the bone marrow. Instead, the harvested marrow—cleansed by soybean lectin—was then reintroduced into the patients. These treatments have shown some very good results.

The soybean lectin also contains estrogen-related compounds genistein and daidzein. These compounds not only help balance the effect of a woman's estrogen levels but also contain other properties that can help reduce the blood supply to tumor cells.

Soybeans in all forms are beneficial to Type A and Type AB as a general cancer preventative. The vegetable proteins in soy are easier for these blood types to use, and so it is strongly suggested that these blood types reexamine any aversion they may have to tofu and tofu products. Think of tofu not only as a food, but as a powerful medicine.

Japanese women have such a low incidence of breast cancer because the use of tofu and other soy products is still high in the overall Japanese diet. As the diet becomes more Westernized, it is possible that we will see a proportionate rise in certain forms of cancer. One study of Japanese immigrant women living in San Francisco showed that they had twice the rate of breast cancer as their cousins living in Japan—no doubt due to a change in dietary habits.

PEANUTS

The peanut agglutinin has also been found to contain a specific lectin sensitive to breast cancer cells, particularly the medullary form. The peanut lectin shows activity to a lesser degree against all other forms, including intraductal, lobular, and scirrhous breast cancers. This connection is probably true of other Type A–like cancers.

Eat fresh peanuts with the skins still on them (the skins, not the shells). Peanut butter is probably not a good source of the lectin, as the majority of commercial brands are too processed and homogenized.

Amaranth
The grain amaranth contains a lectin that has a specific affinity to colon cancer cells. It programs the cancer cells to kill themselves, a process known as apoptosis.

Mushrooms and Fava Beans
Commercial (silver dollar) mushrooms and fava beans contain lectins that react and suppress the T antigen. If you have a history of colon polyps, which are often a precancerous condition, you may want to increase your consumption of these foods. An amazing series of studies have shown that these lectins actually reverse many of the precancerous changes in the colon, reprogramming cells to change back to a more normal state.

Lentils
The lectin found in common domestic brown or green lentils (*Lens culinaris*) shows a strong specific attraction for lobular, medullary, intraductal, and stromal forms of breast cancer and is likely to affect other A-like cancers.

Lima Beans
Lima bean lectin is one of the most potent agglutinants of all Type A cells, cancerous or not. When you're healthy, lima beans will hurt you— so they shouldn't be part of a prevention strategy. However, if you are suffering from an A-like cancer, eat the lima beans. The lectin will agglutinate untold numbers of cancer cells. It will also destroy some perfectly innocent and upstanding Type A cells, but the exchange is worth it.

Wheat Germ
Wheat germ agglutinin shows a great affinity for Type A cancers. It is concentrated in the seed coating of the wheat, the outer husk that is usually discarded. Unprocessed wheat bran will provide the most significant quantity of the lectin, although you can also use commercial wheat germ preparations.

SNAILS

If you're Type A or Type AB, order escargots the next time you dine at a fancy French restaurant. Consider it medicine packaged in a glamorous, delicious form. The edible snail, *Helix aspersa/pomatia*, is a powerful breast cancer agglutinin, capable of determining whether cancerous cells will metastasize to the lymph nodes.

Unless the thought of eating snails disgusts you (and really, they're quite delicious), what harm can it do? A colleague of mine from Italy once showed me a fifteenth-century manuscript that advised medieval physicians "to have the woman eat snails should she have crablike scarring of the breast."

Other Strategies

TAKE CARE OF YOUR LIVER AND COLON

Women should be aware that the liver and colon are two major sites where estrogens can be degraded—if their functions are disturbed, the levels of estrogen throughout the body can rise. Elevated estrogen activity can stimulate the growth of cancerous cells.

Adopt a high-fiber diet to increase the levels of butyrate in the colon wall cells. Butyrates, as you may recall, promote the normalization of tissue.

ANTIOXIDANTS

Vitamin antioxidants have been studied for breast cancer and have been shown to be not very effective in preventing the disease. Vitamin E and beta-carotenes don't deposit in high enough concentrations in breast tissue to effect positive change. Plant-based antioxidants do seem to make some difference but must be combined with supplemental sources of vitamin C to synergize for greatest effect.

Yellow onions contain very high levels of quercetin, an especially potent antioxidant. Quercetin has none of the estrogenizing activity of vitamin E and is hundreds of times stronger than vitamin antioxidants. It is available as a supplement in many health food stores.

Women with a risk factor for breast cancer who are considering or are on estrogen-replacement therapy should use phytoestrogens derived from natural products instead of synthetic estrogens. Plant-based estrogens contain high levels of estriol, a weaker form of the estrogen hormone than estradiol, which is manufactured synthetically. Estriol seems to lower your chances of developing breast cancer. The synthetics increase the risk. Tamoxifen, an estrogen-blocking drug prescribed to breast cancer patients with estrogen-sensitive breast tumors, is itself a weaker form of estrogen. Genistein is an estrogen-related compound found in the soybean lectin. This phytoestrogen inhibits angiogenesis, interfering with the production of new blood vessels needed to feed the growth of cancerous tumors.

SPROUTED VEGETABLES

Sprouting vegetables unlock powerful medicines hidden within them. This is especially true if the vegetables are part of the cruciferous family, which when sprouted liberate large amounts of a powerful anticancer molecule known as sulforaphane. Sulforaphane has well-researched effects on DNA, encouraging its proper repair and controlling how genes are expressed in response to environmental stimulation.

GENERAL PALLIATIVES

Exercise frequently. Get adequate rest. Have adequate creative expression in your life. Avoid known pollutants and pesticides. Eat your fruits and vegetables. Don't use antibiotics indiscriminately. If you get sick, allow your immune system to fight off the illness. You'll be much healthier if you do, rather than relying excessively on flu shots or antibiotics. They suppress your immune system's natural responses, which can be very powerful if given the chance.

CASE HISTORY: ADVANCED BREAST CANCER
JANE, AGE 50; BLOOD TYPE AB

When I first saw Jane in my office, she had already had a mastectomy and several rounds of chemotherapy for an infiltrating ductal breast cancer that extensively seeded into the lymph nodes. At the time of her initial diagnosis, Jane had two separate tumors on her left breast—one 4 centimeters and the other 1.5 centimeters. No one was holding out any great hope for her long-term survival.

I put Jane on the modified cancer diet for Type AB, with an emphasis on soy; I had her pneumovaxed; and I put her on the botanical protocol I use for Type As with breast cancer. Her tumor marker, CA15-3, which was 166 when she came in (normal is less than 10) dropped to 87 within three months and to 34 within four months of following my protocol. I recommended that she go see Georg Springer in Chicago to see if she could get into his vaccine study, which she did.

To this day all signs, including bone scans, look promising, although because Jane is a Type AB, I would be hesitant to pronounce her cured at this point. Only time will tell.

Cancer prevention and natural immune-system enhancement offer the brightest hope for the future. Genetic research is bringing us ever closer to being able to understand—perhaps someday even control—the cellular workings of these astounding machines that we call our bodies.

Cancer has long been among the most dreaded diseases of mankind. We seem powerless to protect ourselves and those we love from its clinging and relentless grip. Blood type analysis allows us a deeper understanding of our susceptibilities. By consciously examining our exposures to both environmental and dietary carcinogens and changing some of our lifestyle and food choices, we can minimize the effects of cell damage.

Blood type analysis also provides a way to enhance the ability of the immune system to search out and destroy cancerous and mutated cells while they are few in number. Cancer patients can use their knowledge of blood type to fully develop the capabilities of their immune systems to fight the disease. They can also gain a greater understanding of the mechanisms involved in the growth and spread of cancer.

The treatments for cancer are still far from perfect, although many people have been saved by the latest advances in therapy and scientific medical knowledge. For those of you with cancer and for those of you who have a family history of cancer, the advice is clear: Change your diet, change your attitudes, and start using antioxidant supplements. If you follow these suggestions you will be able to gain more control and a greater peace of mind. We all dread this horrible disease, but we can take positive action against it.

FURTHER READING ABOUT YOUR
BLOOD TYPE AND CANCER

Three books in my Blood Type Diet series can give you more detailed information about your blood type and cancer:

- *Live Right 4 Your Type: The Individualized Prescription for Maximizing Health, Metabolism, and Vitality in Every Stage of Your Life*

- *Eat Right 4 Your Type Complete Blood Type Encyclopedia: The A–Z Reference Guide for the Blood Type Connection to Symptoms, Disease, Conditions, Vitamins, Supplements, Herbs, and Foods*

- *Cancer: Fight It with the Blood Type Diet*

Individuals Evolving Together:

The Next Frontier

T HE HUMAN JOURNEY BEGAN AS THE SUCCESS STORY OF ONE IM-mune system—Type O. Not necessarily the first by molecular design, but certainly the most effective early survivor. It is an ineffable mystery as to precisely why Type A, the first molecular type, seemed to disappear, then resurrect itself as little as 40,000 years ago, but undoubtedly changes in diet, disease, location, and behavior exerted very strong influences. As those influences further evolved, different circumstances in specific parts of the world seemed to favor Type B. Finally, there is Type AB, not a true construct in a developmental sense, but rather the odd attribute only we humans possess of making a different blood type by combining two elemental ones.

We are always learning. Today, thanks to the pioneering work of the Human Genome Project, we are able to map the genetic structure of the human body—to name, gene by gene, chromosome by chromosome, the purpose of each living cell in the grand scheme of some master builder. Thus far, many breakthroughs have come in our understanding of the vast cellular networks of which we are composed—among them, the discovery of a large genetic architecture for breast cancer. Soon we will be able to control our genetic fates as never before.

Or will we?

Our classic understanding of genetic evolution is that it unfolds over long periods of time. However, we now know that genes constantly change, rearrange themselves, and turn each other on and off. Many of these day-to-day changes in gene activity can, under the right circumstances, be passed from one generation to the next. We've also discovered that, despite the vast genetic encyclopedia we've managed to amass, very few single genes do much of anything on their own. Rather, they exist and function in large networks that work more like computers than as simple chemical reactions.

Yet there is one gene system that continues to defy easy characterization: the blood types. When I first began to be interested in blood type chemistry, many of my colleagues advised me to find something more modern, more cutting edge. After all, they would say, "What is left to find out about blood type?" One colleague put it more succinctly, saying, "Peter, interest in the blood types went out with women's high-button shoes."

Yet, nowadays, you cannot go a week without seeing a new research paper linking blood type to a new disease or a new finding about the microbiome or a new aspect of our physiology. As I write this, blood type is a very hot research topic.

Yet I sometimes shake my head when an article comes out that purports to have discovered a new link between blood type and some disease. Very often these same conclusions were arrived at many decades ago. It seems our newfound medical interest in blood types comes with a certain historical amnesia about the important work done by many of the early pioneers.

The Revolution Continues

WHERE DOES the power of life come from? What propels us and compels us to survive?

Our blood. Our life force.

There have been recent outbreaks of rare viruses and infectious diseases, such as Ebola, which have challenged us anew. We are more conscious than ever of diseases that seem to defy medical intervention.

Will our bodies produce answers to the challenges posed by the unknown?

This is what we face:

- Increasing ultraviolet radiation caused by the depletion of the ozone layer
- Increased pollution of our air and water
- Depletion of water resources across the globe
- Increasing food contamination
- Overpopulation and famine
- Infectious diseases beyond our power to control
- Unknown plagues emerging from all of the above

We will survive. We have always survived. What form that survival will take, and what the world and its stresses will be like for the survivors, we do not know.

Perhaps, in the future, our scientific knowledge will finally allow us to gain dominion over the worst impulses of humanity, and civilization will be able to rouse itself from the suicidal impulses that seem to impel it to doom.

Our knowledge is truly vast, and there is every reason to hope that the finest and most altruistic minds and spirits of our age might focus on a way to deal with the realities of our world—violence, war, crime, ignorance, intolerance, hatred, and disease—and thus pull us out of this toxic spiral.

Nothing is complete. This world and our purpose in it is an ever-changing equation of which each of us is momentarily an integral part. The revolution continues with us or without us. Time sees us only as a blink of the eye, and it is this impermanence that makes our lives so precious.

By sharing my father's fascination with and my scientific knowledge of the Blood Type Diet, I hope to make a positive impact on the life of everyone who examines this book. Let's take a moment to luxuriate in our individuality: to study and celebrate what makes each one of us unique. All that it requires is a willingness to expand our horizon beyond simple, one-size-fits-all solutions, overextrapolations, and generalizations.

It will require a bit more work, but this vision holds the key that opens the door to our self-realization.

Like my father before me, I am a practicing naturopathic physician. I have dedicated myself to the pursuit of naturopathic knowledge and research, and this work has been my passion for many years. It began as a gift from my father and became, for me, a gift to my father. The Blood Type Diet is the revolutionary breakthrough that will change the way you eat and live.

Blood Type Charts

Type O

The Hunter

Strong
Self-Reliant
Leader

STRENGTHS	WEAKNESSES	MEDICAL RISKS	DIET PROFILE	WEIGHT-LOSS KEY	SUPPLEMENTS	EXERCISE REGIMEN
Hardy digestive tract	Intolerant to new dietary and environmental conditions	Blood clotting disorders	High protein (meat, fish)	Avoid: wheat, corn, kidney beans, navy beans, lentils, cabbage, Brussels sprouts, cauliflower, mustard greens	Vitamin B Vitamin K Calcium Iodine Licorice Kelp	Intense physical exercise, such as
Strong immune system		Inflammatory diseases (arthritis)	Vegetables Fruit			Aerobics Martial arts
Natural defenses against infections	Immune system can be *over*active and attack itself	Low thyroid production	Limited: grains, beans, legumes			Contact sports Running
System designed for efficient metabolism and preservation of nutrients		Ulcers Allergies		Aids: kelp, seafood, salt, liver, red meat, kale, spinach, broccoli		

Type A

The Cultivator

Settled
Cooperative
Orderly

STRENGTHS	WEAKNESSES	MEDICAL RISKS	DIET PROFILE	WEIGHT-LOSS KEY	SUPPLEMENTS	EXERCISE REGIMEN
Adapts well to dietary and environmental changes	Sensitive digestive tract	Heart disease	Vegetarian (vegetables, tofu, beans, legumes, grains)	Avoid: meat, dairy, kidney beans, lima beans, wheat	Vitamin B₁₂	Calming, centering exercises, such as
		Cancer			Folic acid	
	Vulnerable immune system, open to microbial invasion	Anemia			Vitamin C	Yoga
						Tai chi
Immune system preserves and metabolizes nutrients easily		Liver and gallbladder disorders	Seafood	Aids: vegetable oil, soy foods, vegetables, pineapple	Vitamin E	
			Fruit		Hawthorn	
		Type 1 diabetes			Echinacea	
					Quercetin	
					Milk thistle	

Type B

The Nomad

Balanced
Flexible
Creative

STRENGTHS	WEAKNESSES	MEDICAL RISKS	DIET PROFILE	WEIGHT-LOSS KEY	SUPPLEMENTS	EXERCISE REGIMEN
Strong immune system	No natural weaknesses, but imbalance causes tendency toward autoimmune breakdowns and rare viruses	Type 1 diabetes	Balanced omnivore	Avoid: corn, lentils, peanuts, sesame seeds, buckwheat, wheat	Magnesium	Moderate physical, with mental balance, such as
Versatile adaptation to dietary and environmental changes		Chronic fatigue syndrome	Meat (no chicken) Dairy Grains		Licorice	
		Auto-immune disorders (ALS, lupus, multiple sclerosis)	Beans Legumes Vegetables Fruit	Aids: greens, eggs, venison, liver, licorice tea	Ginkgo Lecithin	Hiking Cycling Tennis Swimming
Balanced nervous system						

Type AB

The Enigma

Rare
Charismatic
Mysterious

STRENGTHS	WEAKNESSES	MEDICAL RISKS	DIET PROFILE	WEIGHT-LOSS KEY	SUPPLE-MENTS	EXERCISE REGIMEN
Designed for modern conditions	Sensitive digestive tract	Heart disease	Mixed diet in modera-tion (meat, seafood, dairy, tofu, beans, legumes, grains)	Avoid: red meat, kidney beans, lima beans, seeds, corn, buckwheat	Vitamin C	Calming, centering exercises, such as
		Cancer			Hawthorn	
Highly tolerant immune system	Tendency for over-tolerant immune system, allowing microbial invasion	Anemia			Echinacea	Yoga
					Valerian	Tai chi
Combines benefits of Type A and Type B			Vegetables	Aids: tofu, seafood, dairy, greens, kelp, pineapple	Quercetin	Combined with moderate physical such as
			Fruit		Milk thistle	
	Reacts negatively to A-like and B-like conditions					Hiking Cycling Tennis

Results
Matter

WHEN I FIRST SET UP MY WEBSITE COMMUNITY AT DADAMO.COM, I launched a Blood Type Diet Results Database, allowing people to record their results on the diet in their own words. I've found that few things are as convincing as the experiences of real people telling their stories. Here is a selection from the database. You might recognize yourself in these stories!

Blood Type O

YOUNG MALE

Before I began, I was an overweight, fatigued vegetarian, and constantly coming down with various illnesses. After hearing and reading a bit about the diet, I began eating meats (particularly lean reds) and fish, and modified my other eating habits according to the plan. Over the past year and a half (when I began modifying my diet), I have had no significant illnesses, I've lost weight, I have constant energy, and I have a better sense of well-being. I have even felt a greater hormonal drive. My life has really taken a 180-degree turn since I began the diet.

YOUNG WOMAN

I had reached the point where it seemed to me that all food was poisonous to me. I was very ill at least twice a day, lived on Imodium to get through a day at work. I was also being treated for several health problems with traditional medicine. My gallbladder was removed, my high blood pressure was out of control and I had a minimally functioning thyroid. Within a week of changing to the Type O Diet, I noticed significant improvement. All intestinal pain/IBS was eliminated. I was still being treated for high blood pressure and low thyroid activity, but they were finally able to regulate both. I lost some weight, but the big change was in my general well-being and energy levels. People who had known me previously and had watched me day after day struggle to find something to eat that wouldn't half kill me and were aware of my general weakness, fatigue, and extremely low energy levels were dumbfounded. I became like a teenager again.

MIDDLE-AGED FEMALE

I have tried vegetarianism for a while and, until now, never understood why my health failed to improve, nor why I failed to lose a significant amount of weight. I was diagnosed as a type 2 diabetic about a year ago, and controlling my blood glucose level has been a struggle, to say the least. Having tried just about everything else, I decided to give Dr. D'Adamo's dietary advice a chance. I'm excited to experience more energy and lower blood glucose levels after following the Type O diet for a mere few weeks. Also, I have eliminated indigestion, heartburn and flatulence by simply avoiding wheat and corn products.

YOUNG MALE

Before I started the diet, I suffered from acid reflux, edema and burning bowel elimination. I have eliminated or cut back on all the foods on the Type O avoid list, save for my coffee and an occasional mixed drink. I also engaged in aerobics and weight lifting 3–5 times per week. Since I started the food plan, I have lost over 30 pounds (from 235 to about 197), the acid reflux is gone (I was a cheese binger—I think that had something to do with it) and I no longer spend stupid amounts of money on anti-fungal preparations. This book has changed my life.

YOUNG FEMALE

I noticed immediate changes as my body adjusted. Within 2 months, my patterns of elimination stabilized from chronic daily bouts of alternate diarrhea and constipation to normal elimination without gas and discomfort. My condition was chronic and diagnosed as an "active colon" from the time I was 20. I have experienced virtually none of my past symptoms for almost a year since I have been on the diet.

MIDDLE-AGED MALE

I was a vegetarian for over ten years, which left me with high blood pressure, high blood sugar, and very obese. I had food cravings, and an insatiable appetite. For example, I would crave apple pie à la mode, so I would eat a whole apple pie and a half gallon of vanilla ice cream at one sitting. I could eat a whole thick-crust family-size pizza all by myself at one sitting. Since reading your book, and committing to the diet, I have finally gained control of my appetite and eating habits. I have lost 70 lbs in just 7 months. I stick with beneficial meats, fish, and poultry. Very few carbohydrates. Maybe a small dinner salad, or 2 to 3 tablespoons of steamed rice with the evening meal. I intend to lose about 60 more pounds, as I believe 160 to 170 is about right for me.

YOUNG FEMALE

I had digestive problems for several years, which got progressively worse, and then a friend recommended your book. I was initially skeptical, but also very desperate. I visited my doctor who was not able to offer much help because I couldn't be specific about which foods were making me sick. After eliminating breads and grains from my diet, I immediately lost weight and felt less bloated. I intend to write to my doctor and tell him to read your book cover to cover!

YOUNG FEMALE

I have lost 55 lbs and feel great. I don't have the stomachaches any longer. I don't have to take Pepto any longer and I'm sleeping at night. I have lost inches and have gone down 2 dress sizes. I have made ER4YT a way of life and co-workers and family are interested in the same lifestyle.

YOUNG FEMALE

This book has given me back my quality of life. I was getting terrible headaches that lasted two to five days. I had trouble with arthritis and was getting nowhere with my aerobics workouts as I would need to quit after ten to fifteen minutes. I was beginning to think I would need to give up most aspects of my favorite hobbies, which involve work with my dogs. I almost never get headaches any longer, and when I do, they are manageable. I can get up in the morning and move about without having to limber up. I can run with my dogs in agility for the first time—it is such a thrill for me! I just can't remember the last time I felt this good in general. People ask me often what I have changed and I tell them what a difference the right diet has made for my life. Thanks for helping me help myself!

MIDDLE-AGED MALE

I was 212 pounds, waist size of 42, with high blood pressure, severe sleep apnea, numerous allergies, and an immune system not functioning well. Within one week my blood pressure returned to normal 120/80 (WITHOUT MEDICATION)! My allergies also disappeared this first week. It has now been almost 10 months and I now weigh 179, waist size is now 37, blood pressure is still at 120/80 and my severe SLEEP APNEA is GONE! I no longer need to use my CPAP (constant air pressure machine) to enable me to breathe while sleeping. I went through the entire winter without any flu, colds or any other sickness for the first time in years.

Blood Type A

MIDDLE-AGED FEMALE

I immediately noticed that my asthma was under control with less need for medication. I could take much deeper breaths without wheezing. It was noticed by my friends and family members as well. In general, I had more energy, no more elimination problems, and my mood swings disappeared, as pointed out by one of my daughters. I've also shed unwanted pounds without any effort, just following the A diet plan. I can't thank you enough for this new lease on life.

YOUNG FEMALE

I have suffered with Rheumatoid Arthritis for a year and a half. I stopped taking all medication and began the Blood Type Diet only. After 2 months, I felt as good as I did on the anti-inflammatory and immune-suppressant medications. Swelling of joint tissue in elbow has disappeared. The medication did not reduce this swelling at all. Nothing else could contribute to this change. I am very careful about trying one thing at a time. I am very pleased and recommend this diet to everyone who has any type of health concern.

MIDDLE-AGED MALE

I am a practicing chiropractor in New York who uses the Blood Type Diet for my patients. I was initially introduced to the Blood Type Diet approximately 2 years ago while attempting to research a practical, baseline diet for personal use. After experiencing significant benefits from applying its suggestions, I began to recommend it to my patient base cautiously, in order to evaluate their response and achieve a wider opinion base regarding benefits, etc. The response was, and has been, overwhelmingly positive. I, thus far, have well over 300 patients on the diet, as their baseline nutritional program, and have seen all varieties of ailments resolve through the application of its principles. I am greatly appreciative, both personally and professionally, for the material contained in the book and would like to thank you for this truly significant body of information.

MIDDLE-AGED FEMALE

I have asthma and frequent respiratory infections. Since following the Type A diet, my nighttime wheezing is nearly gone and I wake up feeling more rested as a result. I have also lost 8 pounds with little effort—just eliminated all dairy products and have virtually stopped eating meat. I occasionally "sneak" a small bit of white meat turkey into a stir-fry, but ordinarily stick to the wide variety of soy products as a source of protein. In general, I think I am feeling better since trying the Type A diet. My cholesterol has also gone from 200 to 171 in the past two months, and my good cholesterol is now at 59.

YOUNG MALE

I found this diet to be very easy to follow and with a lot of results. I not only lost 35 pounds in 8 months, but my asthma and allergy symptoms are way under control with no need to take drugs. I'm really happy with this diet and would share my experience at any time.

YOUNG FEMALE

I suffered from terrible allergies; after a week on the diet they were completely gone. I have lost 25 pounds in two months. I feel great and my self-esteem is growing every day.

MIDDLE-AGED MALE

I feel like I am no longer being poisoned by my diet. My weight continues to drop steadily as the fat burns off. Virtually everything in my former diet was wrong for Type A.

GERIATRIC MALE

Pain from arthritis in joints of fingers, hips, entirely alleviated. Muscle tightness reduced substantially. General sense of well-being. Eliminated need for allopurinol for gout without any recurring incident.

Blood Type B

MIDDLE-AGED MALE

I became vegetarian over twenty years ago. I had occasional digestive problems before that time, but things only became worse over the past twenty years. Many well-intentioned people suggested that I try this food or that. Nothing worked. Out here in California, my lifetime home, foods containing corn, tomatoes and avocados are very popular. I dropped those ingredients and added Kefir. That was a bit over a year and a half ago. MY LIFE IS NOW TURNED AROUND! "Significant" does not adequately describe my feeling. I would tend more towards "miracle."

MIDDLE-AGED FEMALE

I had seen a rheumatologist for extremely painful arthritis in my hips and knees. Also had difficulty in other joints—but these were worst. After about 30 days of avoiding the foods I should avoid and focusing on those recommended, I began to notice significant pain relief. Now, I have virtually no arthritis pain—additionally, I have lost a significant amount of weight. (I had lost weight before, however, and still had the arthritis. The exciting difference to me is the pain-free state I now enjoy!)

MIDDLE-AGED FEMALE

My husband and I are both Bs. My hypoglycemia disappeared almost overnight and my husband's sinuses cleared and his snoring stopped. Our diet was full of wheat bran, grains, pastas and chicken (i.e., the Food Guide Pyramid). We've made our own pyramid, but it looks more like a rectangle! I'm a registered/licensed dietitian specializing in complementary care so I see lots of chronic pain and inflammatory conditions that allopathic medicine hasn't helped. Without exception, my clients experience dramatic improvement in less than thirty days—most have decreased pain in 7–10 days! Their physicians ask them how they were able to decrease their pain meds or how did their cholesterol drop 150 points (!) and they are amazed at the results. So am I. I will continue to follow and recommend ER4YT to everyone. My dad, at 65, says he feels so good he feels guilty (but he gets over it!).

MIDDLE-AGED MALE

I have no more heartburn since I started this diet one year ago. That is just one of the many benefits I have experienced. I thank the lord for all your research to good health.

YOUNG FEMALE

My endometriosis has not given me any problem for over 9 months. I only have flare-ups when I go off the diet. I have also lost 40 pounds.

MIDDLE-AGED MALE

Weight since late December has gone from 304 to 285. Energy seems to be greater; I feel more "motivated" at times. Heartburn has gone away completely (those damn tomatoes were my favorite food, too). I no longer have the desire to eat between meals—and my meals are smaller, too. Odd . . . I am 90% on the diet; 10% off (simply for mental health . . . ice cream is a medicine, you know).

MIDDLE-AGED FEMALE

My physician told me about your book and gave me a printed summary of the do's and don'ts. I have tried for 8 years to lose weight since I quit smoking. Now I understand that all of the Weight Watchers meals have chicken and/or pasta. No wonder I couldn't succeed. I have lost 30 pounds since January 1 and best of all, I don't feel deprived. My rings actually fell off my fingers, and I have joyfully needed to get a new wardrobe since all of my clothes are now too big. There are so many good things that I like on my beneficial list that it's easy to stick to it. My sister and her husband bought the book last weekend and literally gave away all of their food and purchased according to their respective blood types. After 2 days, my brother-in-law says he feels noticeably better. There are 4 women in my office who are now on the program and we share experiences and all are losing weight and feeling good.

Blood Type AB

YOUNG FEMALE

I have been suffering from many health problems for the past 5+ years and have gotten increasingly worse over the past 2. The most prevalent are a digestive disorder that was moderate to severe, weight that I could not lose even with the most extreme of diets and exercise, and that I was severely exhausted. I spent many hours with my doctor having multiple tests performed and nothing would come of the weight problem—they just assumed that I was not trying as hard as I said I was. As for the digestive I was diagnosed as having IBS and micro-scopic colitis. I have been on the ER4YT diet for about 6 weeks and feel like an entirely new person. I have had no digestive problems (ex-cept for the few meals I had an item that is on my avoid list to eat). I have an energy level I did not know was possible for me and I have begun losing weight. The part I like about my weight loss is that I can feel it is a healthy loss that feels right. I am not tired or hungry and I feel healthy.

MIDDLE-AGED MALE

Weight loss was only the most dramatic change/improvement; I lost 20 lbs in 3–4 months following the diet closely without ever being hun-gry or without energy. Those around me are very impressed by this change. I am also impressed by the improvements in my psychological well-being, better elimination with less volume and never a bloated feeling, almost total non-use of antacid products that I was using regu-larly, and a sort of muting of hunger pangs between meals. My wife and I might consume half a loaf of bread during preparation of dinner and now don't eat anything before. I also feel that the diet is a major element along with other lifestyle changes that have allowed me to "tune in" to my bodily processes and states that I was not aware of before.

YOUNG FEMALE

Benefits: Weight Loss. 15 pounds in the first month, elimination of chicken, reduction of corn. Lifelong Acne: Ended with elimination of chicken. Monthly ear infections: Ended in first month. Hay fever: re-duced in first month, but not eliminated until diet followed perfectly in 9 months. I no longer have to take allergy pills for the first time in 10 years! Problem foods that had a direct impact in order of impor-tance: Chicken, Corn, Butter, Coconut, Duck, Shrimp (I am from the Philippines). I now maintain my ideal weight (105 pounds) with no conscious effort on my part except to follow the diet, which is easy because when I deviate my sinuses go crazy immediately. I have sold at least 10 books for you. Thank you. In observing the people who have followed the diet, I see the strongest improvement in allergies (hay fever, asthma) rather than weight loss. I understand the economic reasons for promoting your program as a "diet" but its biggest impact seems to be on health.

MIDDLE-AGED FEMALE

I was 40+ pounds overweight and experiencing worsening asthmatic conditions over the last 2 years. I tried all manner of drugs: no help. I tried acupuncture and Chinese herbs, which helped some. Your diet + natural supplements to build my immune system have changed my life. I've lost 30 pounds so far. I'm not taking any drugs and have had no asthma symptoms in 4 months. Adjusting to the diet was difficult at first, but now I find it simple and I find I'm satisfied; i.e.: not always craving something to eat. Thank you for your work; it's nothing short of amazing.

YOUNG FEMALE

The biggest change for me was the complete balancing of my blood sugar. Before the diet, I had trouble eating any fruit because it would just send my blood sugar for a roller coaster ride. Now as long as I follow the diet, my blood sugar is beautifully balanced and I have twice the energy. Another side benefit, my hands and nails have dramatically improved (strong nails, no problem with cuticles and hangnails).

Common
Questions

IT HAS BEEN MY EXPERIENCE THAT MOST PEOPLE RESPOND WITH GREAT enthusiasm and curiosity when they learn about the Blood Type Diet. Yet it is far easier to embrace a provocative idea than it is to immerse oneself in the gritty details.

The Blood Type Diet is revolutionary and as such requires many fundamental adjustments. Some people find it easier than others, depending on how much they're already living according to the needs of their blood type. Most of the questions people ask me have similar themes. I've included the most common ones here. They may help you get a clearer sense of what this diet will mean for you.

Where does my blood type come from?

Blood is universal, yet it is also unique. Like the color of your eyes or hair, your blood type is determined by two sets of genes—the inheritance you receive from your mother and father. It is from those genes commingling that your blood type is selected, at the moment of your conception.

Like most genes, some blood types are dominant over others. In the cellular creation of a new human being, Type A and Type B are dominant over Type O. If at conception the embryo is given an A allele (an alternate form of a gene) from the mother and an O allele from the father, the infant will be Type A, although it will continue to carry the father's O allele unexpressed in its DNA. When the infant grows up and passes these alleles to its offspring, half of the alleles will be for Type A blood and half will be for Type O blood.

Because A and B alleles are equally strong, you are Type AB if you received an A allele from one parent and a B allele from the other. Finally, because the O allele is recessive to all the others, you are Type O only if you receive an O allele from each parent.

It is possible for two Type A parents to conceive a child who is Type O. This happens when the parents each have one A allele and one O allele and each passes the O allele on to the offspring. In the same way, two brown-eyed parents can conceive a blue-eyed offspring if each carries the recessive gene for blue eyes.

Blood type genetics can sometimes be used to help determine the paternity of a child. There is one catch, however. Blood type can prove only that a man is not the father of a child. It cannot be used to prove that a man is the child's father (although newer DNA technology can do that). Consider this sample paternity case: An infant is Type A, the mother is Type O, and the man alleged to be the father is Type B. Because both A and B alleles are dominant to O, the child's father could not be Type B. Think about it. The child's A allele could not have come from the father, who, because he is Type B, would have either two B alleles or a B allele and an O allele. Nor could the A gene have come from the mother, because people with Type O blood always carry two O alleles. The A allele had to come from someone else. These were the exact circumstances surrounding the famous paternity suit against Charlie Chaplin in 1944. Unfortunately, Chaplin was subjected to a tumultuous trial, because the use of blood type to determine paternity was not yet acceptable in a California court of law. Even though blood type had clearly shown that Chaplin was not the father of the child, the jury still decided in favor of the mother, and he was forced to pay child support.

How do I find out my blood type?

To find out your blood type, you can donate blood or you can call your doctor to see if your blood type is in your medical file. If you'd like to test your own blood type, you can do so by ordering a finger-stick test. You can also order a saliva test to find out your secretor status. See Appendix F for details.

Do I have to make all of the changes at once for my Blood Type Diet to work?

No. On the contrary, I suggest you start slowly, gradually eliminating the foods that are not good for you and increasing those that are highly beneficial. Many diet programs urge you to plunge in headfirst and radically change your lifestyle immediately. I think it's more realistic and ultimately more effective if you engage in a learning process. Don't just take my word for it. You have to learn it in your body.

Before you begin your Blood Type Diet, you may know very little about which foods are good or bad for you. You're used to making your choices according to your taste buds, family traditions, and fad diet books. Chances are you are eating some foods that are good for you, but the Blood Type Diet provides you with a powerful tool for making informed choices every time.

Once you know what your optimal eating plan is, you have the freedom to veer from your diet on occasion. Rigidity is the enemy of joy; I certainly am not a proponent of it. The Blood Type Diet is designed to make you feel great, not miserable and deprived. Obviously, there are going to be times when common sense tells you to relax the rules a bit—like when you're eating at a relative's house.

I'm Blood Type A and my husband is Blood Type O. How do we cook and eat together? I don't want to prepare two separate meals.

My wife, Martha, and I have exactly the same situation. Martha is Type O and I am Type A. We find that we can usually share about two-thirds of a meal. The main difference is in the protein source. For example, if we make a stir-fry, Martha might separately prepare some chicken, while I'll add cooked tofu. We have also found that many Type O and Type A foods are beneficial for both of us, so we emphasize those foods. For example, we might have a meal that includes salmon, rice, and broccoli. It has become relatively easy for us because we are quite familiar with the specifics of each other's Blood Type Diet. It will help you to spend some time getting familiar with your spouse's food lists. You can even make a separate list of foods that you can share. You might be surprised at how many there are.

People worry a lot about what they fear will be impossible limitations on the Blood Type Diet. But think about it. There are more than 200 foods listed for each diet—many of them compatible across the board. Considering that the average person eats only about 25 foods, the Blood Type Diets actually offer more, not fewer, options.

For extra tips, check out our companion cookbook, *Cook Right 4*

Your Type and the four *Eat Right for Your Type* personalized cookbooks. Also, check out the website 4yourtype.com.

My family is Italian, and you know the kinds of foods we like to eat. Being Type A, I don't see how I can still enjoy my favorite Italian foods—especially, no tomato sauce!

We tend to associate ethnic foods with one or two of the most commonly available—like spaghetti with meatballs and tomato sauce. But the Italian diet, like most others, includes a wide variety of different foods. Many southern Italian dishes, usually prepared with olive oil instead of heavy sauces, are wonderful choices for both Type A and Type AB. Instead of a plate of pasta drenched in red sauce, try the more delicate flavors of olive oil and garlic, a complex pesto, or a light white wine sauce. Fresh fruits or flavorful but light Italian ices are preferable to rich pastries.

My seventy-year-old husband has a history of heart problems and has had bypass surgery. He still has a hard time staying away from the wrong foods. He's Type B and I think the Type B Diet would be perfect for him. But he's very resistant to diets. Is there a good way to introduce the diet without a lot of fuss?

It isn't easy to radically change your diet at age seventy, which is probably why your husband has had so much trouble eating healthily, even after surgery. Rather than nagging, which is usually counterproductive, begin to gradually incorporate the beneficial Type B foods into his diet, while slowly eliminating those that aren't good for Type B. It's likely that your husband will develop preferences for the good foods as his digestive tract adjusts to their positive qualities.

Why do you list different portion recommendations according to ancestry?

The portion listings according to ancestry are merely refinements to the diet that you may find helpful. In the same way that men, women, and children have different portion standards, so too do people according to their body size and weight, geography, and cultural food preferences. These suggestions will help you until you are comfortable enough with the diet to naturally eat the appropriate portions.

The portion recommendations also take into account specific problems that people of different ancestries tend to have with food. African Americans, for example, are often lactose intolerant, and most Asians are unaccustomed to eating dairy foods, so they may have to introduce these foods slowly to avoid negative reactions.

I'm allergic to peanuts, but you say they're a highly beneficial food for my blood type. Are you saying I should eat them? I'm Type A.

No. Type A has plenty of great protein sources without peanuts. These allergic reactions are generated by the immune system, which creates antibodies that resist the food and are not related to your blood type. Again, you don't need to include peanuts in your diet, especially if you are highly allergic to them and eating them would endanger your health. However, you may find that you tolerate them quite well once you've adjusted to the Type A Diet.

I'm Type B and my meat choices are very strange to me. It seems like all I can eat are lamb, mutton, venison, and rabbit—which I never eat. Why no chicken?

The elimination of chicken is the toughest adjustment for most people I've treated who are Type B. Not only is chicken a protein staple of many ethnic groups, but most of us have been conditioned to think that chicken is healthier than beef and other meats. Once again, however, there is no single rule that works for everyone. Chicken contains a lectin in its muscle meat that is very detrimental to Type B. On the brighter side, you can eat turkey and a wide variety of seafood.

What does neutral *mean? Are these foods good for me?*

The three categories are designed to help you focus on the foods that are most and least beneficial to you, according to your blood type reactions to certain lectins. The highly beneficial foods act as medicine;

the foods to avoid act as poison. The neutral foods simply act as foods. While the neutral foods may not have the special health benefits of some other foods, they're certainly good for you in the sense that they contain many nutrients that your body needs.

Must I eat all of the foods marked "highly beneficial"?

It would be impossible to eat everything on your diet! Think of your Blood Type Diet as a painter's palette from which you may choose colors in different shades and combinations. However, do try to reach the weekly amount of the various food groups if possible. Frequency is probably more important than the individual portion sizes, so if you are Type O and have a very small build, try to have animal protein five to seven times a week but cut back on the portions, perhaps eating 2 to 3 ounces instead of 4 to 5 ounces. This ensures that the most valuable nutrients will continue to be delivered into the bloodstream at a constant rate.

Is food combining helpful on the Blood Type Diet?

Some diet plans recommend food combining, which involves eating certain food groups in combination for better digestion. Many of these plans are full of bunk and hokum, with a lot of unnecessary rules and regulations. Perhaps the only real food-combining rule is to avoid eating animal proteins, such as meats, with large amounts of starches, such as breads and potatoes. This is important because animal products are digested in the stomach in a high-acid environment, while starches are digested in the intestines in a high-alkaline environment. When these foods are combined, the body alternately nibbles at the protein, then the starch, then back to the protein, then back to the starch; not a very efficient method. By keeping these food groups separated, the stomach can concentrate its full functions on the job at hand. Substitute low-starch, high-fiber vegetable side dishes, such as greens. Protein-starch avoidance doesn't apply to tofu and other vegetable proteins, which are essentially predigested.

What should I do if a "food to avoid" is used in small amounts in a recipe?

That depends on the severity of your condition or the degree of your compliance. If you have food allergies or colitis, you may want to practice complete avoidance. Many high-compliance patients avoid these foods altogether, although I think this might be too extreme. Unless they suffer from a specific allergic condition, it won't hurt most people to occasionally eat a food that is not on their diet.

Will I lose weight on the Blood Type Diet?

I have included specific recommendations for weight loss, which have been developed for each blood type. Your personalized Blood Type Diet is tailor-made to eliminate any imbalances that lead to weight gain. If you follow your Blood Type Diet, your metabolism will adjust to its normal level, and you'll burn calories more efficiently; your digestive system will process nutrients properly and reduce water retention. You'll lose weight immediately.

In my practice, I've found that most of my patients who have weight problems also have a history of chronic dieting. One would think that constant dieting would lead to weight loss, but that's not true if the structure of the diet and the foods it includes go against everything that makes sense for your specific body.

In our culture, we tend to promote one-size-fits-all weight loss programs, and then we wonder why they don't work. The answer is obvious! Different blood types respond to food in different ways. In conjunction with the recommended exercise program, you should see results very quickly.

Do calories matter on the Blood Type Diet?

As with most general diet issues, concerns about calories are automatically taken care of by following your specific Blood Type Diet. Most new patients who follow the guidelines concerning diet and exercise lose some weight. Some people even complain that they are losing too much weight. There is an adjustment period on this diet, and over time you'll be able to find the food amounts that suit your needs. However, the charts in each food category give you a place to start.

It's important to be aware of portion sizes. No matter what you eat, if you eat too much of it you'll gain weight. This probably seems so obvious that it doesn't even bear mentioning, but overeating has become one of America's most difficult and dangerous health problems. Millions of Americans are bloated and dyspeptic because of the amounts of food they eat. When you eat excessively, the walls of your stomach stretch like an inflated balloon. Although stomach muscles are elastic and were created to contract and expand, when they are grossly enlarged, the cells of the abdominal walls undergo a tremendous strain. If you are eating until you feel full, and you normally feel sluggish after a meal, try to reduce your portion sizes. Learn to listen to what your body is telling you.

I have heart problems and I've been told to totally avoid any fat and cholesterol. I'm Type O. How can I eat meat?

First, realize that it is grains, not meats, which are the cardiovascular culprits for Type O. This is especially interesting because almost everybody who has attempted or is attempting to prevent heart disease is advised to go on a diet based largely on complex carbohydrates!

For Type O, a high intake of certain carbohydrates, usually wheat breads, increases the triglyceride and insulin levels. In response, your body stores more fat in the tissues, and fat levels are elevated in the blood. For Type O, high triglycerides are double the risk factor for heart disease compared to high cholesterol.

Also bear in mind that your blood cholesterol level is only moderately controlled by the dietary intake of foods that are high in cholesterol content. Approximately 90 percent is actually controlled by the manufacture and metabolism of cholesterol in your liver.

I'm Type O and don't want to eat much fat in my diet. What do you suggest?

A high-protein diet does not automatically mean one that is high in fat, especially if you avoid heavily marbleized meats. Although more expensive, try to find free-range meats that have been raised without the excessive use of antibiotics and other chemicals. Our ancestors consumed rather lean game or domestic animals that grazed on alfalfa and other grasses; today's high-fat meats are produced by using high amounts of corn feed.

If you can't afford or can't find free-range meats, choose the leanest cuts available and remove all excess fat before cooking. Type O also has many other good protein choices that are naturally lower in fat—such as chicken and seafood. The fat in the oil-rich fish is composed of omega-3 fatty acids, which seem to promote lower cholesterol and healthier hearts.

How can I be sure to buy the most natural and the freshest foods?

Fortunately, in the last decade, natural and fresh foods, which were once available only in health food stores, have become increasingly available in supermarkets. Natural food markets and farmers' markets have sprung up in many communities. Fresh food home delivery stores bring the best ingredients right to your door. Health food stores themselves have been transformed, providing a wide variety of products and delicious prepared foods. You can even shop for whole foods online.

Are organic foods more healthy than nonorganic foods?

A good rule of thumb is to use organic vegetables if they are not exorbitantly priced. They do taste better and are more healthy. However, if you are on a fixed income and cannot find competitively priced organic produce, high-quality, properly cleaned, fresh nonorganic produce will do just fine.

More and more supermarkets seem to be stocking organic produce, mostly from California, a state with specific laws concerning the use of the term *organic*. It is interesting that in one supermarket in my neighborhood, organic vegetables and fruits are displayed next to the nonorganic versions and are priced identically! I suspect that market pressures will continue to push more and more vegetable and fruit growers toward the organic way, if for no other reason than the cost of commercial fertilizers, made from petrochemicals, will eventually make them more expensive to produce than naturally grown products.

Will eating canned food hurt my diet?

Commercially canned foods, subject to high heat and pressure, lose most of their vitamin content, especially the antioxidants, such as vitamin C. They do retain the vitamins that are not heat sensitive, such as vitamin A. Canned foods are typically lower in fiber than their fresh counterparts and higher in salt, usually added to offset the loss of flavors in production. Canned foods are often soggy, with little of the "life" we find in fresh fruits and vegetables, and contain few natural enzymes (which are destroyed by the canning process); thus they should be used sparingly, if at all. You pay much more per weight for canned food and don't get back much in return.

Other than fresh, frozen foods are your best second bet. Freezing does not change the nutritional content of the food very much (its preparation before freezing may), although the taste and texture are often blunted.

Why is stir-frying so beneficial?

The quick frying of Asian-style cooking is healthier than deep frying. Less oil is used, and the oil itself, typically sesame oil, is more resistant to high temperatures than are safflower or canola oil. The idea behind stir-frying is to quickly braise the food on its outside, which has the added effect of sealing in flavors.

Most types of meals can be prepared in this manner using a wok. The deep, cone-shaped design of the wok concentrates the heat at a small area at its base, which allows food to be cooked there and then moved to the cooler edges of the pan. Wok cooking usually mixes vegetables and seafoods or meats. Cook the meats and vegetables that require longer heating first, then move them to the outside of the pan, adding the vegetables that require less cooking to the center.

Steaming vegetables is also a quick and effective method of cooking and helps keep the nutrients in the food. Use a simple steamer basket, purchased at any hardware or department store, fitted inside a large pot filled with water to the level of the basket bottom. Add vegetables, cover and heat. Don't cook until soggy! Crisp means better taste, better texture, and better nutrition.

Should I take a multivitamin every day on the Blood Type Diet?

If you are in good health and are following your Blood Type Diet, you shouldn't really need a supplement, although there are many possible exceptions. Pregnant women should supplement their diet with iron, calcium, and folic acid. Most women also need extra calcium—especially if their diet doesn't include many dairy foods.

Those engaged in heavy physical activity, people in stressful occupations, the elderly, those who are ill, heavy smokers—all should be on a supplementation program. More specific details are available in your individual Blood Type Diet.

How important are herbs and herbal teas?

The importance of herbs and herbal teas depends on your blood type. Type O responds well to soothing herbs, Type A to the more stimulating ones, and Type B does quite nicely without most of them. Type AB should follow the herbal protocols given for Type A, with the added proviso that Type AB shuns those herbs that both Type A and Type B are asked to avoid.

Why are vegetable oils so limited on the Blood Type Diet? I thought all vegetable oils were good for you.

What you've probably heard is advertisers hawking the news that vegetable oils have no cholesterol. Well, that's not news to anyone with even a modicum of knowledge about nutrition. Plants and vegetables do not manufacture cholesterol, which is found only in products derived from animals. Your cholesterol-free oil may have little else to recommend it.

Oils are very blood type specific, and you'll need to consult the recommendations for your type. I prefer to use olive oil as much as possible in cooking. I believe that olive oil has proven to be the most tolerated and beneficial of fats. As a monounsaturated oil it seems to have positive effects on the heart and arteries. There are many different blends of olive oil available. The finest quality is the extra-virgin grade. It is slightly greenish in color and almost odorless—although when gently heated, the perfume of the olives is sensational. Olive oil is usually cold-pressed rather than extracted using heat or chemicals. The less processed an oil is, the better its quality.

Tofu seems like a very unappealing food. Must I eat it if I'm Type A?

Many Type A and Type AB people are initially resistant to the idea that they make tofu a staple of their diets. Well, tofu is not a glamour food. I admit it. When I was an impoverished Type A college student, I ate tofu with vegetables and brown rice almost every day for years. It was cheap, but I actually liked it.

I think the real problem with tofu is the way it is usually displayed in the markets. Tofu—in soft or hard cakes—sits with its other tofu friends in a large plastic tub, immersed in cold water. Thankfully, tofu has grown more common as an ingredient in foods, and many restaurants regularly serve up delicious dishes whose main protein is tofu.

If you are going to use tofu, it is best cooked and combined with vegetables and strong flavors that you enjoy, such as garlic, ginger, and soy sauce. Tofu is a nutritionally complete food that is filling and extremely inexpensive. Type A take note: The path to your good health is paved with bean curd!

I've never heard of many of the grains you mention. Where do I find out more?

If you're looking for alternative grains, health food stores are a bonanza. In recent years, many ancient grains, largely forgotten, have been rediscovered and are now being produced. Examples of these are amaranth, a grain from Mexico, and spelt, a variation of wheat that seems to be free of the problems found with whole wheat. Try them! They're not bad. Spelt flour makes a hearty, chewy bread that is quite flavorful, while several interesting breakfast cereals are now being made with amaranth. Another alternative is to use sprouted-wheat breads, sometimes referred to as Manna or Essene bread, as the gluten lectins found principally in the seed coat are destroyed by the sprouting process. These breads spoil rapidly and are usually found in the refrigerator cases of health food stores. They are a live food, with many beneficial enzymes still intact. Beware of commercially produced sprouted wheat breads, as they usually have a minority of sprouted wheat and a majority of whole wheat in their formulas. Sprouted bread is somewhat sweet tasting, as the sprouting process also releases sugars, and it is moist and chewy. This bread makes wonderful toast.

I'm Type A and I've been a runner for many years. Running seems to be a great way to reduce stress. I'm confused about your advice that I shouldn't exercise heavily.

There is a great deal of evidence that your blood type informs your unique reaction to stress, and that Type A tends to do better with less intense exercise. My father observed this thousands of times in his 35 years studying the connection. However, there is much we don't yet know, so I would hesitate to say absolutely that you shouldn't run.

I would ask you to reevaluate your health and energy levels. I often have patients who say things like, "I've always been a runner," or "I've always eaten chicken," as if that were all the proof they needed that an activity or a food was beneficial. Often, these very people are suffering from an assortment of physical problems and stresses that they've never thought to associate with specific activities or foods. You may be a Type A with a twist—one who thrives on intense physical activity—or you may discover that you're running on empty.

Should I avoid genetically engineered (GMO) food?

Yes! Genetic engineering often involves moving lectin molecules from one species to another. Because lectins are the molecules that interact with our blood types, an okay food can easily become one to avoid. Currently, because GMO content is not required to be listed on the food label, the only way to safely avoid GMO foods is to choose organic.

Why should all blood types avoid pork?

Hog is very A-like immunologically, which makes it an avoid food if you happen to have antibodies to the Blood Type A antigen, like Type B and Type O do. Paradoxically, hog also has an antibody (isohemagglutinin) in its tissues that reacts to the A antigen, so it should be avoided for this reason by Type A and Type AB as well. A surprising number of people carry antibodies in their blood type to pork products.

You mentioned that most Native Americans are Type O. I was wondering (being a Type O) about the use of corn because many tribes have used that as a staple.

Corn is a sacred food in many Native American cultures. Unfortunately, that doesn't make it any better as a health choice! A good example of the effect in adding corn into the diet of Type O Native Americans can be observed in the bone remains of the Indiana Mound Building cultures. We can exactly trace the introduction of corn into their diet after their long history as hunter-gatherers, by the marked change in their bone structure. Before corn became a staple, the bones show little arthritis or thinning; after corn was introduced, bone deformation began, including major changes to the teeth structure and jaw (periodontal disease). In addition, maize stimulates a very rapid and powerful glycemic response, so it may be that the switch to a maize-based diet from a hunter-gatherer way of life may have been responsible for a precipitous increase in diabetes. If corn lectins are problematic for Type O, they are even more serious as a hemagglutinin in Type B and Type AB individuals.

Aside from blood type principles, from a general health standpoint, are there any food choice tips?

Organic produce, organic dairy, and free-range meats are recommended. Genetically altered foods (which includes virtually all nonorganic soybeans), hydrogenated oils (margarine), partially hydrogenated oils, and artificial additives (sweeteners, colors, aromas, and flavors) should be avoided. Smoked and fried foods are not recommended. Oils should be purchased and stored in lightproof containers and preferably refrigerated after opening. White flour and sugars should be eaten rarely, if at all. MSG should not be used. Avoid aluminum cookery (it can contaminate your food with aluminum), and microwaves (they change the molecular structure of foods in unknown ways) for cooking.

One of my friends sees a naturopathic doctor who claims that naturopathic philosophy is based exclusively on vegetarian diets.

This association is so ingrained in the belief systems of some individuals that to even suggest that appropriate consumption of animal foods might actually enhance some individuals' health places me somewhere between public enemy number one and the devil in the eyes of several of my critics. Furthermore, veganism, which rejects all animal-based foods, even eggs and dairy, has been gaining popularity at a rapid pace—and that trend seems particularly prominent among millennials.

Often a good question to ask is, what does the evidence show? Naturopathic medicine developed from the water cure movement of Europe. Theodor Hahn is credited as being the first to integrate vegetarian dietary principles into the water cure movement. He was convinced that a meat-free diet would prolong life. In fact he was so convinced of the value of a vegetarian diet that he spent a great deal of his professional life writing books and pamphlets on the subject and was the editor of a magazine called the *Vegetarian*. He died of colon cancer at the age of 59. The point is, before you make a decision to adopt a particular diet, understand your reasons—apart from vague claims—and look at the evidence. If your goal is a long and healthy life, don't base your choices on someone's philosophy, but on what will help you reach that goal. I like a quote from the Talmud, an ancient rabbinical text, that pretty much sums it up: "Feed me in ways that are convenient for me."

How can it be that wheat isn't good for anyone? Hasn't it been a staple in the human diet for thousands of years?

Wheat, as we know it today, is not the same as it was when humans first started eating it. The genetics of wheat show that its development has been very complex. Today's grain is derived from three groups of wheat. Through natural crossings, mutations, and natural selection, these have evolved into all the many varieties of wheat grown worldwide.

In essence, the hard wheat that we eat nowadays has a protein content as high as 13 percent, versus the more ancient wheats, which had a protein content of, at most, about 2 percent. Increasing the protein content has had the effect of making wheat a viable source of protein for many people around the world, but this has also increased the allergenic (gliadin-, gluten-, and lectin-containing), proinflammatory, and metabolic-blocking portions of the plant almost sevenfold.

Aside from the underinvestigated metabolic effects of wheat lectin, classic hypersensitivity to wheat is found in many infants and adults. Reactions are often localized in the GI tract. In a study of asthma patients, 46 percent of children and 34 percent of adults were found to have immunoglobulin E (IgE) to wheat as tested by Pharmacia CAP System. In another study, specificity for wheat allergen using the same system was 98 percent. Wheat allergy was found to cause a persistent food hypersensitivity in 75 percent of atopic dermatitis patients. In 102 children who had grass pollen allergies, 12 percent were found to be allergic to wheat.

I appear to be allergic or reactive to a highly beneficial food. What do I do?

Don't eat it. In the event that your body has been altered by drugs, surgery, or disease, you may have different tolerances for food. The best thing to do in this situation is avoid the allergy-causing food and the other avoid foods for your blood type. Choose as many beneficial and neutral foods as possible. This sensitivity may change over time.

Are there any healthy sugars or sweeteners for my blood type?

Refined sugar is considered as addictive as a drug and potentially as detrimental to your health. Yet, according to the U.S. Department of Agriculture, the average American consumes between 150 and 170 pounds of refined sugar each year! It is clear that collectively we have a serious habit to kick. Sure, there are plenty of sugar-free sweetener alternatives on the market, but those chemically created artificial sweeteners are even more toxic than refined sugar. Ending your sugar addiction doesn't mean that you have to stop enjoying a hint of sweetness—it just requires that you find healthier alternatives. Fortunately, there are some all-natural, blood-type-friendly options.

Agave nectar is a honey-like sweetener made from the sap found in the core of the agave plant. It's sweeter than table sugar, so you can use less to get the same results, while at the same time boosting your recommended daily allowance of vitamins and minerals: It has trace amounts of calcium, iron, potassium, and magnesium. Agave nectar also has a lower glycemic index than table sugar, so it won't cause a spike in blood sugar levels. It's neutral for all blood types and both secretors and non-secretors.

Raw organic local honey contains trace amounts of niacin, riboflavin, thiamin, vitamin B_6, and free-radical-fighting antioxidants, and, some studies show, may help alleviate seasonal allergies. If you're trying to lose weight, there's good news for you; honey's low glycemic index helps keep sugar levels in check, and it's 50 percent sweeter than refined sugar, so you'll be satisfied with less. It's neutral for all blood type secretors, but should be avoided by Type O and Type AB non-secretors.

Pure maple syrup can be used as a sugar substitute in baking. Research shows that maple syrup also has some health benefits, including promoting cardiovascular health and boosting the immune system. It's neutral for all blood type secretors but should be avoided by Type O and Type AB non-secretors.

Molasses is the product of the refining of sugar cane and sugar beets; the juice squeezed from these plants is boiled to a syrupy mixture from which sugar crystals are extracted. The remaining brownish-black liquid is molasses. Molasses is a popular sweetener in baking and can also be used as a syrup on pancakes and waffles. Its health benefits include a high iron content as well as vitamin B_6, magnesium, calcium, and more antioxidants than any other natural sweetener. It's beneficial for Type A secretors and neutral for all the other blood types.

Stevia is the powdered extract of the plant *Stevia rebaudiana*, an herb indigenous to Paraguay and Brazil. While this zero-calorie sugar substitute tastes just like table sugar, it won't cause a spike in blood sugar levels. When using stevia, note that it is 200 to 400 times sweeter than sugar and you should use far less when baking or stirring it into coffee or tea. Health benefits include phytochemical compounds that help control blood sugar, cholesterol, and blood pressure. It's neutral for most blood types, but should be avoided by Type B secretors and Type O non-secretors.

Glossary
of Terms

ABO BLOOD GROUP SYSTEM: THE MOST IMPORTANT OF THE BLOOD-TYPING systems, the ABO blood group is the determinant for transfusion reactions and organ transplantation. Unlike the other blood-typing systems, the ABO blood types have far-ranging significance other than transfusion or transplantation, including the determination of many of the digestive and immunological characteristics of the body. The ABO blood group is made up of four blood types: O, A, B, and AB. Type O has no true antigen but carries antibodies to both A and B blood. Type A and Type B carry the antigen named for their blood type and make antibodies to each other. Type AB does not manufacture any antibodies to other blood types because it has both A and B antigens. Anthropologists use the ABO blood types extensively as a guide to the development of early peoples. Many diseases—especially digestive disorders, cancer, and infection—express preferences among the ABO blood types.

Agglutinate: Derived from the Latin word for "to glue." The process by which cells are made to adhere to one another, usually through the actions of an agglutinin, such as an antibody or a lectin. Certain viruses and bacteria also are capable of agglutinating blood cells. Many agglutinins, particularly food lectins, are blood type specific. Certain foods clump only the cells of one blood type but do not react with the cells of another type.

Allele: An alternative form of a gene, such as the blood type alleles, A, B and O.

Anthropology: The study of humankind in relation to distribution, origin, and classification. Anthropologists study human evolution, human physical characteristics, the relationships among ethnic groups, the interaction between the environment and society, and ancient and modern culture. ABO blood types have been extensively used by anthropologists in the study of early human populations.

Antibody: A class of chemicals, called the immunoglobulins, made by the cells of the immune system to specifically tag or identify foreign material within the body of the host. Antibodies combine with specific markers—antigens—found on viruses, bacteria, or other toxins and agglutinate them. The immune system is capable of manufacturing millions of different antibodies against a wide variety of potential invaders. Individuals of Type O, Type A, or Type B blood carry antibodies to other blood types. Type AB, the universal recipient, manufactures no antibodies to other types.

Antigen: Any chemical that causes the immune system to generate an antibody in response to it. The chemical markers that determine blood type are considered blood type antigens because other blood types may carry antibodies to them. Antigens are commonly found on the surface of germs, and are used by the immune system to detect foreign material. Specialized antigens are often made by cancer cells and are called tumor antigens. Many germs and cancer antigens are clever impersonators that can mimic the blood type of the host in an effort to escape detection by the immune system.

Antioxidants: Vitamins that are believed to strengthen the immune system and prevent cancer by fighting off toxic compounds (called free radicals) that attack cells. Vitamins C and E and beta-carotene are believed to be the most powerful antioxidants.

Cro-Magnon: The first truly modern human. Cro-Magnon migrated extensively from Africa into Europe and Asia. A master hunter, Cro-Magnon led a largely hunter-gatherer existence. Most of the digestive characteristics of people with Type O blood are derived from Cro-Magnon.

Differentiation: The cellular process by which cells develop their specialized characteristics and functions. Differentiation is controlled by the genetic machinery of the cell. Cancer cells, which often have defective genes, usually de-evolve and lose many of the characteristics of a normal cell, often reverting to earlier embryologic forms long repressed since early development.

Gene: A component of the cell that controls the transmission of hereditary characteristics by specifying the construction of a particular protein or enzyme. Genes are composed of long chains of deoxyribonucleic acid (DNA) contained in the chromosomes of the cell nucleus.

Indo-European: An early white people who migrated westward to Europe from their original homelands in Asia and the Middle East in 7,000 to 3,500 B.C.E. The Indo-Europeans were probably the progenitors for Type A blood in western Europe.

Ketosis: A state that is achieved with a high-protein, low-carbohydrate diet. The high-protein diets of our early Type O ancestors forced the burning of fat for energy and the production of ketones—a sign of rapid metabolic activity. The state of ketosis allowed early humans to maintain high energy, metabolic efficiency, and physical strength—all qualities needed for hunting game.

Lectin: Any compound, usually a protein, found in nature that can interact with surface antigens found on the body's cells, causing them to agglutinate. Lectins are often found in common foods, and many of them are blood type specific. Because cancer cells often manufacture copious amounts of antigens on their surface, many lectins will agglutinate them in preference to normal cells.

Microbiome: The collection of microorganisms that make up your internal ecosystem. The health of the microbiome depends on an abundance of healthy bacteria.

Mucus: Secretions manufactured by specialized tissues, called mucous membranes, which are used to lubricate and protect the delicate internal linings of the body. Mucus contains antibodies to protect against germs. In secretors, large amounts of blood type antigens are secreted in mucus, which serves to filter out bacteria, fungi, and parasites with opposing blood type characteristics.

Naturopathic doctor (ND): A physician trained in natural healing methods. Naturopathic doctors receive four-year postgraduate training at an accredited college or university, and function as primary-care providers.

Neolithic: The period of early human development characterized by the development of agriculture and the use of pottery and polished tools. The radical change in human lifestyle, from the previous hunter-gatherer existence, probably was a major stimulus to the development of Blood Type A.

Panhemagglutinins: Lectins that agglutinate all blood types. An example is the tomato lectin.

Polymorphism: Literally means "many shapes." A polymorphism is any physical manifestation within a species of living organisms that is variable through genetic influence. The blood types are a well-known polymorphism.

Phytochemical: Any natural product with specific health applications. Most phytochemicals are traditional herbs and plants.

Triglycerides: The body's fat stores, also contained in the bloodstream. High triglycerides, or high blood fats, are considered a risk for heart disease.

Notes on the
Anthropology
of Blood Type

ANTHROPOLOGY IS THE STUDY OF HUMAN DEVELOPMENT AND DIFFER-
ences, both cultural and biological. For our purposes, we can look at
the way the field is divided into two categories: cultural anthropology,
which looks at the manifestations of culture, such as language and
ritual, and biological anthropology, the study of the evolutionary biology of our species, *Homo sapiens*. Biological anthropologists attempt to
trace human historical development through hard scientific methods,
such as examining the blood types. A central task in biological anthropology has been to document the sequence of how the human line
evolved from early nonhuman primate ancestors. The use of blood types
to study early societies has been termed paleoserology, the study of
ancient blood.

Biological anthropology is also concerned with how humans adapted
to environmental pressures. Traditional biological anthropology relied
heavily on the measuring of skull shape, stature, and other physical characteristics. Blood type became a powerful tool for this type of analysis
in the 1950s, as emphasis shifted to genetic characteristics, such as blood
types and other genetic markers. A. E. Mourant, a physician and anthropologist, published two key works, *Blood Groups and Diseases* (1978) and
Blood Relations: Blood Groups and Anthropology (1983), that collected much
of the available material on the subject.

In addition to Mourant, I've used a variety of other source material for
this appendix, including earlier anthropology sources such as William
Boyd's *Genetics and the Races of Man* (1950), and a series of studies that were
published in various journals of forensic medicine from 1920 to 1945.

It is possible to map the occurrence of the various blood groups in
ancient populations by blood typing grave exhumations. Small amounts
of blood type materials can be reconstituted from the remains and the

blood type determined. By studying the blood types of human populations, anthropologists gain information about that population's local history, movement, intermarriage, and diversification.

Many national and ethnic groups have unique blood type distributions. In certain more isolated cultures, a clear majority of one blood type over another can still be seen. In other societies, it may be more evenly distributed. In the United States, for example, the equal rates of Type O and Type A blood reflect masses of immigration.

The United States also has a higher percentage of Blood Type B than the western European countries, which probably reflects the influx of more eastern nationalities.

For the purpose of this analysis, we can divide humankind into two basic clusters—Ethiopian and Palearctic. The Palearctic can be further broken down to Mongolians and Caucasians, although most people lie somewhere in between. Each race is physically characterized by its environment and occupies distinct geographic areas. Ethiopians, probably the oldest race, are dark-skinned Africans, inhabiting the southern third of Arabia and sub-Saharan Africa. The Palearctic region is made up of Africa north of the Sahara; Europe; and most of Asia, including India, Southeast Asia, and southern China but with the exception of southern Arabia.

The roughest guesswork places the beginnings of human migration from Africa to Asia at about 1 million years ago. In Asia, most likely, the modern *Homo sapiens* species split from a trunk of the ancestral Ethiopians into the Caucasians and Mongolians, but we know almost nothing about when or why it occurred.

Each of the basic races has its own homeland—a geographic area where it is preeminent. The Ethiopian homeland was Africa; the Caucasian, Europe and northern Asia; and the Mongolian, central and southern Asia. There may be more physical differences between Africans and the other races, but the blood type differences between Caucasians and Mongolians are more clear-cut—a good reason to reexamine racial stereotypes.

Although we trace the numerical predominance and ascent of Type O blood back to early prehistory, it still remains a very workable chemistry, largely because of its simplicity and the fact that animal protein diets still account for a great portion of the world's current food intake.

The first attempt at using blood type to describe ethnic and nationality characteristics was undertaken by a husband-and-wife team of physicians, the Hirszfelds, in 1918. During World War I both had served as doctors in the Allied armies that had concentrated in the area of Salonika, Greece. Working with a multinational force, the Hirszfelds systematically blood-typed large numbers of refugees of different ethnic backgrounds, also recording their race and nationality. Each group contained at least five hundred subjects.

The Hirszfelds found, for example, that the rate of Blood Type B ranged from a low of 7.2 percent of the population of English subjects to a high of 41.2 percent in Indians, and that western Europeans in general had a lower incidence of Type B than Balkan Slavs, who had a lower incidence than Russians, Turks, and Jews, who again had a lower occurrence than Vietnamese and Indians. The distribution of Blood Type AB essentially followed the same pattern, with a low of 3 to 5 percent in western Europeans and a high of 8.5 percent in Indians.

In subcontinental India, Type AB makes up 8.5 percent of the population—remarkably high for a blood type that typically averages between 2 and 5 percent worldwide. This prevalence of Type AB is probably due to subcontinental India's location as an invasion route between the conquered lands to the west and the Mongolian homelands to the east.

Blood Type O and Type A were essentially the reverse of Type B and Type AB. The percentage of Type A remained fairly consistent (40 percent) among Europeans, Balkan Slavs, and Arabs, while being quite low in West Africans, Vietnamese, and Indians. About 46 percent of the English population tested were Type O, which accounted for only 31.3 percent of the Indians tested.

Modern analysis (largely the result of records kept by blood banks), encompasses the blood types of more than 20 million individuals from around the world. Yet these large numbers can do no more than confirm the original observations of the Hirszfelds. No scientific journals saw fit to publish their material at that time. For a while, the Hirszfelds' study languished in an obscure anthropology journal; for more than 30 years this fascinating and important work was overlooked.

Apparently, there was little interest in using this knowledge of the blood types as an anthropological probe into the history of humanity.

Recent work by Dr. Luigi Cavalli-Sforza at Stanford University has tracked the genetic movement of ancient humans, using even more sophisticated methods based on the new DNA technology. Many of his findings have confirmed the earlier observations of Mourant, the Hirszfelds, Snyder, and Boyd concerning the distribution of blood types worldwide.

The Blood Type Support Community

Discover Your Blood Type

It is difficult to begin a diet based on blood type if you are not aware of your own type. In Europe, blood type is something almost everyone knows, but here in the United States, unless we need a transfusion, we can go our entire lives without knowing what blood type we are. What follow are several simple ways to find out your blood type:

1. Donate blood. Not only are you providing a critical service to the community but this is a free and simple way to find out what blood type you are. To find your local donation center, visit the American Red Cross website's Give Blood page (redcrossblood.org).
2. Purchase a blood-typing kit from D'Adamo Personalized Nutrition (4yourtype.com), under "Books and Tests." The kit is inexpensive and simple to do in your own home.
3. Next time you visit your doctor for a blood workup, ask him or her to add blood typing to the blood test protocol.

Secretor Status

If you do not know your secretor status and want to further refine your personalized profile, you can purchase a Secretor Status Collection Kit from D'Adamo Personalized Nutrition (4yourtype.com).

Center of Excellence in Generative Medicine

The Center of Excellence in Generative Medicine (COEGM) is a collaboration between Peter D'Adamo and the University of Bridgeport (UB) to create a frontiers-focused biomedical initiative without parallel in any other medical school. The COEGM combines patient care, clinical research, and hands-on teaching opportunities for students of the university's health sciences program. It is also home to Dr. D'Adamo's clinical practice and uses his state-of-the-art bioinformatic software programs like SWAMI GenoType and Opus23. For information and appointments for either private practice patients or clinic-shift patients, please contact the center at:

Center of Excellence in Generative Medicine
115 Broad Street
Bridgeport, CT 06604
203-366-0526
generativemedicine.org

For All Things Peter D'Adamo—dadamo.com

One of the longest-running websites on the Internet, dadamo.com is the home page for the community of "netizens" who follow the work of Dr. Peter D'Adamo. This easy-to-navigate site is chock-full of helpful tools, blogs, and one of the warmest, most welcoming chat forums to be found. Newbies are welcome to this moderated, family-friendly community.

D'Adamo Personalized Nutrition—North American Pharmacal, Inc.

For information on the Blood Type Diet, individualized supplements, and testing kits, please contact Dr. D'Adamo at:

D'Adamo Personalized Nutrition
North American Pharmacal, Inc.

149 Water Street
South Norwalk, CT 06854
203-761-0042
203-761-0043 FAX
Toll-free: 1-877-ABO-TYPE (226-8973)
4yourtype.com

The Official Blood Type Diet Phone App

The Official Blood Type Diet App for Android and iPhones and tablets lists beneficial, neutral, and avoid foods for each of the four blood types. Handy for grocery shopping, eating in restaurants, and meal planning. On the go or at home, you can always be sure you are eating right for your type. Simply select your blood type and start choosing foods for your type categorized in the handy food lists. Know your secretor status or want to learn more about it? It's an option in the app. Content includes the following:

1. Blood type and secretor status selector
2. Food lists with blood type–specific values
3. Family food list, which combines common foods for multiple blood types to make food prep easier
4. Shopping list, with ability to choose your own or combine the family list for multiple blood types
5. Email the shopping list directly from the app
6. Food search function
7. Information on each blood type
8. Dietary supplement information
9. Recipe access (Internet connection required)

Personalized Living Blog— northamericanpharmacal.com/living

Find inspiration, recipes, helpful tips and tools, success stories, and support on the only blog dedicated to personalized living.

The Blood Type Diet Community
on Social Media

Facebook: facebook.com/drpeterdadamo
Twitter: @peterdadamo
Instagram: @eatright4yourbloodtype
Pinterest: pinterest.com/right4yourtype

The Scientific
Evidence

RATHER THAN FILL THIS BOOK WITH ENDLESS FOOTNOTES, I'VE COL-
lected the most important influences on the work and listed them here
where they might be most easily referred to. They are grouped into
several categories and listed alphabetically by author.

Blood Types, General Information

American Association of Blood Banks. *Technical Manual.* 10th ed. 1990.

D'Adamo, P. "Gut Ecosystems III: The ABO and Other Polymorphic Systems." *Townsend Letter for Doctors*, August 1990.

D'Adamo, P., and G. Kelly. "Metabolic and Immunologic Consequences of ABH
Secretor Status." *Alternative Medicine Review*, August 6, 2001, pp. 390–405.

Marcus, D. M. "The ABO and Lewis Blood-Group System." *New England
Journal of Medicine* 280 (1969): 994–1005.

Blood Types and Anthropology

Boyd, W. C. *Genetics and the Races of Man: An Introduction to Modern Physical
Anthropology.* Boston: Little, Brown, 1950.

Brues, A. M. "Stochastic Tests of Blood Selection in the ABO Blood Groups."
American Journal of Physical Anthropology 21 (1963): 287–99.

Childe, V. G. *Man Makes Himself.* London: Watts, 1936.

Coon, C. S. *The Races of Europe.* New York: Macmillan, 1939.

Gates, R. R. *Human Ancestry.* Cambridge: Harvard University Press, 1948.

Hirszfeld, L., and H. Hirszfeld. "Serological Differences Between the Blood
of Different Races" *Lancet* 2 (1919): 675–79.

Livingstone, F. R. "Natural Selection, Disease and Ongoing Human Evolution, as Illustrated by the ABO Groups." n.d., n.p.

McNeill, W. H. *Plagues and Peoples.* New York: Doubleday/Anchor, 1975.

Mourant, A. E. *Blood Relations: Blood Groups and Anthropology.* Oxford: Oxford University Press, 1983.

Mourant, A. E., A. C. Kopec, and K. Domaniewska-Sobczak, *Blood Groups and Diseases.* 4th ed. Oxford: Oxford University Press, 1984.

Muschel, L. "Blood Groups, Disease and Selection." *Bacteriological Review* 30, no. 2 (1966): 427–41.

Race, R. R., and R. Sanger. *Blood Groups in Man.* Oxford: Blackwell Scientific, 1975.

Sheppard, P. M. "Blood Groups and Natural Selection." *British Medical Bulletin* 15 (1959): 132–39.

Soulsby, E. J. L. "Antigen-Antibody Reactions in Helminth Infections." *Advances in Immunology* 2 (1963): 265–308.

Wyman, L. C., and W. C. Boyd. "Blood Group Determinations of Prehistoric American Indians." *American Anthropologist* 39 (1937): 583–92.

Wyman, L. C., and W. C. Boyd. "Human Blood Groups and Anthropology." *American Anthropologist* 37 (1935): 181–200.

Blood Types and Lectins

D'Adamo, P. "Gut Ecosystems II: Lectins and Other Mitogens." *Townsend Letter for Doctors*, 1991.

Freed, D. L. J. "Dietary Lectins and Disease." *Food Allergy and Intolerance* (1987): 375–400.

Freed, D. L. J. "Lectins." *British Medical Journal* 290 (1985): 585–86.

Helm, R., and A. Froese. "Binding of the Receptors for IgE by Various Lectins." *International Archives of Allergy and Applied Immunology* 65 (1981): 81–84.

Macholz, R. *The Lectins: Properties, Functions and Applications in Biology and Medicine.* New York: Harcourt Brace Jovanovich/Academic Press, 1986.

Nachbar, M. S., et al. "Lectins in the United States Diet: A Survey of Lectins in Commonly Consumed Foods and a Review of the Literature." *American Journal of Clinical Nutrition* 33 (1980): 2338–45.

Nachbar, M. S., et al. "Lectins in the U.S. Diet: Isolation and Characterization of a Lectin from the Tomato (*Lycopersicon esculentum*)." *Journal of Biological Chemistry* 255 (1980): 2056–61.

Norn, S., et al. "Intrinsic Asthma and Bacterial Histamine Release via Lectin Effect." *Agents and Action* 13, nos. 2–3 (1983): 210–12.

Sharon, N., and H. Lis. "The Biochemistry of Plant Lectins (Phytohemaglu-tinins)." *Annual Review of Biochemistry* 42 (1973): 541–74.

Sharon, N., and H. Lis. "Lectins: Cell-Agglutinating and Sugar-Specific Pro-teins." *Science* 177 (1972): 949–59.

Shechter, Y. "Bound Lectins That Mimic Insulin Produce Persistent Insulin-Like Effects." *Endocrinology* 113 (1983): 1921–26.

Triadou, N., and E. Audron. "Interaction of the Brush-Border Hydrolases of the Human Small Intestine with Lectins." *Digestion* 27 (1983): 1–7.

Uhlenbruck, G., et al. "Love to Lectins: Personal History and Priority Hys-terics." *Lectins and Glycoconjugates in Oncology.* New York: Springer-Verlag, 1988.

Ulmer, A. J., et al. "Stimulation of Colony Formation and Growth Factor Production of Human T Lymphocytes by Wheat Germ Lectin." *Immunol-ogy* 47 (1982): 551–56.

Wagner, H., et al. "Immunostimulant Action of Polysaccharides (Heterogly-cans) from Higher Plants." *Arzneimittelforschung* 34 (1984): 659–61 [Ger-man abstract in English].

Waxdal, M. J. "Isolation, Characterization and Biological Activities of Five Mitogens from Pokeweed." *Biochemistry* 13 (1974): 3671–75.

Zafriri, D., et al. "Inhibitory Activity of Cranberry Juice on Adherence of Type 1 and Type P Fimbriated *Escherichia coli* to Eucaryotic Cells." *Anti-microbial Agents and Chemotherapy* 33 (1989): 92–98.

Disease Associations with Blood Type

Addis, G. J. "Blood Groups in Acute Rheumatism." *Scottish Medical Journal* 4 (1959): 547.

Aird, I., et al. "The Blood Groups in Relation to Peptic Ulceration and Car-cinoma of Colon, Rectum, Breast, and Bronchus." *British Medical Journal* (1954): 315–42.

Alexander, K., L. McClure, V. Wadley, et al. "ABO Blood Type, Factor VIII, and Incident Cognitive Impairment in the REGARDS Cohort." *Neurol-ogy* 83 (2014): 1271–76.

Allan, T. M., and A. A. Dawson. "ABO Blood Groups and Ischaemic Heart Disease in Men." *British Heart Journal* 30 (1968): 377–82.

Billington, B. P. "A Note on the Distribution of ABO Blood Groups in Bronchi-ectasis and Portal Cirrhosis." *Australian Annals of Medicine* 5 (1956): 20–22.

"Blood-Groups and the Intestine." *Lancet* 7475 (1966): 1232–1233 [Editorial].

Buchanan, J. A., and E. T. Higley. "The Relationship of Blood-Groups to Disease." *British Journal of Experimental Pathology* 2 (1921): 247–55.

Buckwalter, J. A., et al. "ABO Blood Groups and Disease." *Journal of the American Medical Association* (1956): 1210–15.

Buckwalter, J. A., et al. "Ethnologic Aspects of the ABO Blood Groups: Disease Associations." *Journal of the American Medical Association* (1957): 327–29.

Camps, F. E., and B. E. Dodd. "Frequencies of Secretors and Non-Secretors of ABH Group Substances Among 1,000 Alcoholic Patients." *British Medical Journal* 4 (1969): 457–59.

Camps, F. E., and B. E. Dodd. "Increase in the Incidence of Non-Secretors of ABH Blood Group Substances Among Alcoholic Patients." *British Medical Journal* 1 (1967): 30–31.

D'Adamo, P. "Blood Types and Diseases, A Review." Clinical Rounds Presentation, Bastyr University, 1982.

D'Adamo, P. "Combination Naturopathic Treatment of Primary Biliary Cirrhosis." *Journal of Naturopathic Medicine* 4, no. 1 (1993): 24–25.

D'Adamo, P., and E. Zampieron. "Does ABO Bias in Natural Immunity Imply an Innate Difference in T-Cell Response?" *Journal of Naturopathic Medicine* 2 (1991): 11–17.

De Marco, M., and A. Venneri. "'O' Blood Type Is Associated with Larger Grey-Matter Volumes in the Cerebellum." *Brain Research Bulletin* (2015).

Fraser Roberts, J. A. "Blood Groups and Susceptibility to Disease: A Review." *British Journal of Preventative & Social Medicine* 11 (1957): 107–25.

Fraser Roberts, J. A. "Some Associations Between Blood Groups and Disease." *British Medical Bulletin* 15 (1959): 129–33.

Harris, R., et al. "Vaccinia Virus and Human Blood-Group-A Substance." *Acta Genetica* 13 (1963): 44–57.

Havlik, R., et al. "Blood-Groups and Coronary Heart-Disease." *Lancet* 7614 (1969): 269–70.

Hein, H. O., et al. "Alcohol Consumption, Lewis Phenotypes, and Risk of Ischaemic Heart Disease." *Lancet* 341 (1993): 392–96.

"An Insight Is Gained on How Ulcers Develop." *New York Times*, December 17, 1993.

Koskins, L. C., et al. "Degradation of Blood Group Antigens in Human Colon Ecosystems." *Journal of Clinical Investigation* 57 (1976): 74–82.

Langman, M. J. S., et al. "ABO and Lewis Blood-Groups and Serum-Cholesterol." *Lancet* (1969): 607–9.

Lim, W., et al. "Association of Secretor Status and Rheumatic Fever in 106 Families." *American Journal of Epidemiology* 82 (1965): 103–11.

McConnell, R. B., et al. "Blood Groups in Diabetes Mellitus." *British Medical Journal* 1 (1956): 772–76.

McDuffie, F., and E. Kabat. "The Behavior in the Coombs Test of Anti-A and Anti-B Produced by Immunization with Various Blood Group A and B Substances and by Heterospecific Pregnancy." *Journal of Immunology* 77 (1956): 61–71.

Martin, N. G., et al. "Do the MN and JK Systems Influence Environmental Variability in Serum Lipid Levels?" *Clinical Genetics* 24 (1983): 1–14.

Myrianthopoulos, N. C., et al. "The Relation of Blood Groups and the Secretor Factor to Amyotrophic Lateral Sclerosis." *American Journal of Human Genetics* 19 (1967): 607–16.

"O! My Aching Stomach!" *Witby Republican*, December 12, 1993.

Ratner, J. J., et al. "ABO Group Uropathogens and Urinary Tract Infection." *American Journal of Medical Science* 292 (1986): 84–92.

Roath, S., et al. "Transient Acquired Blood Group B Antigen Associated with Diverticular Bowel Disease." *Acta Haematologica* 77 (1987): 188–90.

Saarloos, M. N., T. F. Lint, and G. T. Spear. "Efficacy of HIV-Specific and 'Antibody-Independent' Mechanisms for Complement Activation by HIV-Infected Cells." *Clinical and Experimental Immunology* 99, no. 2 (1995): 189–95.

Springer, G. F. "Relation of Blood Group Active Plant Substances to Human Blood Groups." *Acta Haematologica* 20 (1958): 147–55.

Springer, G. F., and R. E. Horton. "Erythrocyte Sensitization by Blood Group-Specific Bacterial Antigens." *Journal of General Physiology* 47 (1964): 1229–49.

Struthers, D. "ABO Groups of Infants and Children Dying in the West of Scotland (1949–51)." *British Journal of Preventive & Social Medicine* 5 (1951): 223–28.

Young, V. M., H. C. Gillen, and J. H. Akeroyd. "Sensitization of Infant Red Cells by Bacterial Polysaccharides of *Escherichia coli* during Enteritis." *Journal of Pediatrics* 60 (1962): 172–76.

Blood Types and Cancer

Aird, I., et al. "The Blood Groups in Relation to Peptic Ulceration and Carcinoma of Colon, Rectum, Breast and Bronchus." *British Medical Journal* 2 (1954): 315–21.

Aird, I., et al. "A Relationship Between Cancer of the Stomach and the ABO Blood Groups." *British Medical Journal* 1 (1953): 799–801.

Aird, I., et al. "ABO Blood Groups and Cancer of Oesophagus, Cancer of Pancreas, and Pituitary Adenoma." *British Medical Journal* 1 (1960): 1163–66.

Bazeed, M. A., et al. "Effect of Lectins on KK-47 Bladder Cancer Cell Line." *Urology* 32 (1988): 133–35.

Boland, C. R. "Searching for the Face of Neoplasia." *Journal of Clinical Gastroenterology* 10, no. 6 (1988): 599–604.

Brooks, S. A., and A. J. C. Leathem. "Predictive Value of Lectin Binding on Breast-Cancer Recurrence and Survival." *Lancet* 1, no. 8541 (1987): 1054–56.

Brooks, S. A., and A. J. C. Leathem. "Prediction of Lymph Node Involvement in Breast Cancer by Detection of Altered Glycosylation in the Primary Tumor." *Lancet* 8759, no. 338 (1991): 71–74.

Cameron, C., et al. "Acquisition of a B-Like Antigen by Red Blood Cells." *British Medical Journal* 2, no. 5140 (1959): 29–32.

D'Adamo, P. "Possible Alteration of ABO Blood Group Observed in Non-Hodgkin's Lymphoma." *Journal of Naturopathic Medicine* 1 (1990): 39–43.

Dahiya, R., et al. "ABH Blood Group Antigen Expression, Synthesis, and Degradation in Human Colonic Adenocarcinoma Cell Lines." *Cancer Research* 49, no. 16 (1989): 4550–56.

Dahiya, R., et al. "ABH Blood Group Antigen Synthesis in Human Colonic Adenocarcinoma Cell Lines." *Proceedings of the Annual Meeting of the American Association of Cancer Research* 30 (1989): A1405 [Abstract].

Davis, D. L., et al. "Medical Hypothesis: Xenoestrogens As Preventable Causes of Breast Cancer." *Environmental Health Perspectives* 101, no. 5 (1993): 372–77.

Feinmesser, R., et al. "Lectin Binding Characteristics of Laryngeal Cancer." *Otolaryngology Head Neck Surgery* 100, no. 3 (1989): 207–9.

Fenlon, S., et al. "Helix Pomatia and Ulex Europeus Lectin Binding in Human Breast Carcinoma." *Journal of Pathology* 152 (1987): 169–76.

Kvist, E., et al. "Relationship Between Blood Groups and Tumors of the Upper Urinary Tract." *Scandinavian Journal of Urology and Nephrology* 22, no. 4 (1988): 289–91.

Langkilde, N. C., et al. "Binding of Wheat and Peanut Lectins to Human Transitional Cell Carcinomas." *Cancer* 64, no. 4 (1989): 849–53.

Lemon, H. "Clinical and Experimental Aspects of Anti-Mammary Carcinogenic Activity of Estriol." *Frontiers of Hormone Research* 5 (1978): 155–73.

Lemon, H. "Pathophysiologic Considerations in the Treatment of Menopausal Patients with Oestrogens: The Role of Oestriol in the Prevention of Mammary Carcinoma." *Acta Endocrinologica Supplementum* 233 (1980): 17–27.

Marth, C., and G. Daxenbichler, G. "Peanut Agglutinin Inhibits Proliferation of Cultured Breast Cancer Cells." *Oncology* 45 (1988): 47–50.

De Marco, M., and A. Venneri. "'O' Blood Type Is Associated with Larger Grey-Matter Volumes in the Cerebellum." *Brain Research Bulletin* 116 (2015): 1–6.

Morecki, S., et al. "Removal of Breast Cancer Cells by Soybean Agglutinin in an Experimental Model for Purging Human Marrow." *Cancer Research* 48 (1988): 4573–77.

Motzer, R. J., et al. "Blood Group-Related Antigens in Human Germ Cell Tumors." *Cancer Research* 48, no. 18 (1988): 5342–47.

Murata, K., et al. "Expression of Blood Group-Related Antigens, ABH, Lewis A, Lewis B, Lewis X, Lewis Y, Ca19-9 and CSLEX1 in Early Cancer, Intestinal Metaplasia and Uninvolved Mucosa of the Stomach." *American Journal of Clinical Pathology* 98 (1992): 67–75.

Osborne, R. H., and F. V. DeGeorge. "The ABO Blood Groups in Neoplastic Disease of the Ovary." *American Journal of Human Genetics* 15 (1963): 380–88.

Renton, P. H., et al. "Red Cells of All Four ABO Groups in a Case of Leukemia." *British Medical Journal* (1962): 294–97.

Roberts, T. E., et al. "Blood Groups and Lung Cancer." *British Journal of Cancer* 58, no. 2 (1988): 278 [Letter].

Romodanov, S. A., et al. "Efficacy of Chemo and Immunochemistry in Neuro-Oncological Patients with Different ABO System Blood Group." *Zhurnal Voprosy Neĭrokhirurgii Imeni NN Burdenko* 53, no. 1 (1989): 17–20.

Stachura, J., et al. "Blood Group Antigens in the Distribution of Pancreatic Cancer." *Folia Histochemica et Cytobiologica* 27, no. 1 (1989): 49–55.

Springer, G., et al. "Blood Group MN Antigens and Precursors in Normal and Malignant Human Breast Glandular Tissue." *Journal of the National Cancer Institute* 54, no. 2 (1975): 335–39.

Springer, G., et al. "T/Tn Antigen Vaccine Is Effective and Safe in Preventing Recurrence of Advanced Breast Cancer." *Cancer Detection and Prevention* 19 (1995): 374–80.

Tryggvadottir, L., et al. "Familial and Sporadic Breast Cancer Cases in Iceland: A Comparison Related to ABO Blood Groups and Risk of Bilateral Breast Cancer." *International Journal of Cancer* 42, no. 4 (1988): 499–501.

Tzingounis, V. A., et al. "Estriol in the Management of the Menopause." *Journal of the American Medical Association* 239, no. 16 (1978): 1638–41.

Wolf, G. T., et al. "A9 and ABH Antigen Expression Predicts Outcome in Head and Neck Cancer." *Proceedings of the Annual Meeting of the American Association of Cancer Research* 30 (1989): A902.

Acknowledgments

THERE ARE MANY PEOPLE TO THANK, AS NO SCIENTIFIC PURSUIT IS solitary. Along the way, I have been driven, inspired, and supported by all of the people who placed their confidence in me. In particular, I give deep thanks to my wife, Martha Mosko D'Adamo, for her love and friendship; my daughters, Claudia and Emily, who inspire and challenge me to be a better man; my parents, James D'Adamo Sr., ND, and Christiana, for teaching me to trust in my intuition; and my brother, James D'Adamo Jr., for believing in me.

I am also more grateful than I can express to:

Catherine Whitney, my writer, who imparted a style and organization to the raw material characteristic of a true wordsmith.

Gail Winston, the editor who long ago, out of the clear blue sky, rang me up and asked me if I wanted to write a book about natural medicine.

My literary agent, Janis Vallely, who saw the promise of my work and didn't allow it to languish somewhere in a dusty file cabinet; Amy Hertz, my original editor at Riverhead/Putnam, whose vision turned manuscript into the rich and important document I believe it has now become; Denise Silvestro, who continued to shepherd the book at Berkley; and Tom Colgan and Allison Janice, who guided the 20th-anniversary edition.

I am also thankful to:

Dorothy Mosko, for her invaluable assistance in the preparation of the early manuscript.

Scott Carlson, my former assistant, who never missed a UPS pickup.

Carolyn Knight, RN, my former right-hand nurse and expert phlebotomist.

Jane Dystel, Catherine's literary agent, whose advice was always on target.

Paul Krafin, who lent his sharp writing and editing skills to the revision process.

Dina Khader, MS, RD, CDN, who helped with the recipes and meal planning.

The physicians, staff, residents and students at the Center of Excellence in Generative Medicine at the University of Bridgeport in Connecticut for reawakening my love of clinical medicine.

Javier Caceres and Bill Weksner for their vigilant proofreading. Melissa Cybart for managing my hectic and ever-changing schedule.

John Schuler, who designed the illustrations.

Last, I thank all the wonderful patients, who in their quest for health and happiness chose to honor me with their trust, as well as all the wonderful people on dadamo.com forums and message boards who over the years have built an enduring community, and to whom I am profoundly grateful.

Index